Current Cancer Research

Series Editor

Wafik El-Deiry

More information about this series at http://www.springer.com/series/7892

Sandip Pravin Patel • Razelle Kurzrock
Editors

Early Phase Cancer Immunotherapy

Springer

Editors
Sandip Pravin Patel
Division of Hematology/Oncology
Department of Medicine
University of California, San Diego
Moores Cancer Center
La Jolla, CA, USA

Razelle Kurzrock
Division of Hematology/Oncology
Department of Medicine
University of California, San Diego
Moores Cancer Center
La Jolla, CA, USA

ISSN 2199-2584 ISSN 2199-2592 (electronic)
Current Cancer Research
ISBN 978-3-319-63756-3 ISBN 978-3-319-63757-0 (eBook)
DOI 10.1007/978-3-319-63757-0

Library of Congress Control Number: 2017956906

Printed on acid-free paper

This Springer imprint is published by Springer Nature
The registered company is Springer International Publishing AG
The registered company address is: Gewerbestrasse 11, 6330 Cham, Switzerland

Preface

Immunotherapy: Transforming Cancer Care

> *1986: "Cancer is a wound that never heals"; 2017: " The patient is both the host and the treatment for their cancer."*

While connoting both the social as well as biological consequences of an entity that has plagued mankind for millennia, this sentiment recognizes the central role of the immune system in wound healing, or, in this context, tumor elimination. The critical role that the immune system plays in tumor regression, and therapeutic strategies harnessing the host immune response against tumor, have been recognized since the advent of Coley's toxin over a century ago—based on observations that patients with severe postoperative skin infections after their sarcoma surgery would spontaneously achieve cancer remission. Bacillus Calmette–Guérin (BCG) vaccine has shown durable efficacy in localized bladder cancer with reported responses in metastatic cancers as well. Decades of innovation in medical science would be required to further refine cancer immunotherapy for clinical use.

More recently, an improved understanding of the various immune cells within the tumor microenvironment has revealed the importance of immunomodulatory pathways in tumor control and rejection. Both the innate and adaptive arms of the immune system are crucial to tumor control and rejection. The importance of T cell-mediated rejection of tumor was first harnessed in the form of cytokine therapy, in particular interleukin-2, as a therapeutic agent in metastatic melanoma and renal cell carcinoma. Subsequently, advances in cell processing led to the advent of autologous tumor-infiltrating lymphocyte therapy with initial responses in melanoma and subsequently other tumor types. Similarly, immune checkpoint blockade targeting inhibitory T cell axes such as CTLA-4 and PD-1/PD-L1 have revolutionized oncology and can result in durable responses in tumor types ranging from melanoma to lung cancer to Hodgkin lymphoma, among others.

The promise of immunotherapy in achieving long-lasting remissions in advanced disease has unleashed a torrent of drug development, focusing in particular on novel combinatorial immunotherapeutic strategies. Distinct from chemotherapy and targeted therapy in drug development, response kinetics, toxicity, and biomarker science, early phase clinical trials of cancer immunotherapy have numerous unique characteristics in trial design that are as paradigm shifting as the agents themselves. For example, radiographic pseudoprogression can be seen due to initial immune infiltration of tumor, which, if not appreciated, can result in premature discontinuation of therapy and an incorrect assessment of therapeutic efficacy. Also of importance, residual radiographic lesions may represent inactive cancer or immunologic scars of phagocytosed tumor. Durable stable disease can also be observed resulting in substantial clinical benefit to the patient. This data may not be sufficiently appreciated in early phase clinical trials powered by response rates based on early assessments of tumor shrinkage, relative to often major improvements in symptoms and longer-term survival.

Classes of Cancer Immunotherapy

- Vaccines
  - Peptide/Protein/Tumor cell lysates
  - Viral
  - Dendritic Cell
  - Oncolytics
- Small molecule agonists and inhibitors
  - IDO
  - TGF-beta
- Cytokines
  - IL-2
- Immune checkpoint modulation
  - CTLA-4
  - PD-1, PD-L1
  - TNFSRF agonists
- Cellular therapy
  - CARs, TCRs
  - NK cell

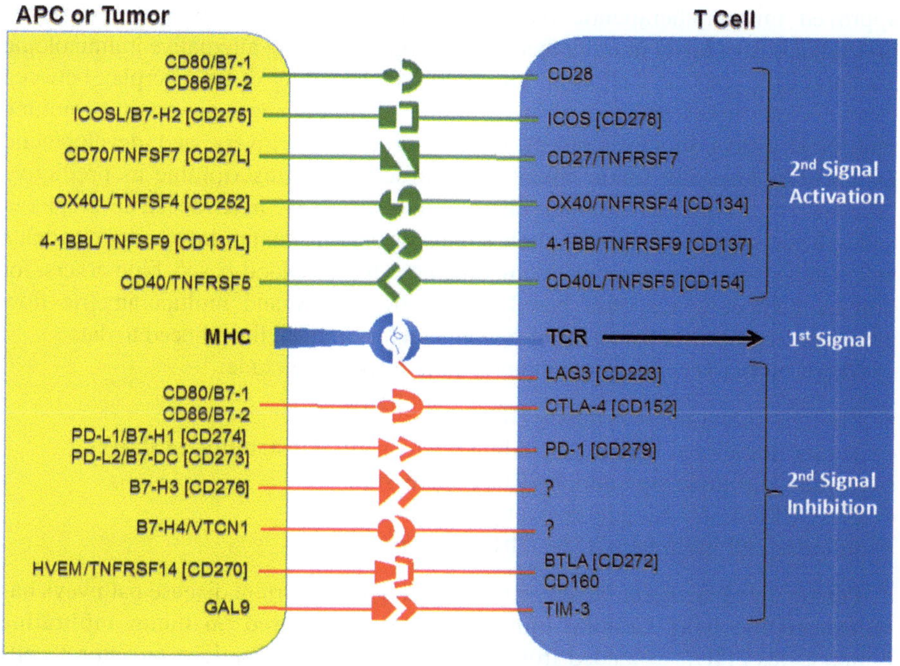

Furthermore, conventional dose-limiting toxicities for early phase clinical trials of cytotoxic chemotherapy based on relatively common cytopenias or end-organ toxicity that are dose-dependent are exceeding rare with immunotherapy. Instead, rarer immune-related adverse events with delayed toxicity kinetics or severe cytokine release syndrome may be observed with the clinical utilization of immune checkpoint blockade and cellular therapy, respectively. These rare and delayed phenomena place heightened importance on pharmacokinetic and pharmacodynamics biomarkers to determine safe dosing, and novel clinical trial designs to best ascertain safe dosing schema for these novel agents. Nuances may exist even within similar pathways—for example dose-dependent immune related adverse events based on increased weight-based dosing of anti-CTLA-4 targeted agents, but similar efficacy and toxicity across dose ranges of anti-PD-1/PD-L1 targeting therapies that result in the latter being more amenable to fixed dosing schema. Dosing of cellular therapeutics such as CAR T-cells may be dependent not only on antecedent conditioning chemotherapy, but on nuances of co-stimulatory factors, individual variances in cell harvest, and ratios of immune cell populations. Whether acting on extant immune cells within the tumor microenvironment via immune checkpoint blockade, or via exogenously engineered cellular therapeutics, novel clinical trial designs to allow for the early investigation of these pharmacodynamically atypical agents are needed.

The advent of next-generation sequencing has revolutionized genomically-based precision medicine, currently utilized and integrated into clinical practice. To date, the use of PD-L1 immunohistochemistry represents the state-of-the-art in clinically approved immunotherapeutic biomarker science. However, with an improved understanding of novel immunotherapeutic targets affecting alternative immunologic axes and cell types, as well as an improved understanding of the interplay between cancer neoantigens and the adaptive immune system, next-generation immune multiplex assays in development will foster drug discovery and development. Diagnostics assaying tumor mutational burden and transcriptome as predictive biomarkers of response to immune checkpoint blockade are in advanced development and will add substantially to the clinical diagnostic armamentarium to ensure patients are matched to their optimal immunotherapy. Novel blood-based biomarkers for immunotherapeutic response based on cell-free DNA and multiparametric flow cytometry represent active areas of research and an unmet clinical need to date.

Major biomarkers for immunotherapeutic response include:

- PD-L1 immunohistochemistry (IHC)
- Tumor mutational burden (including microsatellite instability, MSI-H)
- Immune infiltrate signature by RNA expression
- PD-L1/PD-L1/JAK2 genomic amplification
- Immune cell infiltrate (CD8+, Th1, memory)

Personalized medicine based on the targeting of important disease pathways has reinvented the field. Cellular immunotherapeutics, based on tumor infiltrating lymphocytes (TILs) expanded from the tumor or chimeric antigen receptor T cells (CAR-T) targeting extracellular cancer targets represent personalized immunotherapy—a form of therapy in which a patient's own cells are mobilized in a manner to fight their particular cancer, and can result in durable remissions. Novel therapeutic targets and cellular engineering methods that maximize efficacy while ameliorating serious toxicities are undergoing rapid clinical development, with the need for equally novel clinical trial designs given the promise of the agents. Given the personalized nature of these cellular therapeutics, paired with currently onerous costs, novel trial designs and regulatory pathways will be needed to ensure continued innovation in this space.

Combinations of immunotherapy with existing cancer approaches has led to novel observations on classical cancer therapeutics. Radiation, typically considered a form of tumor ablative therapy, can be harnessed to modify a tumor microenvironment and unleash cancer neoantigens in combination with immune checkpoint blockade—effectively converting radiation into a cancer vaccination modality. Similarly, cytotoxic chemotherapy can result in immunogenic cell death and heightened efficacy in combinations with immune checkpoint blockade. Efforts to combine these therapies while minimizing autoimmune toxicity and antagonistic chemotherapeutic effects on immune cells are under active clinical investigation. Finally, combinations of targeted therapy and immune checkpoint blockade can result in tumor killing and neoantigen release, as well as cell signaling modulation that can foster enhanced efficacy of immunotherapeutics. Such combinations can harness the relatively rapid response kinetics of targeted therapeutics with the potential for long-term durable benefit from the engendered immune response and sustained with immune checkpoint blockade.

Combinations of immunotherapeutics, in particular immune checkpoint blockade, have resulted in durable responses in melanoma as well as in non-small cell lung cancer, among other tumor types. An improved understanding of the tumor microenvironment and mechanisms of immune tolerance have led to the mechanistic-based use of immunotherapeutics in Hodgkin lymphoma and Merkel cell carcinoma. Further insights and therapies targeting novel immune cell types and pathways will be required in order to expand the promise of immunotherapy beyond the currently known histologies and molecularly-defied cohorts.

With the advent of an ever-expanding cadre of immunotherapeutics, early phase clinical trials investigating these agents will have to be as novel as the immunotherapeutics themselves. Many of the unique challenges related to the investigation of cancer immunotherapy are intertwined with their mechanism of action and inexorably linked to their efficacy. Ultimately, immunotherapeutics are based on the premise that the host immune system can successfully reject tumors—in other words, *the patient is both the host and the treatment for their cancer*. With a growing arsenal of promising immunotherapeutic agents, the inexorable goal of healing the wound that is cancer seems ever closer and reinforces a message well-known to family, friends, and caregivers of those fighting cancer—the most important aspect of any cancer therapy is already within the patient.

La Jolla, CA, USA

Sandip Pravin Patel
Razelle Kurzrock

Contents

Chapter 1
Primer on Cancer Immunotherapy and the Targeting of Native Proteins

Valentin Barsan and Paul C. Tumeh

Abstract Immunotherapy has notable potential for achieving durable clinical responses in many cancer types. The ability to readily measure the genomic landscape and infiltrating immune spectra of individual patient tumors offers mechanistic insights for combination therapy selection. Immunotherapeutic approaches through immune checkpoint blockade or stimulation, immune cell therapies, as well as tumor vaccination are being studied as mono and combination therapy in multiple cancer types. Uniquely, many immunotherapies target "native" self-proteins and thus herald a paradigm shift in cancer management in which the drug target is no longer an oncogenic protein but rather a normal signal that impacts the interactions of myriad immune cell types with both cancerous and normal cells. Native proteins in immunology are found in multiple isoforms with distinct interaction partners and at heterotypic transient cellular interfaces. Methods for evaluating the presence and function of native proteins for therapeutic targeting necessitates resolving for tumor–immune cellular interactions to understand which cell type is expressing which native protein isoform in the contextual (variably inflamed) tumor microenvironment. Just as tumor genomics has facilitated the selection of targeted therapies, precision immuno-oncology necessitates a comprehensive understanding of the immune system and the native proteins that govern its coordinated behavior. This primer on the relevant immunobiology, its clinical assessment, and therapeutic implications establishes a framework for conceptualizing the clinical advances in cancer immunotherapy that are the focus of this volume.

Keywords Immuno-oncology • Immunogenomics • Cancer immunotherapy • Checkpoint blockade • Immunobiology • Tumor biology • Adaptive immunity • Native proteins

V. Barsan, MD (✉)
UC San Diego School of Medicine, Moores Cancer Center, Valentin Barsan, MD, USA
e-mail: vbarsan@ucsd.edu

P.C. Tumeh, MD
BioGraph 55, Inc., San Francisco, CA, USA
e-mail: paul.tumeh@biographicpharma.com

S.P. Patel, R. Kurzrock (eds.), *Early Phase Cancer Immunotherapy*,
Current Cancer Research, DOI 10.1007/978-3-319-63757-0_1

1.1 An Intersection of Oncology and Immunology

The tissues that form human organs are composed primarily of two symbiotic cellular components: the parenchyma and the stroma. The parenchyma establishes unique tissue function whereas the stroma comprises an admixture of resident tissue cells (fibroblasts, dendritic and mast cells), vascular and lymphatic endothelial cells, inflammatory cells (lymphocytes, macrophages, myeloid cells), regenerative mesenchymal stem cells, as well as structural matrix proteins and proteoglycans [1]. Healthy tissues maintain a dynamic balance of these composite cellular and structural components across time and despite environmental stressors to achieve resilient "youthful" organ function. However, genomic instability (germline and somatic variants) in cells results in the development of cancer hallmarks [2] and the accompanying loss and compromise of normal tissue function at which time patients present for clinical consultation. Beyond "driver" mutations [3] that establish key mechanisms for neoplastic progression, nonsynonymous somatic mutations (that alter the amino acid sequences of the proteins encoded by the altered genes) can encode the aberrant translation of a diverse set of peptide "neoantigens" that, when recognized as foreign, triggers tumor immunogenicity [4]. Rudolph Virchow first proposed a link between inflammation and cancer in the 1860s when he observed leukocytes infiltrating neoplastic tissues [5]. A century later, it was postulated that lymphocytes can recognize and eliminate aberrant cells [6, 7]. More recently, "immunoediting" has been proposed as an active process in which immune cells both eliminate cancerous cells through immuno-recognition yet simultaneously promote neoplastic progression secondary to collateral inflammation [8]. Each patient's cancer is therefore wholly unique – an evolutionary outcome of successive neoplastic cellular divisions within distinct tumor microenvironments shaped through time as much by the patient's immune system as by successive therapeutic interventions.

The presence, subtype, location, and density of infiltrating immune cells in the tumor microenvironment characterize the degree of tumor inflammation. Diverse immune cell subtypes of varying immune "fitness" within each tissue stroma [9] and in the lymphatic system facilitate the intricate intercellular processes of discriminating self from nonself. Feedback control through suppression of inflammation is equally important in tuning the nature of the immune response to counter neoplastic cellular behaviors with sufficient, yet limited, on-target responses. Cancer immunotherapy and autoimmunity are thus finely related and likely coexist along a clinical spectrum in which the discriminate recognition of self from nonself determines the efficacy and toxicity profile of immunotherapeutics. Cancer immunotherapy therefore entails harnessing the power of the immune system to eliminate cancerous cells while preserving the integrity and function of otherwise healthy tissue. Historically speaking, the cancer drug development paradigm has entailed designing one drug to target one protein which is usually mutated and specific to a tumor type. The paradigm shift in cancer immunotherapy extends beyond targeting immune cells instead of cancerous cells. Rather, coordinating tumor immunity entails targeting native nonmutated proteins instead of oncogenes. These native proteins are expressed by different immune cell types of varying fitness, in multiple isoforms (with distinct interaction partners), across discrete tissue compartments, and at heterotypic and transient cellular interfaces. Therapies that target the immune system are thus fundamentally different in biologic mechanism, pharmacokinetics, and clinical application than therapies that target key cancer pathways. Conversely, therapies that target driver mutations in oncogene pathways of cancer cells can inadvertently dampen critical intracellular pathways in immune cell activation.

Targeting native proteins introduces a level of biologic and clinical complexity with which we have limited experience in oncology. Methods for evaluating the presence and function of native proteins necessitate resolving for tumor–immune cellular interactions to understand which cell type is expressing which native protein isoform in what contextual (inflamed or noninflamed) tumor microenvironment. Just as each cancer has a distinct mutational landscape so too each patient presents with a unique immune system whose fitness is shaped by genetics, age, vaccination and pathogen exposure history, as well as the environment. For example, epidemiologic studies associate the development of mumps in childhood with protection against ovarian cancer ostensibly due to primed immune surveillance [10]. Important environmental influences on the immune system and cancer progression are intuitive yet complexly interrelated. These include diet and exercise that can modulate gut/airway/skin microbiomes, UV/airborne/ingested carcinogens, and infectious exposures. In health, the immune cells can recognize both pathogens (i.e., viruses, bacteria, fungi, and parasites) as well as mutated cells to effectuate a targeted cytotoxic response with limited collateral inflammatory damage to surrounding tissues. When the immune system cannot effectively discriminate between self and nonself, autoimmune diseases (such as rheumatoid arthritis, diabetes, lupus) develop. The balance between self-tolerance and autoimmunity thus underpins the mechanisms by which immunotherapies have been applied to treat cancer. Our deepening understanding of the immune system at a molecular level has led to broad therapeutic advances in immunomodulatory monoclonal antibodies, cellular therapies, and vaccination strategies that are now being studied in all cancer types alongside conventional approaches of surgery, chemotherapy, and radiation. Understanding when, where, and how the diverse cells of the immune system interact to mount a coordinated cytotoxic immune response against cancer establishes the foundation for implementing these insights in clinical settings.

1.2 Innate and Adaptive Immunity

An effective and specific cytotoxic immune response against a tumor is coordinated by multiple cross-priming agonist and antagonist signals coordinated between varied cells of the innate and adaptive immune systems [11, 12]. These systems are comprised of more than 200 immune cells types and more than 300 immune cell state

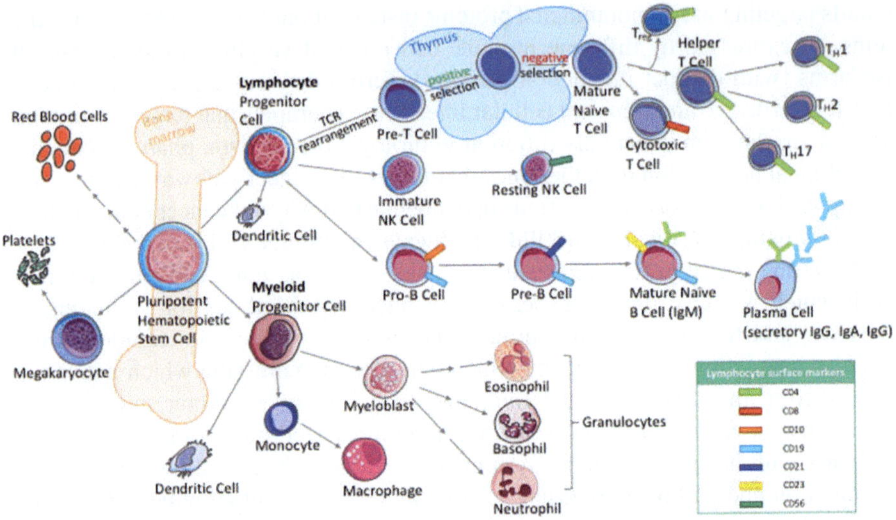

Fig. 1.1 Immune cell growth and differentiation. Cells of the immune system differentiate across myeloid or lymphoid lineages from hematopoietic stem cell precursors in the bone marrow. Hundreds of additional cell types and intermediate states exist. Partial maturation of T cells in the thymus and B cells in the bone marrow is followed by further differentiation in peripheral lymphoid tissues throughout development. Lymphocytes are commonly characterized by the surface expression of cluster of differentiation (CD) markers as well as the types of cytokines or antibodies produced

transitions [13]. All cells of the immune system differentiate (that is, increasingly functionalize) across myeloid or lymphoid lineages from hematopoietic stem cell precursors in the bone marrow (Fig. 1.1). Cells of the myeloid lineage include red blood cells, platelets, granulocytes (eosinophils, neutrophils, basophils), mast cells, and macrophages. Cells of the lymphoid lineage include natural killer (NK) cells, T cells (γδ, NK, $CD4^+$ and $CD8^+$ subsets), and B cells. Antigen-presenting dendritic cells may derive from either myeloid or lymphoid lineages. The myeloid and lymphoid lineages are functionally characterized by innate or adaptive cellular behaviors. The *innate* component includes most immune cells of the myeloid compartment as well as NK cells whereas the *adaptive* component consists solely of lymphoid (B and T) cells and their myriad subtypes. Partial maturation of T cells in the thymus and B cells in the bone marrow in utero is followed by further differentiation in peripheral lymphoid tissues after birth and attainment of immunocompetency under antigenic stimulus. Immune cells and their degree of differentiation are commonly characterized by expression of surface clusters of differentiation (CD) or the types of cytokines they secrete. Adaptive immunity is defined by the ability to discern and remember immunologic threats based on foreign, mutated, or atypically expressed antigens. At baseline, both components of the immune system are "on alert" until a threat has been identified at which time, rapid innate immune activation occurs and primes an adaptive response. Because each major immune cell type has an active and a regulatory form, the balance between these states characterizes the quality of an immune response.

Cells of the *innate* immune system use generic methods to recognize foreign pathogens based on nonspecific and nonhuman molecular patterns such as single-stranded RNA or lipopolysaccharide. Germline-encoded non-self-reactive receptors on neutrophils, macrophages, natural killers, and mast cells respond to generalized pathogen-associated molecular patterns (PAMPs) such as mannose receptors or toll-like receptors shared by many classes of microbes [14]. Innate cells such as macrophages and neutrophils migrate into tissues though expression of high-affinity integrin, kill microbes through phagocytosis and reactive oxygen species (triggered by interferon-γ), induce inflammation (through tumor necrosis factor, IL-1 and IL-6), activate T cells and NK cells (through IL-12), and initiate tissue repair (through secretion of immunosuppressive interleukins, TGF-ß, and fibroblast growth factors). Innate immunity defense mechanisms further include the complement cascade and inflammation. The complement system is comprised of nine major factors (C1 to C9), most of which are pro-enzymes present in normal serum and not increased by antigenic stimulation. The complement cascade facilitates inflammation, leukocyte recruitment, anaphylatoxin production, mast cell degranulation, opsonization for phagocytosis, secondary signals for B-cell activation, and the formation of membrane attack complexes against pathogenic cells. Tissue inflammation stimulates the adaptive immune response, enables the elimination of invasive foreign pathogens through controlled passage of immune cells, and initiates tissue repair.

Tissue inflammation also influences the resident cells within a tumor microenvironment. In an environment of chronic inflammation, myeloid cell differentiation can be skewed [15] toward the expansion of myeloid-derived suppressor cells (MDSCs). MDSCs are a heterogeneous subpopulation of immune cells (including macrophages, neutrophils, and dendritic cells) with potent immunosuppressive functions. Whereas M1 macrophages release interferon-γ and are responsible for phagocytosis, M2 macrophages release cytokines (IL-4, IL-10, TGF-ß) that curtail inflammatory responses and foster immune tolerance [16]. Macrophages also serve as important regulators of tumor angiogenesis by producing various pro-angiogenic molecules such as erythrocyte growth factor (EGF) and vascular endothelial growth factor (VEGF). Tumors can foster immuno-tolerance in the microenvironment through the manipulation of cytokines (increased secretion of IL-6, IL-10, and TGF-ß; consumption of IL-2) that encourage infiltration of inhibitory immune cells such as MDSCs and regulatory T cells (Tregs). Several therapeutic approaches (PDE5 inhibitors, COX-2 inhibitors, ARG1 inhibitors, bisphosphonates, gemcitabine, and paclitaxel, among others) play a complementary role in promoting antitumor immune responses by inhibiting the function or proliferation of MDSCs [17]. Immune cells also acquire distinct metabolic characteristics [18] that influence the plasticity of their immunological phenotypes and functions.

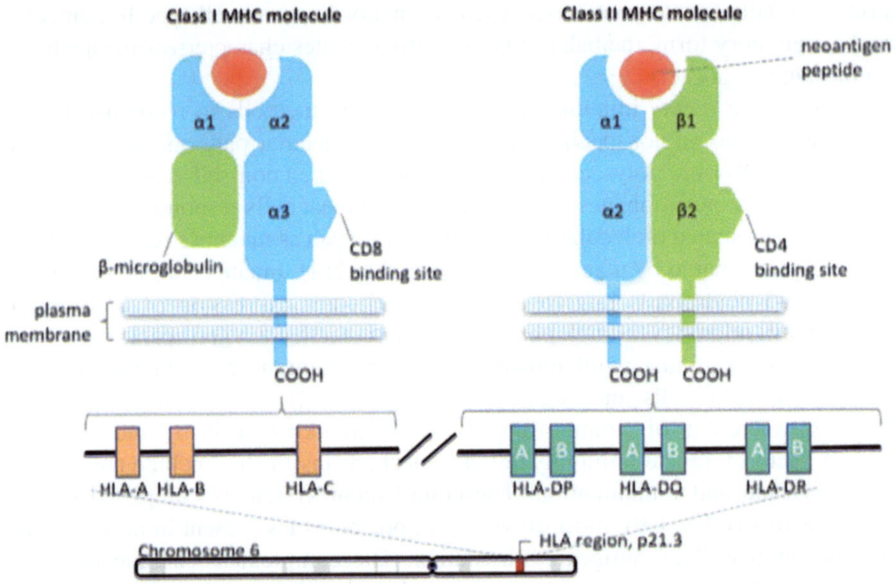

Fig. 1.2 Class I and Class II MHC Molecules. The maternal and paternal HLA haplotypes are located at chromosome 6, on the short arm at position p21.3, and encode the genes for MHC. HLA haplotypes are codominantly expressed. Both MHC Class I and MHC Class 2 consist of an alpha (heavy) and a beta (light) chain. The class I HLA molecule contains an alpha chain anchored to the cell membrane. The peptide antigen of 8 to 11-mer amino acids (red) is presented in a groove formed from a pair of alpha-helicies on a floor of antiparallel beta strands. The class I alpha chains are coded for by genes within the MHC (e.g., HLA-A, HLA-B), whereas the beta chain, beta-2 microglobulin, is encoded on chromosome 15, not in the MHC. The class II HLA molecule is MHC-encoded by both alpha and beta chains each anchored to the cell membrane without beta2-microglobulin. The peptide antigen of ~15-mer amino acids is presented in a groove formed from a pair of alpha helices on a floor of antiparallel beta strands. Class II antigens are constitutively expressed on B cells, dendritic cells, and monocytes and can be induced during inflammation on many other cell types that normally have little or no expression. Genes within the MHC (e.g., HLA-DP/Q/R) code for both chains

1.3 Orchestrating Adaptive Immunity

All human cells express a cell-surface major histocompatibility complex (MHC) that is genetically encoded by the human leukocyte antigen (HLA) locus. HLAs are inherited as haplotypes from both parents and expressed co-dominantly as MHC on all cells (Fig. 1.2). The MHC thus functions as an authenticating cell surface complex that physically presents peptides to adaptive immune cells [19] and enables the immune system to distinguish between self and nonself. HLA typing has thus enabled the matching of transplanted organs [20] and cells to minimize rejection. The HLA locus contains more than half of the four to five million single nucleotide polymorphisms (SNPs) in each individual genome [21]. This genomic variability implies enormous diversity in any given patient's relative immune fitness and susceptibility to immunologic disorders or infectious agents. MHC diversity explains why tissue transplantation remains so challenging and perhaps as well why autoimmune and infectious susceptibilities cluster by subtype. Proteins encoded by the three key MHC class I genes (HLA-A, HLA-B, and HLA-C) are present on the surface of most cells to present peptides that are internally processed and exported from inside the cell. MHC class I thus facilitates immune surveillance of intracellular pathogens or aberrant proteins. Cells that do not express MHC are indiscriminately attacked by NK cells of the innate immune system. Downregulation of MHC by cancer cells suggests a therapeutic utility of NK cell therapy [22]. The six main MHC class II genes (HLA-DPA, HLA-DPB, HLA-DQA, HLA-DQB, HLA-DRA, and HLA-DRB) encode cell-surface proteins that display peptides derived from circulating, extracellular proteins to the immune system. MHC class II molecules are expressed only on antigen-presenting cells (APCs), such as dendritic cells.

APCs are activated by recognition of antigens that bind surface MHC which induces downregulation of cell-adhesion molecules to facilitate migration from the tissue of residence to a lymph node for antigen presentation to residing adaptive immune T and B lymphocytes. APCs serve as the critical link for priming the adaptive immune cells. Dendritic cells and macrophages are "professional" APCs and critically link the innate and adaptive immune systems. Since their discovery in 1973 [23], dendritic cells have been shown to develop from either myeloid or lymphoid hematopoietic lineages which thereby creates distinctive subsets of dendritic cells that have discreet functions tuned by their tissue of residence and microenvironment (these nuances are especially relevant in vaccine development). The main dendritic subtypes include plasmacytoid DCs (pDCs) and conventional DCs (cDCs). Both pDCs and cDCs are comprised of additional subtypes that have discrete morphology, tissue distribution, surface marker expression, and cytokine production which consequently lead to distinct pathways to T-cell activation. Also, tumor-associated macrophages are ontogenetically diverse [24] and specially tuned to the function of their host tissue. APCs such as dendritic cells or macrophages phagocytose (engulf) and process antigens released from tumor cells to present them to T and B cells. Engagement of the T- or B-cell receptor with MHC peptide is a necessary first step in lymphocyte cell activation. The complementarity determining region (CDR) determines the specificity of a lymphocyte receptor to its cognate antigen. T lymphocytes express clonal T-cell receptors (TCRs) on their surface that recognize antigenic peptides presented by host cells whereas B-cell receptors (BCRs) are secreted as soluble antibodies (immunoglobulins) upon antigen recognition. Lymphocyte receptors also exhibit tremendous genetic diversity to enable the recognition of so many potential antigens presented by MHC. The generation of diverse TCRs and BCRs begins with immature T and B lymphocytes through VDJ recombination, a process in which *germline* DNA is spliced to recombine noncontiguous variable (V), diversity (D), and joining (J) region gene segments and collectively encode the complementarity determining region 3 (CDR3) [25] of a given naïve (antigen inexperienced) lymphocyte. Diversity of the CDR3 region is increased by the deletion and template-independent insertion of nucleotides at the V-D and D-J junctions and further through somatic hypermutation in the BCR.

These receptors recognize residues of peptide antigens in MHC as well as polymorphic residues of the MHC molecule itself. An estimated 100,000–750,000 peptide-MHC class I complexes are expressed for each allelic product (HLA-A and HLA-B loci) [26], and each individual carries ~10^7 different TCRs [27] each detecting up to 10^6 variations of a given peptide sequence [28].

Immature T and B cells must subsequently demonstrate the ability to discern between harmful and innocuous antigens through a tolerance process prior to their release into circulation. B or T cells optimally recognize only one antigen. Developing T cells undergo tolerance and maturation in the thymus whereas B cells do so in the bone marrow. To establish immunologic tolerance in these organs, immature T and B cells undergo positive selection (weak receptor interaction with self-antigen allows for cell survival) and negative selection (lymphocytes that bind too strongly to self-antigens are signaled to die). Randomly generated TCRs and BCRs recognizing endogenously expressed self-epitopes (peptide/MHC "ligandomes") are variably pruned in the thymus [29] and marrow [30], respectively, during their development to limit immunological self-destruction. Mature lymphocytes continuously recirculate between blood and peripheral lymphoid tissues, localizing and extravasating into tissues when guided by chemokine gradients from tissue-resident sentinel innate immune cells. The patient's adaptive immune cells are thus finely tuned within a discrete range of binding affinities – a process that when disrupted can result in autoimmunity or when engineered ex vivo enables potent cellular therapies. Paradoxically, self-reactive adaptive immune cells theoretically comprise an autogenous source of potential anticancer activity. Autoimmunity eliminates cancerous cells.

Through interaction with APCs, the lymphoid cells of the *adaptive* immune system evolve with exquisite specificity to surface and soluble antigens through selective clonal expansion of T and B lymphocytes. The tumor draining lymph node is a more immuno-active microenvironment in which high throughput antigen exposure by APCs to standby lymphocytes occurs. In lymph nodes, naïve T and B cells recognize tumor antigens and can become activated. The mode of cancer cell death (apoptosis versus necrosis) influences the degree and quality of antigen spreading [31], in which previously intracellular immunogenic antigens are released because of cell lysis [32] thereby broadening antitumor responses to additional antigens. T cells exert immune effects through cellular interactions whereas B cells become activated upon antigen recognition to differentiate into antibody-producing plasma cells. Secreted antibody subtypes (immunoglobulins) are frequently measured in infectious diseases as titers and clinically indicate primary versus repeat/historical antigen exposures. B-cell homing areas enable rapid antibody secretion and are found primarily in the splenic follicles, marrow pulp, lymph nodes, and mucosal-associated tissues. Mature B cells are educated (antigen-specific) APCs that present to effector CD4 T cells via MHC-II, who will in turn activate B cells to undergo "class switching" and "affinity maturation" to produce clonal circulating antibodies of varying kinetics and increasing potency. A rapid adaptive immune response is initiated by T and B cells if the presented antigen has been recognized previously.

Both tumor and transplant rejection are mediated mainly by cytotoxic T lymphocytes. T-cell activity is controlled by a combination of antigen-specific signals from the TCR as well as antigen-independent signals from myriad co-receptors [33]. The TCR binds specific short stretches of amino acids (i.e., peptides) presented by MHC molecules located on all host cells, and notably APCs (Fig. 1.3). VDJ recombination produces a TCR that is composed of two different proteins chains (α and ß whose ratios change throughout cellular maturation as well as in diseased states) and CD3 which encodes an invariant transmembrane protein complex that relays surface signals for secretion of pro-inflammatory cytokines such as IL-12 and interferon gamma. The MHC molecules expressed in the thymus restrict a mature T cell to a predetermined spectrum of antigens. Each T cell expresses monoclonal membrane-bound TCRs that all recognize the same specific peptide/MHC complex during physical contact between the T cell and an APC (MHC class II) or any host cell (MHC class I). T-cell subtypes are characterized broadly by their co-receptors: CD4 on helper and regulatory T cells is specific for MHC class II whereas CD8 on cytotoxic T cells is specific for MHC class I. The subtypes of effector $CD4^+$ and $CD8^+$ T cells are often characterized by the specific cytokines (interleukins) produced upon their activation. Activated $CD8^+$ (killer) T cells engage in direct cytotoxic activity whereas activated $CD4^+$ (helper) T cells support other lymphocytes, for example, by promoting the maturation of B cells into plasma cells and memory B cells and activating cytotoxic T cells and macrophages. To mount an effective immune response beyond activation through MHC-peptide and TCR binding, T cells require additional costimulatory signals. A critical priming costimulatory signal in naïve T cells is CD28, which binds to B7-1 and B7-2 (CD80/86) on the APC [34]. Without CD28:B7 interaction, the naïve T cell remains anergic (refractory to activation or unresponsive). The most differentiated effector and memory (antigen-experienced) T cells [35] are least dependent on costimulatory signals due to avidity maturation that reduces the activation threshold of these subtypes.

Once activated, T cells reduce expression of CD28 and upregulate surface immune checkpoint molecules which are native proteins that facilitate feedback inhibition and limit cytotoxic activity. Unrestrained T-cell activation would otherwise lead to malignant proliferation or autoimmune disease. CTLA-4 is one such *inducible* surface checkpoint molecule that is upregulated on T cells after activation, has higher affinity for the ligands CD80 and CD86, and is also constitutively expressed on a variety of Tregs [36]. CTLA acts as an "off switch" when bound to CD80 or CD86 on the surface of APCs. CTLA-4 blockade hence produces both a direct enhancement of T-cell effector function and a concomitant inhibition of regulatory T-cell activity [37]. Programmed cell death-1 (PD-1) is expressed later and functions as an inhibitory homologue of CD28 following T-cell activation. A key mechanism by which cancer cells diffuse the host immune response is the upregulation of PD-1 that bind to PD-1 on tumor-specific CD8+ T cells [38] as well as NK T cells and B cells. PD-1 is a member of the extended CD28/CTLA-4 family of T-cell regulators that is highly expressed on *activated* T cells whose two ligands PD-L1 and PD-L2 have been found to be expressed as immuno-escape behaviors of several cancers. PD-L1 and PD-L2 are also expressed on cells of the immune system

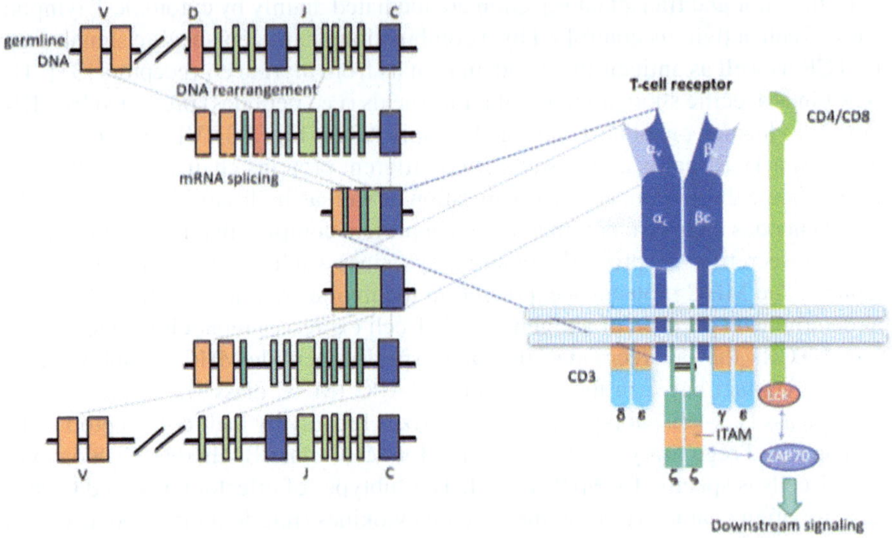

Fig. 1.3 The T cell receptor. The mature T cell heterodimer consists of alpha- and beta-subunit chains that are formed by rearranged germline DNA of variable (V), diversity (D), joining (J), and constant (C) regions. The TCR alpha chain is generated by VJ recombination, whereas the beta chain is generated by VDJ recombination. Signalling is initiated by aggregation of TCR by MHC-peptide complexes on APC. Costimulation is required from CD4 on helper-T cells or CD8 on cytotoxic T cells. The intracytoplasmic region of the TCR is too short to transduce a signal from the cell surface so CD3 facilitates signalling through the TCR. Once MHC-peptide binds the TCR, lymphocyte cell-specific protein tyrosine kinase (Lck) is activated and phosphorylates tryosine residues within the immunoreceptor tyrosine-based activation motifs (ITAMs) of the CD3 and zeta chains, enabling zeta chain-associated protein kinase 70 (ZAP-70) recruitment to the TCR which triggers downstream signaling events required for T cell activation

(upregulated on macrophages and DCs in response to bacterial lipopolysaccharide as well as activated T, B, and NK cells). PD-L1 can also interact (like CTLA-4) with the CD80 receptor on T cells, sending a further immunosuppressive signal. In addition, PD-L1 is also expressed constitutively on nonlymphoid tissues such as the heart, lung, placenta, and skeletal muscle where it may serve to downregulate TCR signaling in PD-1+ cytotoxic T-lymphocytes and therefore protect against autoimmune-mediated tissue damage. Multiple additional co-receptors that modulate T-cell activation and inhibition have become the central focus of checkpoint blockade or stimulation (Fig. 1.4). The activation of T-cell subtypes is dependent on the balance of antagonist (e.g., CTLA-4, PD-1, LAG3, TIM3) and agonist native proteins (e.g., GITR, OX40, ICOS) on *both* the APC and T cells [33]. The therapeutic targeting these native proteins implies modulating complex cellular interactions both within the tumor bed and in lymphoid organs where APCs and T cells interact to amplify immune responses. Antibodies that mimic or block the effect of these checkpoint or agonist receptors or ligands aim to enhance the immune response against tumor cells. Chronic recognition of an antigen (such as that present in a malignant clone or in a chronic viral infection) may lead to feedback inhibition on effector T-cell function, resulting in a phenotype termed "exhaustion" [39]. Several therapeutic strategies aim to revitalize exhausted T cells. The plurality of inducible signaling molecules that exist as native proteins across diverse immune cell subtypes underscores the challenge in developing a comprehensive understanding of tumor–immune cell interactions.

1.4 Immunobiology of Cancer Immunotherapy

The cancer immunity cycle [40] and the cancer-immune set point [41] have established the conceptual frameworks through which tumor-specific T cells amplify a highly specific, cytotoxic, and clonal response to tumor neoantigens after priming by APCs. In a dynamic multidirectional process, immune cells interact in three distinct tissue compartments: the tumor microenvironment (TME), the draining lymph nodes, and the bloodstream. Each environment can be theorized to exhibit unique biology of variable diagnostic and therapeutic utility. In the tumor bed, resident APCs such as dendritic cells initiate an immune response through maturation to present antigens from the TME, in the form of peptide–MHC molecule complexes, to naïve (antigen inexperienced) T cells in secondary lymphoid tissues [42] such as the draining lymph node. There, T cells are activated when their surface TCRs recognize the cognate peptide-MHC-I on the APC. Now-primed effector and regulatory T cells traffic into the tumor by extravasation from blood vessels as triggered by chemokine gradients of tissue inflammation and TME endothelial upregulation of selectins. Cancer cells evade immune regulation by disrupting this cycle through multiple mechanisms including downregulation of MHC/antigen presentation, expression of inhibitory cell surface molecules that inhibit cytotoxic T cells (PD-L1, FasL), and upregulation of inhibitors of apoptosis (Bcl-XL, FLIP). Checkpoint inhibitors have been developed and approved for various tumor types with the objective of reducing the effector T-cell threshold for activation and thereby facilitating more sensitive immunogenicity (i.e., autoimmunity) preferably towards neoplastic cells that appear more foreign [43]. PD-1 and CTLA-4 antibody-based therapies appear to have broad spectrum antineoplastic activity and may well serve as a backbone therapy [44, 45] in immuno-oncology. However, the spatiotemporal differences between PD-1 and CTLA-4 checkpoints in the tumor microenvironment and germinal lymph tissues imply variable downstream immunomodulatory consequences that depend on the composition of differential immune cell infiltrates as well as a plurality of local factors [46]. Because of their nuanced effector functions, the same immune cell types and cytokines may promote or prevent tumor formation depending on the biological (i.e., tissue and TME) context in which they act.

Inflamed tumors are characterized by the presence of tumor-infiltrating lymphocytes (TILs) whose differential and dynamic representations, relative densities, and spatial distributions form the antitumor immune response [47, 48], and these factors have predictive clinical value [49, 50]. Tumor infiltration with $CD8^{+}$ T cells and an

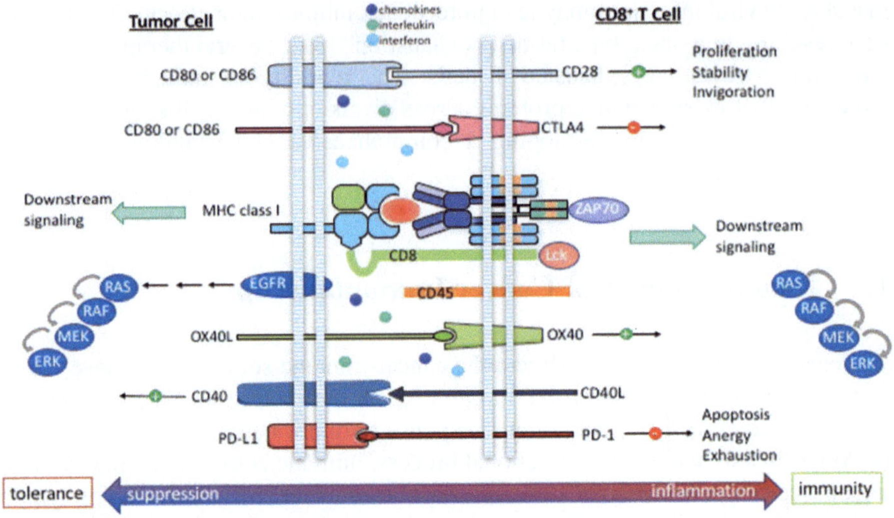

Fig. 1.4 The summative effects of co-stimulatory and inhibitory interactions regulate T cell responses. T cells activate downstream signaling to these ligand-receptor interactions only if they first recognize the cognate MHC-antigen through the TCR. Ligands can bind multiple receptors (with distinct kinetics of expression) giving rise to costimulatory or inhibitory signals amidst a milieu of circulating chemokines, interferons, and interleukins. Costimulatory receptors are often expressed on naïve and resting T cells whereas inhibitory receptors are upregulated only after T-cell activation to facilitate feedback inhibition. There are common pathways within both tumor and immune cells that may have variably suppressive or inflammatory effects depending on summative signals and tissue contexts

associated chemokine/interferon gene signature has been correlated with favorable clinical outcomes to checkpoint blockade, and this phenotype can be influenced by specific oncogene pathways activated within the TME as well as by host commensal microbiota that synergistically activate the immune system. The tissue-specific architecture of different cancer types reveals a range of somatic mutations [51, 52] as well as inflammatory landscapes [53, 54] from very focal expansion of TILs within tumor islets to diffuse inflammation throughout the tumor stroma. Spatial relationships are key to understanding cellular interactions within unique TMEs. Pleotropic stromal determinants further nuance tumor–immune cellular interactions and intercommunications in the tumor microenvironment [41, 55, 56], and multiple immunosuppressive factors may mediate intrinsic resistance to immunotherapy [57, 58]. T cells are inhibited in the TME by surface membrane native proteins (checkpoints: PD1, CTLA4, LAG3, TIM3, BTLA, Adenosine A2AR), soluble factors, and metabolic alterations (IL10, TGFbeta, adenosine, IDO, arginase) [59], as well as inhibitory cells (cancer-associated fibroblasts, Tregs and Bregs, MDSCs, tumor-associated macrophages). The milieu required for optimal functioning of the immune system is thus defined by summative effects of antigen-presenting cells, immuno-modulating cytokines, and optimal surface molecule expression by both tumor cells and infiltrating lymphocytes.

Cancer progression (immune escape) relies on the exhaustion or suppression of antitumor immune activity which can be attributed to both sustained immune cell presence as well as the presence of regulatory lymphocyte subtypes [60]. Certain mutations in cancer cells are more strongly immunogenic (a subject of concerted research), and some cancers attempt to discard those mutations, which renders them resistant to therapies that boost the immune system [61]. Additional mechanisms of evading immune recognition include loss or somatic mutations of HLA haplotypes or JAK1/JAK2 genes [62, 63] that disrupt antigen presentation as well as upregulation of alternate immune checkpoints [64]. Clonal evolution of a primary cancer and the epithelial-to-mesenchymal transition that coordinates metastasis [65] can be promoted by immune cells [66] in inflammatory TMEs. Tumors can evolve to physically exclude immune cells as commonly seen in melanoma liver metastases and colorectal cancers [67, 68]. Inclusion of some immune cells can even promote tumor growth. For example, recruitment of macrophages via cytokines promotes epidermal growth factor (EGF) production, which nurtures tumor growth while macrophage digestion of the surrounding stroma enables tumor metastasis. Targeting macrophages and/or other protumorigenic immune cells may thus alter the TME and extend the cytotoxic properties of $CD8^+$ T cells. Epigenetic regulation of cellular transcription is an additional mechanism for immune escape within the TME. Histone deacetylation and methylation can inhibit both the expression of T-cell stimulating ICAM1, CD80, CD86 as well as dampen neoantigen peptide-MHC loading [69].

Fundamentally, a functional antitumor T-cell response results in the production of IFNγ which facilitates effector functions as well as induces PD-L1 that mediates adaptive resistance [70]. Interferon and interleukin signaling convergence [71–73] most proximately explains the summative functional orientation of lymphocyte cytotoxicity within the TME. The summative quality of peptide–MHC–TCR interactions and TCR signaling in multiple anticancer T-cell clones directed against cancer antigens is subject to dynamic regulation by native co-stimulatory and co-inhibitory proteins. Cytokines dynamically regulate checkpoint expression [74] at nodes of the cancer-immunity cycle and therefore further modulate T-cell responses. Immunotherapies targeting native proteins such as molecular checkpoints thus have variable effects within a patient's primary tumor, across any metastatic sites, throughout the lymphoid structures in which immune responses are organized, and subsumed into the patient's systemic immunity. The relationship between tumor-specific antigens, the ratios of immune cell types targeting those epitopes, and the native proteins that orchestrate their interfaces may best capture the dynamisms of tumor evolution and immune response.

The intrinsic nature of many tumor antigens limits host antitumor responses since such "neoantigens" are often aberrantly expressed self-proteins that are merely subtle alterations of the normal protein. Mutations generate a range of immunogenic neoantigens. For example, insertions and deletions (indels) may make more foreign-looking peptides than SNVs whereas silent mutations may go unnoticed by the immune system since the encoded amino acid is not changed. Moreover, binding affinity of neoantigens to MHC may not correlate as strongly to immunogenicity as binding stability [75] of peptide-MHC with the TCR. The net mutational load of a tumor theoretically increases the probability that an antigenic peptide is presented, recognized, and targeted by the adaptive immune system. Mutations are acquired through either exogenous exposure to mutagens (i.e., radiation, carcinogens, or oncogenic viruses) or endogenous mechanisms that abrogate the integrity of DNA replication (i.e., mismatch repair deficiency) [76, 77]. Accordingly, different tumor types have characteristic mutational frequencies and patterns [78, 79] whose antigenic load arises from viral or genomic variants that encode ostensibly immunogenic peptides for MHC presentation and variable T-cell binding avidity [80–82]. The mutational load across tumor types is highly variable. However, the quantity of neoantigens may not directly correlate with their quality (i.e., immunogenicity) or specificity. For example, pediatric and hematological cancers have the lowest mutation rates (approximately one mutation per megabase for chronic lymphocytic leukemia) compared with cancers exposed to environmental mutagens that randomly increase the mutation burden, such as melanoma and lung cancer (~15 mutations per megabase for melanoma). In more mutated tumors, immunosurveillance may be especially prevalent. For example, a 200-fold increase in risk of nonmelanoma skin cancers was demonstrated in renal transplant patients, highlighting a curious role for cancer immunosurveillance at sites exposed to highly mutagenic UV radiation [83]. Most tumor antigens are presumably weakly immunogenic as they often appear related to host antigens and lack "danger signals" such as PAMPs. Virally mediated cancers (up to 25% of human cancers) contain foreign pathogen antigens, and therefore, have distinct mechanisms for inducing immune responses beyond mutational load. Patients exhibit a spectrum of susceptibilities to infectious, autoimmune, and cancer-immune processes based on their immune fitness. Clinical measurements of immune function inform disease pathogenesis and treatment optimization.

1.5 Biomarkers and Diagnostics in Immuno-oncology

Biomarker methods help explain cellular functions and relationships in tumor immunology and immuno-genomics [84, 85]. Immune monitoring is needed for comprehensive assessment of the immune status in patients and to establish biomarkers of diagnosis, prognosis, and response to therapy. The standard of care diagnostic workup in cancer has progressed from stage (radiographic imaging) and grade (histology) to encompass myriad molecular features that are either pathognomonic for diagnosis or prognosticating for disease risk. Consensus guidelines (such as those set forth by NCCN, CAP, ASCO, ESMO, etc.) are continuously updated to broaden clinical utility of companion and complementary diagnostic biomarkers. The pathologist's assessment of a tumor specimen can involve a range of methods that assay the biologic continuum from DNA to RNA to protein alongside complementary immunoassays that measure patient's immune responses. Proteomic considerations are uniquely important in immuno-oncology diagnostics since the targeting of native proteins implies understanding their cellular localization, splice and isoform variations, signaling pathways, post-translational modifications, and interaction networks and complexes. Tumor samples can be evaluated for clinical biomarkers through multiparametric immunohistochemistry, fluorescence in situ hybridization (FISH), gene expression profiling, polymerase chain reaction (PCR), and next generation sequencing (NGS). The resident immune cells of tumor specimens and lymph tissues may be studied through multiparameter flow cytometry to ascertain the functional orientation of lymphocytes through surface CD markers. Increased numbers of T-cell infiltrates within the tumor microenvironment have been associated with improved survival in several tumors types, including colorectal cancer and ovarian cancer [86, 87].

Multiple levels of post-transcriptional regulation imply that the relationship between RNA expression and protein abundance are often not linear. The primary (DNA), secondary (RNA), tertiary (peptide), and quaternary (cellular) levels of structure imply emergent properties at each scale. Hence, the co-evaluation of biomarkers in a sample helps elucidate functional relationships of gene and regulatory networks. Proteomic data are generally obtained using "shotgun proteomics" in which the combination of liquid chromatography (LC) and tandem mass spectrometry (MS/MS) identifies peptides by matching MS/MS spectra against theoretical spectra of all candidate peptides represented in a reference protein sequence database. This approach is limited since all protein-coding sequences in the genome are not known nor accurately annotated. Thus, distinct protein products of gene models are uncharacterized in protein reference databases (such as Ensembl, RefSeq, or UniProtKB) and, consequently, mutated native proteins and alternative splice forms are not being routinely measured.

The large majority of mutations in human tumors are unique to the individual tumor, necessitating the identification of mutations that can form neoantigens within clinically actionable timeframes using NGS and bioinformatics [88]. The clinically relevant types of genomic alterations (single nucleotide variants, insertions and deletions, amplifications, and gene fusions) each pose different diagnostic challenges beyond variable tumor purity in most clinical specimens [89]. PCR amplification and counting methods are limited by cost and throughput necessitating a compromise between a limited number of genes assayed in a large cohort or all coding genes sequenced in a small number of samples. Over the past decade, NGS has dramatically scaled our ability to sensitively and comprehensively identify mutations. The sensitivity of sequencing-based approaches is determined by the sequencing methods (amplicon vs enrichment library preparation) and read depth required to detect variants at clinically significant variant allele frequencies. Owing to the high sensitivity of NGS, rigorous analytical and clinical validations have been necessary to establish the accuracy and reproducibility of NGS panels that precedes their routine clinical use. Whole exome and whole transcriptome sequencing methods have broadened the measurable content beyond gene panels to enable identification of specific tumor neoantigens [90]. Detected neoantigens, when qualified by host HLA allotype (i.e., are presented by host MHC) may reveal not only the tumor "mutanome" but more specifically which mutated peptides are most immunogenic for focusing the immune response through various therapeutic strategies including cellular therapies and tumor- or patient-specific cancer vaccines. Concordance across neoantigen profiling methods has been limited by variations in exome capture methods, DNA and RNA target enrichment, sequencing depth, bioinformatics for variant calling, intracellular neoantigen processing and MHC binding predictors, filtering for expression, and ranking criteria of vaccine peptides based on myriad criteria [85]. Large series of epitopes are being evaluated for their recognition by T cells from multiple independent T-cell repertoires to methodically examine the mechanisms of neoantigen presentation and T-cell recognition. Strong neoantigen-MHC binding, however, does not necessarily equate to strong immunogenicity since binding affinity and binding stability have different consequences on immune cell responses. Validation of immunogenic neoantigens through functional assays remains a limiting step for translating in silico predictions into the clinic. Functional assays of immunogenicity include ELISPOT, flow cytometry, capillary chromatography, tandem mass spectrometry workflows, and proteomics [91, 92].

Common methods for studying TME heterogeneity (IHC and flow cytometry) rely on a limited repertoire of phenotypic markers. Deconvolution algorithms applied to bulk tumor RNA-seq or methylation data can resolve aggregate transcripts into their relative TIL constituents [93] to identify cell types involved in immunoediting. These methods are beginning to demonstrate clinical relevance since a priori knowledge of the densities and types of TILs [94] helps characterize the TME per the degree of immune cell polarization towards inflammatory or immunosuppressive cell types. RNA-seq deconvolution algorithms aim to enumerate (immune and tissue) cell subsets from tissue expression profiles and are predicated on applications of machine learning such as classification and regression, position-specific scoring matrices, support vector machines, hidden Markov models, and artificial neural networks. These methods still require extensive further validation in mixed tissues and clinical samples. Myriad additional computational genomics tools have been developed to mine tumor immunologic and genomic data effectively and provide novel mechanistic insights, predictive biomarkers, and therapeutic targets [95]. The clinical utility of gene signature-based methods, however, strongly depends on the fidelity of reference profiles that deviate in cells undergoing heterotypic interactions, phenotypic plasticity, or disease-induced dysregulation. Transcriptional signatures reflective of T-cell orientation, exhaustion, and memory differentiate activation states and proliferation of key subsets of exhausted T cells defined by co-expression patterns such as T-bet or eomesodermin (eomes) in combination with PD-1 [96–98]. Intra- and inter-patient sample variability in immune cell subset composition, inter-patient genetic variability, as well as prior and concurrent treatment medications are all clinical parameters that confound our ability to establish validated assays to generate biomarker data sets.

Longitudinal monitoring of response to immunotherapies presents additional opportunities for understanding mechanisms. Immunotherapies such as checkpoint blockade enable the mounting of a measurable antitumor immune response over variable clinical timeframes. The conventional Response Evaluation Criteria In Solid Tumors (RECIST) using radiographic methods (e.g., CT and MRI) must account for psuedoprogression in which tumors appear to grow radiographically secondary to inflammation [99, 100]. Owing to the inter and intra-tumoral heterogeneity [101] in metastatic disease, serial or functional imaging [102] such as anti-CD8 immuno-PET of multiple discrete lesions may be necessary to represent immunodynamics across multiple sites. Radiographic assessment thus contextualizes the relationships between circulating biomarkers and tumor inflammation through the course of therapy. Pharmacodynamic biomarkers for dose selection and toxicity anticipation are the basis of ongoing investigation. Unlike small-molecule-targeted agents such as Raf/MEK/PI3K inhibitors that block detectable signals in tumor cells, the targeting of native proteins does not infer an obvious signal for measurement of response. Considerable research is underway to understand and optimize proximal biomarkers unequivocally reflecting dose-dependent native protein target inhibition for immunotherapies. Immunodynamics measurement through complementary and mechanistic approaches [103, 104] will enable the implementation of novel endpoints in efficacy, dose selection, treatment sequencing, and toxicity.

Peripheral monitoring of tumor and immune biomarkers through blood draw is desirable because of the relative ease and standardization of sample collection as well as the ability to trend circulating tumor variants, immune cell subtypes, and pharmacodynamics over time. Existing peripheral monitoring approaches include flow cytometry for minimal residual disease, circulating tumor and exosomal DNA and RNA sequencing to monitor variant allele frequencies, circulating tumor cell isolation for expression analysis, tetramer assays for trending clonal evolution of antigen-specific T cells, and measurement of plasma cytokines and chemokines through ELISPOT assays. Circulating tumor DNA tests have been shown to provide complementary information to that found in primary tissue biopsies [105]. Peripheral evaluation of checkpoint blockade has revealed temporal variance in the differential leukocyte composition and markers of T-cell functionality such as clonality and expression of ICOS on sorted peripheral immune cell subtypes [106, 107]. Analysis of the T-cell receptor repertoire (such as by deep sequencing of the Vβ CDR3 region) has proven increasingly cost-effective and useful for clonality assessment and minimal residual disease detection. T-cell clonality in immuno-oncology enables the tracking of clonal expansion or contraction through serial sampling. Blood sampling also helps establish biomarker baselines for trending key organ function (kidney, liver, etc.) with vigilance towards inflammatory toxicity of immunotherapy such as cytokine release syndrome [108]. The differential immune measurements through blood draw are further confounded by any systemic immune response to opportunistic infections (viral, bacterial, fungal, parasitic) which are more common and can go undetected in immunosuppressed patients. Evaluation of the circulating microbiome through 16sRNA and metagenomic sequencing can measure aggregate effects of therapies on commensal and infectious flora [109–111]. Ongoing efforts are underway to establish the sampling timeframes and mechanistic relationships between circulating biomarkers as a proxy of dynamic antitumor immune activity within the tumor stroma [112, 113].

1.6 Targeting Native Proteins Within Cellular Networks

Treatment complexity is increasing as durable clinical responses require the use of numerous therapies in combination and in sequence [114]. Checkpoint blockade may appear to be the opposite of precision medicine as it can be applied broadly because of the targeting of native proteins. However, we still need biomarkers to understand when and why most patients do not respond while those who do may do so profoundly. Clinical outcomes are influenced by differences in patients' immune repertoires, their capacity to process and present antigens, the "quantity and quality" of tumor antigens generated, as well as the ability of cancer to suppress antitumor immunity. T cells are key effectors [115] and it is hypothesized that T cells can be genetically targeted to any antigen and enhanced to overcome immune escape mechanisms to achieve tumor eradication. As reviewed in this primer, T cells operate within a dynamic network of immune cell subtypes who are systemically under tumor micro-environmental influences and paracrine signals that continuously modulate their functional orientation. Beyond standard approaches of surgery, radiation, and chemotherapy, a variety of approaches to eliciting an antitumor immune response have been developed. These include antitumor antibodies (mono-, bi-, and multispecific), immune checkpoint blockade, T-cell costimulatory agonists, immunomodulators (cytokines, cyclic dinucleotides, IDO inhibitors), toll-like receptor agonists, cancer vaccines and oncolytic viruses, as well as adoptive T and NK cell therapies [116]. Conventional cytotoxic approaches modulate the composition and functional bioactivity of TILs beyond their intended effects on neoplastic cells [117].

The degree of nonlinear thinking required to first perceive and then influence network interactions [118] between immune cells and cancerous ones is central to advances in immuno-oncology. Combination immunotherapies that influence the immune set point may prevent immune escape by targeting complementary mechanisms through which tumor cells avoid elimination by the immune system. Mechanistic synergy can be achieved in: (1) priming – via tumor antigen-expressing dendritic cells or tumor cells transfected with genes that render them immunogenic; (2) amplification – checkpoint blockade or agonistic monoclonal antibodies against costimulatory molecules or immune-potentiating cytokines; and (3) removal of the inhibitions – eliminating mechanisms that self-regulate the strength of the immune response, such as inhibitory receptors or regulatory T cells.

Rational combination strategies must incorporate an understanding of pathway implications in both tumor and immune cell subtypes. The number of therapeutic combinations is exciting because the amount of antitumor activity is unprecedented. Most combinations are currently two drugs, but when adding sequence and dose (which are currently nearly guess work) the combinations become much more complex. Since the receptor occupancy of pembrolizumab (anti-PD-1 monoclonal antibody) is 3–6 months, the concept of monotherapy and sequencing of combinations becomes ever less well defined. Patients may therefore ultimately stratify into checkpoint inhibitor experienced vs checkpoint inhibitor naïve cohorts from a line-of-therapy standpoint. Because of pharmacokinetics and principles of immune memory and regulation, the regimens that will best combine chemotherapy and radiotherapy with immunotherapy are likely not conventional regimens. Improving upon therapy doublets thus requires a comprehensive biomarker strategy. Combination therapies across therapeutic modalities may mitigate toxicity while adding mechanistic synergy. For example, the radiation "abscopal" (off-target) effect is an immunologic-based phenomenon [119] where local treatment leads to a systemic immune response through, presumably, massive neoantigen release, production of IFN-gamma, upregulation of T cells, and immune sensitivity to radiated/injured tissue. Chemotherapy reforms the immune profile since lymphocyte counts decline, then revives through homeostatic proliferation [120], and this leads to a restoration of T-cell responses.

Biomarker strategies must reconcile shared pathways across tumor and immune cells. For example, MEK inhibition of tumor cells also blocks naïve T-cell priming (through interference of the RAS MAP kinase pathway) and causes an increase in incompletely exhausted PD-1^{lo} $CD8^{+}$ T cells in tumors and eventually depletes TILs as tumors relapse. Alternatively, the MAP kinase pathway is only needed for naïve T-cell expansion and differentiation into memory cells, and thus MEK and PD-1L1 may act by preventing rather than reversing T-cell exhaustion [121]. It may therefore be necessary, in some cases, to withhold a MEK inhibitor as the patient responds as this may inhibit immune priming while instead focusing on checkpoint blockade plus monoclonal combination therapies in the BRAF pathway, ß-catenin pathway, or PI3K pathway. The tumor microenvironment (tissue type, proximity to the external world and associated microbiome, vascularity, etc.) will necessitate tissue-specific understanding of how immunotherapies act within certain cancer types beyond the likelihood for generation of immunogenic peptides (TMB) and expression of (inducible) checkpoint antigens. The immunoglobulin isotype of checkpoint blockade monoclonal agents further influences therapeutic antibody function by dictating their structural characteristics and specificity [122]. The type of immune response towards monoclonal antibodies targeted against native proteins can therefore be fine-tuned. Incorporating relevant biologic correlative data will enhance our ability to interpret complex and nuanced clinical responses to drug combinations and can help reduce the likelihood of taking a neutral or antagonistic combination through to phase III. Immune host–microbiota interactions also influence tissue-specific immune fitness (i.e., through gastrointestinal and respiratory flora) and thus systemic immunity. The composition of the microbiome is molded by environmental influences such as diet, exercise, hygiene, and sleep. As cancer patients are often immunosuppressed through chemotherapy which alters the host microbiome [123], antibiotics indiscriminately and broadly eradicate both pathogenic bacteria and commensal flora that may act as an adjuvant to cancer immunotherapy. For example, commensal bacteria have been shown to enhance PD-L1 blockade in murine models [111, 124].

Many have foreseen that checkpoint modulation will supplement chemotherapy as the cornerstone of cancer therapy either directly or after interventions targeting inflammation, by vaccination to boost T-cell repertoires or by adoptive T-cell transfer [125]. Anticipating adaptive resistance followed by immune escape [126, 127], successive therapies must incorporate multiparametric biomarkers that capture the dynamic immunobiology within the tumor microenvironment. Linking adaptive and innate immunity has become a key area of focus in drug development [128]. Through leveraging complementary mechanisms of action, strategies may be devised for rational therapeutic combinations that promote durable immune responses [129]. For example, approaches that promote inflammation of an otherwise noninflamed tumor present as scientifically rational options to be studied as combination partners for checkpoint inhibitors that facilitate adaptive immunoresistance. Mechanistic-based approaches thereby increase the likelihood that effective combinations with acceptable toxicity profiles will progress into phase II/III trials that are prolonged and costly. For example, the recognition that PD-1 and PDL-1 have primary action in the tumor microenvironment whereas CTLA-4 acts in the lymphoid system provides a strong mechanistic basis for testing the combination of nivolumab and ipilimumab for therapeutic synergy [130, 131]. Anti-CTLA4 blockade expands T cells in all compartments of the body (not just those relevant to the cancer), and such global considerations for targeting native proteins are fundamental to understanding clinical responses. With so many therapeutic combinations possible [132], methods to assess the additive benefits of each intervention are needed.

Immunotherapy has catalyzed a change in the delivery of oncology care since the increasing complexity of cancer treatment increases costs. Therefore, optimizing personalized approaches to therapy will be critical to establishing and differentiating clinical value of both diagnostics and therapeutics. It remains to be determined if immunotherapies can advance to even earlier stages of disease such as in the neoadjuvant setting when tumor burden may facilitate enhanced immune system "education." Co-development programs are needed to build upon the historic one drug one protein drug development paradigm. These considerations and their rational implementation into clinical practice are will foster the next wave of advances in cancer immunotherapy.

References

1. Dvorak HF (2015) Tumors: wounds that do not heal-redux. Cancer Immunol Res 3(1):1–11. doi:10.1158/2326-6066.CIR-14-0209
2. Hanahan D, Weinberg RA (2011) Hallmarks of cancer: the next generation. Cell 144(5):646–674. doi:10.1016/j.cell.2011.02.013
3. Bozic I, Antal T, Ohtsuki H, Carter H, Kim D, Chen S, Karchin R, Kinzler KW, Vogelstein B, Nowak MA (2010) Accumulation of driver and passenger mutations during tumor progression. Proc Natl Acad Sci U S A 107(43):18545–18550. doi:10.1073/pnas.1010978107
4. Sjoblom T, Jones S, Wood LD, Parsons DW, Lin J, Barber TD, Mandelker D, Leary RJ, Ptak J, Silliman N, Szabo S, Buckhaults P, Farrell C, Meeh P, Markowitz SD, Willis J, Dawson D, Willson JK, Gazdar AF, Hartigan J, Wu L, Liu C, Parmigiani G, Park BH, Bachman KE, Papadopoulos N, Vogelstein B, Kinzler KW, Velculescu VE (2006) The consensus coding

sequences of human breast and colorectal cancers. Science 314(5797):268–274. doi:10.1126/science.1133427
5. Balkwill F, Mantovani A (2001) Inflammation and cancer: back to Virchow? Lancet 357(9255):539–545. doi:10.1016/S0140-6736(00)04046-0
6. Burnet M (1957) Cancer; a biological approach. I. The processes of control. Br Med J 1(5022):779–786
7. Lawrence HS (1959) Cellular and humoral aspects of the hypersensitive states; a symposium held at the New York Academy of Medicine. In: Symposia of the section on microbiology, the New York Academy of Medicine, vol 9. P.B. Hoeber, New York
8. Schreiber RD, Old LJ, Smyth MJ (2011) Cancer immunoediting: integrating immunity's roles in cancer suppression and promotion. Science 331(6024):1565–1570. doi:10.1126/science.1203486
9. Mackay LK, Kallies A (2017) Transcriptional regulation of tissue-resident lymphocytes. Trends Immunol 38(2):94–103. doi:10.1016/j.it.2016.11.004
10. Cramer DW, Vitonis AF, Pinheiro SP, McKolanis JR, Fichorova RN, Brown KE, Hatchette TF, Finn OJ (2010) Mumps and ovarian cancer: modern interpretation of an historic association. Cancer Causes Control 21(8):1193–1201. doi:10.1007/s10552-010-9546-1
11. Gajewski TF, Schreiber H, Fu YX (2013) Innate and adaptive immune cells in the tumor microenvironment. Nat Immunol 14(10):1014–1022. doi:10.1038/ni.2703
12. Rieckmann JC, Geiger R, Hornburg D, Wolf T, Kveler K, Jarrossay D, Sallusto F, Shen-Orr SS, Lanzavecchia A, Mann M, Meissner F (2017) Social network architecture of human immune cells unveiled by quantitative proteomics. Nat Immunol. doi:10.1038/ni.3693
13. Heng TS, Painter MW, Immunological Genome Project C (2008) The immunological genome project: networks of gene expression in immune cells. Nat Immunol 9(10):1091–1094. doi:10.1038/ni1008-1091
14. Schreibelt G, Tel J, Sliepen KH, Benitez-Ribas D, Figdor CG, Adema GJ, de Vries IJ (2010) Toll-like receptor expression and function in human dendritic cell subsets: implications for dendritic cell-based anti-cancer immunotherapy. Cancer Immunol Immunother 59(10):1573–1582. doi:10.1007/s00262-010-0833-1
15. Gabrilovich DI, Ostrand-Rosenberg S, Bronte V (2012) Coordinated regulation of myeloid cells by tumours. Nat Rev Immunol 12(4):253–268. doi:10.1038/nri3175
16. Laoui D, Van Overmeire E, De Baetselier P, Van Ginderachter JA, Raes G (2014) Functional relationship between tumor-associated macrophages and macrophage colony-stimulating factor as contributors to cancer progression. Front Immunol 5:489. doi:10.3389/fimmu.2014.00489
17. Wesolowski R, Markowitz J, Carson WE 3rd (2013) Myeloid derived suppressor cells – a new therapeutic target in the treatment of cancer. J Immunother Cancer 1:10. doi:10.1186/2051-1426-1-10
18. Biswas SK (2015) Metabolic reprogramming of immune cells in cancer progression. Immunity 43(3):435–449. doi:10.1016/j.immuni.2015.09.001
19. Trowsdale J, Knight JC (2013) Major histocompatibility complex genomics and human disease. Annu Rev Genomics Hum Genet 14:301–323. doi:10.1146/annurev-genom-091212-153455
20. Yang JY, Sarwal MM (2017) Transplant genetics and genomics. Nat Rev Genet doi:10.1038/nrg.2017.12
21. Genomes Project Consortium, Auton A, Brooks LD, Durbin RM, Garrison EP, Kang HM, Korbel JO, Marchini JL, McCarthy S, McVean GA, Abecasis GR (2015) A global reference for human genetic variation. Nature 526(7571):68–74. doi:10.1038/nature15393
22. Dahlberg CI, Sarhan D, Chrobok M, Duru AD, Alici E (2015) Natural killer cell-based therapies targeting cancer: possible strategies to gain and sustain anti-tumor activity. Front Immunol 6:605. doi:10.3389/fimmu.2015.00605
23. Steinman RM, Cohn ZA (1973) Identification of a novel cell type in peripheral lymphoid organs of mice. I. Morphology, quantitation, tissue distribution. J Exp Med 137(5):1142–1162
24. Lavin Y, Mortha A, Rahman A, Merad M (2015) Regulation of macrophage development and function in peripheral tissues. Nat Rev Immunol 15(12):731–744. doi:10.1038/nri3920

25. Tonegawa S (1983) Somatic generation of antibody diversity. Nature 302(5909):575–581
26. Stevanovic S, Schild H (1999) Quantitative aspects of T cell activation--peptide generation and editing by MHC class I molecules. Semin Immunol 11(6):375–384. doi:10.1006/smim.1999.0195
27. Robins HS, Campregher PV, Srivastava SK, Wacher A, Turtle CJ, Kahsai O, Riddell SR, Warren EH, Carlson CS (2009) Comprehensive assessment of T-cell receptor beta-chain diversity in alphabeta T cells. Blood 114(19):4099–4107. doi:10.1182/blood-2009-04-217604
28. Wooldridge L, Ekeruche-Makinde J, van den Berg HA, Skowera A, Miles JJ, Tan MP, Dolton G, Clement M, Llewellyn-Lacey S, Price DA, Peakman M, Sewell AK (2012) A single autoimmune T cell receptor recognizes more than a million different peptides. J Biol Chem 287(2):1168–1177. doi:10.1074/jbc.M111.289488
29. Klein L, Kyewski B, Allen PM, Hogquist KA (2014) Positive and negative selection of the T cell repertoire: what thymocytes see (and don't see). Nat Rev Immunol 14(6):377–391. doi:10.1038/nri3667
30. Tussiwand R, Bosco N, Ceredig R, Rolink AG (2009) Tolerance checkpoints in B-cell development: Johnny B good. Eur J Immunol 39(9):2317–2324. doi:10.1002/eji.200939633
31. Yatim N, Cullen S, Albert ML (2017) Dying cells actively regulate adaptive immune responses. Nat Rev Immunol doi:10.1038/nri.2017.9
32. Srinivasan R, Wolchok JD (2004) Tumor antigens for cancer immunotherapy: therapeutic potential of xenogeneic DNA vaccines. J Transl Med 2(1):12. doi:10.1186/1479-5876-2-12
33. Pardoll DM (2012) The blockade of immune checkpoints in cancer immunotherapy. Nat Rev Cancer 12(4):252–264. doi:10.1038/nrc3239
34. June CH, Ledbetter JA, Gillespie MM, Lindsten T, Thompson CB (1987) T-cell proliferation involving the CD28 pathway is associated with cyclosporine-resistant interleukin 2 gene expression. Mol Cell Biol 7(12):4472–4481
35. Kaech SM, Cui W (2012) Transcriptional control of effector and memory CD8+ T cell differentiation. Nat Rev Immunol 12(11):749–761. doi:10.1038/nri3307
36. Krummel MF, Allison JP (1995) CD28 and CTLA-4 have opposing effects on the response of T cells to stimulation. J Exp Med 182(2):459–465
37. Peggs KS, Quezada SA, Chambers CA, Korman AJ, Allison JP (2009) Blockade of CTLA-4 on both effector and regulatory T cell compartments contributes to the antitumor activity of anti-CTLA-4 antibodies. J Exp Med 206(8):1717–1725. doi:10.1084/jem.20082492
38. Boussiotis VA (2016) Molecular and biochemical aspects of the PD-1 checkpoint pathway. N Engl J Med 375(18):1767–1778. doi:10.1056/NEJMra1514296
39. Wherry EJ (2011) T cell exhaustion. Nat Immunol 12(6):492–499
40. Chen DS, Mellman I (2013) Oncology meets immunology: the cancer-immunity cycle. Immunity 39(1):1–10. doi:10.1016/j.immuni.2013.07.012
41. Chen DS, Mellman I (2017) Elements of cancer immunity and the cancer-immune set point. Nature 541(7637):321–330. doi:10.1038/nature21349
42. Palucka AK, Coussens LM (2016) The basis of oncoimmunology. Cell 164(6):1233–1247. doi:10.1016/j.cell.2016.01.049
43. Blank CU, Haanen JB, Ribas A, Schumacher TN (2016) CANCER IMMUNOLOGY. The "cancer immunogram". Science 352(6286):658–660. doi:10.1126/science.aaf2834
44. Sharma P, Allison JP (2015) Immune checkpoint targeting in cancer therapy: toward combination strategies with curative potential. Cell 161(2):205–214. doi:10.1016/j.cell.2015.03.030
45. Zou W, Wolchok JD, Chen L (2016) PD-L1 (B7-H1) and PD-1 pathway blockade for cancer therapy: mechanisms, response biomarkers, and combinations. Sci Transl Med 8(328):328rv324. doi:10.1126/scitranslmed.aad7118
46. Topalian SL, Drake CG, Pardoll DM (2015) Immune checkpoint blockade: a common denominator approach to cancer therapy. Cancer Cell 27(4):450–461. doi:10.1016/j.ccell.2015.03.001
47. Galon J, Costes A, Sanchez-Cabo F, Kirilovsky A, Mlecnik B, Lagorce-Pages C, Tosolini M, Camus M, Berger A, Wind P, Zinzindohoue F, Bruneval P, Cugnenc PH, Trajanoski Z,

Fridman WH, Pages F (2006) Type, density, and location of immune cells within human colorectal tumors predict clinical outcome. Science 313(5795):1960–1964. doi:10.1126/science.1129139
48. Herbst RS, Soria JC, Kowanetz M, Fine GD, Hamid O, Gordon MS, Sosman JA, McDermott DF, Powderly JD, Gettinger SN, Kohrt HE, Horn L, Lawrence DP, Rost S, Leabman M, Xiao Y, Mokatrin A, Koeppen H, Hegde PS, Mellman I, Chen DS, Hodi FS (2014) Predictive correlates of response to the anti-PD-L1 antibody MPDL3280A in cancer patients. Nature 515(7528):563–567. doi:10.1038/nature14011
49. Tumeh PC, Harview CL, Yearley JH, Shintaku IP, Taylor EJ, Robert L, Chmielowski B, Spasic M, Henry G, Ciobanu V, West AN, Carmona M, Kivork C, Seja E, Cherry G, Gutierrez AJ, Grogan TR, Mateus C, Tomasic G, Glaspy JA, Emerson RO, Robins H, Pierce RH, Elashoff DA, Robert C, Ribas A (2014) PD-1 blockade induces responses by inhibiting adaptive immune resistance. Nature 515(7528):568–571. doi:10.1038/nature13954
50. Galon J, Mlecnik B, Bindea G, Angell HK, Berger A, Lagorce C, Lugli A, Zlobec I, Hartmann A, Bifulco C, Nagtegaal ID, Palmqvist R, Masucci GV, Botti G, Tatangelo F, Delrio P, Maio M, Laghi L, Grizzi F, Asslaber M, D'Arrigo C, Vidal-Vanaclocha F, Zavadova E, Chouchane L, Ohashi PS, Hafezi-Bakhtiari S, Wouters BG, Roehrl M, Nguyen L, Kawakami Y, Hazama S, Okuno K, Ogino S, Gibbs P, Waring P, Sato N, Torigoe T, Itoh K, Patel PS, Shukla SN, Wang Y, Kopetz S, Sinicrope FA, Scripcariu V, Ascierto PA, Marincola FM, Fox BA, Pages F (2014) Towards the introduction of the 'Immunoscore' in the classification of malignant tumours. J Pathol 232(2):199–209. doi:10.1002/path.4287
51. Schneider G, Schmidt-Supprian M, Rad R, Saur D (2017) Tissue-specific tumorigenesis: context matters. Nat Rev Cancer 17(4):239–253. doi:10.1038/nrc.2017.5
52. Chabanon RM, Pedrero M, Lefebvre C, Marabelle A, Soria JC, Postel-Vinay S (2016) Mutational landscape and sensitivity to immune checkpoint blockers. Clin Cancer Res 22(17):4309–4321. doi:10.1158/1078-0432.CCR-16-0903
53. Gentles AJ, Newman AM, Liu CL, Bratman SV, Feng W, Kim D, Nair VS, Xu Y, Khuong A, Hoang CD, Diehn M, West RB, Plevritis SK, Alizadeh AA (2015) The prognostic landscape of genes and infiltrating immune cells across human cancers. Nat Med 21(8):938–945. doi:10.1038/nm.3909
54. Charoentong P, Finotello F, Angelova M, Mayer C, Efremova M, Rieder D, Hackl H, Trajanoski Z (2017) Pan-Cancer immunogenomic analyses reveal genotype-immunophenotype relationships and predictors of response to checkpoint blockade. Cell Rep 18(1):248–262. doi:10.1016/j.celrep.2016.12.019
55. Turley SJ, Cremasco V, Astarita JL (2015) Immunological hallmarks of stromal cells in the tumour microenvironment. Nat Rev Immunol 15(11):669–682. doi:10.1038/nri3902
56. Anderson KG, Stromnes IM, Greenberg PD (2017) Obstacles posed by the tumor microenvironment to T cell activity: a case for synergistic therapies. Cancer Cell 31(3):311–325. doi:10.1016/j.ccell.2017.02.008
57. Zhao X, Subramanian S (2017) Intrinsic resistance of solid tumors to immune checkpoint blockade therapy. Cancer Res 77(4):817–822. doi:10.1158/0008-5472.CAN-16-2379
58. Pitt JM, Vetizou M, Daillere R, Roberti MP, Yamazaki T, Routy B, Lepage P, Boneca IG, Chamaillard M, Kroemer G, Zitvogel L (2016) Resistance mechanisms to immune-checkpoint blockade in cancer: tumor-intrinsic and -extrinsic factors. Immunity 44(6):1255–1269. doi:10.1016/j.immuni.2016.06.001
59. Pickup M, Novitskiy S, Moses HL (2013) The roles of TGFbeta in the tumour microenvironment. Nat Rev Cancer 13(11):788–799. doi:10.1038/nrc3603
60. Hanahan D, Coussens LM (2012) Accessories to the crime: functions of cells recruited to the tumor microenvironment. Cancer Cell 21(3):309–322. doi:10.1016/j.ccr.2012.02.022
61. Anagnostou V, Smith KN, Forde PM, Niknafs N, Bhattacharya R, White J, Zhang T, Adleff V, Phallen J, Wali N, Hruban C, Guthrie VB, Rodgers K, Naidoo J, Kang H, Sharfman WH, Georgiades C, Verde F, Illei P, Li QK, Gabrielson E, Brock MV, Zahnow CA, Baylin SB, Scharpf R, Brahmer JR, Karchin R, Pardoll DM, Velculescu VE (2016) Evolution of neoan-

tigen landscape during immune checkpoint blockade in non-small cell lung cancer. Cancer Discov doi:10.1158/2159-8290.CD-16-0828
62. Shukla SA, Rooney MS, Rajasagi M, Tiao G, Dixon PM, Lawrence MS, Stevens J, Lane WJ, Dellagatta JL, Steelman S, Sougnez C, Cibulskis K, Kiezun A, Hacohen N, Brusic V, Wu CJ, Getz G (2015) Comprehensive analysis of cancer-associated somatic mutations in class I HLA genes. Nat Biotechnol 33(11):1152–1158. doi:10.1038/nbt.3344
63. Zaretsky JM, Garcia-Diaz A, Shin DS, Escuin-Ordinas H, Hugo W, Hu-Lieskovan S, Torrejon DY, Abril-Rodriguez G, Sandoval S, Barthly L, Saco J, Homet Moreno B, Mezzadra R, Chmielowski B, Ruchalski K, Shintaku IP, Sanchez PJ, Puig-Saus C, Cherry G, Seja E, Kong X, Pang J, Berent-Maoz B, Comin-Anduix B, Graeber TG, Tumeh PC, Schumacher TN, Lo RS, Ribas A (2016) Mutations associated with acquired resistance to PD-1 blockade in melanoma. N Engl J Med 375(9):819–829. doi:10.1056/NEJMoa1604958
64. Koyama S, Akbay EA, Li YY, Herter-Sprie GS, Buczkowski KA, Richards WG, Gandhi L, Redig AJ, Rodig SJ, Asahina H, Jones RE, Kulkarni MM, Kuraguchi M, Palakurthi S, Fecci PE, Johnson BE, Janne PA, Engelman JA, Gangadharan SP, Costa DB, Freeman GJ, Bueno R, Hodi FS, Dranoff G, Wong KK, Hammerman PS (2016) Adaptive resistance to therapeutic PD-1 blockade is associated with upregulation of alternative immune checkpoints. Nat Commun 7:10501. doi:10.1038/ncomms10501
65. Lambert AW, Pattabiraman DR, Weinberg RA (2017) Emerging biological principles of metastasis. Cell 168(4):670–691. doi:10.1016/j.cell.2016.11.037
66. Kitamura T, Qian BZ, Pollard JW (2015) Immune cell promotion of metastasis. Nat Rev Immunol 15(2):73–86. doi:10.1038/nri3789
67. Woo SR, Corrales L, Gajewski TF (2015) The STING pathway and the T cell-inflamed tumor microenvironment. Trends Immunol 36(4):250–256. doi:10.1016/j.it.2015.02.003
68. Halama N, Spille A, Lerchl T, Brand K, Herpel E, Welte S, Keim S, Lahrmann B, Klupp F, Kahlert C, Weitz J, Grabe N, Jaeger D, Zoernig I (2013) Hepatic metastases of colorectal cancer are rather homogeneous but differ from primary lesions in terms of immune cell infiltration. Oncoimmunology 2(4):e24116. doi:10.4161/onci.24116
69. Maio M, Covre A, Fratta E, Di Giacomo AM, Taverna P, Natali PG, Coral S, Sigalotti L (2015) Molecular pathways: at the crossroads of cancer epigenetics and immunotherapy. Clin Cancer Res 21(18):4040–4047. doi:10.1158/1078-0432.CCR-14-2914
70. Taube JM, Anders RA, Young GD, Xu H, Sharma R, McMiller TL, Chen S, Klein AP, Pardoll DM, Topalian SL, Chen L (2012) Colocalization of inflammatory response with B7-h1 expression in human melanocytic lesions supports an adaptive resistance mechanism of immune escape. Sci Transl Med 4(127):127ra137. doi:10.1126/scitranslmed.3003689
71. Minn AJ, Wherry EJ (2016) Combination cancer therapies with immune checkpoint blockade: convergence on interferon signaling. Cell 165(2):272–275. doi:10.1016/j.cell.2016.03.031
72. Ji RR, Chasalow SD, Wang L, Hamid O, Schmidt H, Cogswell J, Alaparthy S, Berman D, Jure-Kunkel M, Siemers NO, Jackson JR, Shahabi V (2012) An immune-active tumor microenvironment favors clinical response to ipilimumab. Cancer Immunol Immunother 61(7):1019–1031. doi:10.1007/s00262-011-1172-6
73. Parker BS, Rautela J, Hertzog PJ (2016) Antitumour actions of interferons: implications for cancer therapy. Nat Rev Cancer 16(3):131–144. doi:10.1038/nrc.2016.14
74. Wong MT, Ong DE, Lim FS, Teng KW, McGovern N, Narayanan S, Ho WQ, Cerny D, Tan HK, Anicete R, Tan BK, Lim TK, Chan CY, Cheow PC, Lee SY, Takano A, Tan EH, Tam JK, Tan EY, Chan JK, Fink K, Bertoletti A, Ginhoux F, Curotto de Lafaille MA, Newell EW (2016) A high-dimensional atlas of human T cell diversity reveals tissue-specific trafficking and cytokine signatures. Immunity 45(2):442–456. doi:10.1016/j.immuni.2016.07.007
75. Fritsch EF, Rajasagi M, Ott PA, Brusic V, Hacohen N, Wu CJ (2014) HLA-binding properties of tumor neoepitopes in humans. Cancer Immunol Res 2(6):522–529. doi:10.1158/2326-6066.CIR-13-0227
76. Le DT, Uram JN, Wang H, Bartlett BR, Kemberling H, Eyring AD, Skora AD, Luber BS, Azad NS, Laheru D, Biedrzycki B, Donehower RC, Zaheer A, Fisher GA, Crocenzi TS, Lee

JJ, Duffy SM, Goldberg RM, de la Chapelle A, Koshiji M, Bhaijee F, Huebner T, Hruban RH, Wood LD, Cuka N, Pardoll DM, Papadopoulos N, Kinzler KW, Zhou S, Cornish TC, Taube JM, Anders RA, Eshleman JR, Vogelstein B, Diaz LA Jr (2015) PD-1 blockade in tumors with mismatch-repair deficiency. N Engl J Med 372(26):2509–2520. doi:10.1056/NEJMoa1500596
77. Angelova M, Charoentong P, Hackl H, Fischer ML, Snajder R, Krogsdam AM, Waldner MJ, Bindea G, Mlecnik B, Galon J, Trajanoski Z (2015) Characterization of the immunophenotypes and antigenomes of colorectal cancers reveals distinct tumor escape mechanisms and novel targets for immunotherapy. Genome Biol 16:64. doi:10.1186/s13059-015-0620-6
78. Alexandrov LB, Nik-Zainal S, Wedge DC, Aparicio SA, Behjati S, Biankin AV, Bignell GR, Bolli N, Borg A, Borresen-Dale AL, Boyault S, Burkhardt B, Butler AP, Caldas C, Davies HR, Desmedt C, Eils R, Eyfjord JE, Foekens JA, Greaves M, Hosoda F, Hutter B, Ilicic T, Imbeaud S, Imielinski M, Jager N, Jones DT, Jones D, Knappskog S, Kool M, Lakhani SR, Lopez-Otin C, Martin S, Munshi NC, Nakamura H, Northcott PA, Pajic M, Papaemmanuil E, Paradiso A, Pearson JV, Puente XS, Raine K, Ramakrishna M, Richardson AL, Richter J, Rosenstiel P, Schlesner M, Schumacher TN, Span PN, Teague JW, Totoki Y, Tutt AN, Valdes-Mas R, van Buuren MM, van't Veer L, Vincent-Salomon A, Waddell N, Yates LR, Australian Pancreatic Cancer Genome I, Consortium IBC, Consortium IM-S, PedBrain I, Zucman-Rossi J, Futreal PA, McDermott U, Lichter P, Meyerson M, Grimmond SM, Siebert R, Campo E, Shibata T, Pfister SM, Campbell PJ, Stratton MR (2013) Signatures of mutational processes in human cancer. Nature 500(7463):415–421. doi:10.1038/nature12477
79. Lawrence MS, Stojanov P, Mermel CH, Robinson JT, Garraway LA, Golub TR, Meyerson M, Gabriel SB, Lander ES, Getz G (2014) Discovery and saturation analysis of cancer genes across 21 tumour types. Nature 505(7484):495–501. doi:10.1038/nature12912
80. Snyder A, Makarov V, Merghoub T, Yuan J, Zaretsky JM, Desrichard A, Walsh LA, Postow MA, Wong P, Ho TS, Hollmann TJ, Bruggeman C, Kannan K, Li Y, Elipenahli C, Liu C, Harbison CT, Wang L, Ribas A, Wolchok JD, Chan TA (2014) Genetic basis for clinical response to CTLA-4 blockade in melanoma. N Engl J Med 371(23):2189–2199. doi:10.1056/NEJMoa1406498
81. Van Allen EM, Miao D, Schilling B, Shukla SA, Blank C, Zimmer L, Sucker A, Hillen U, Geukes Foppen MH, Goldinger SM, Utikal J, Hassel JC, Weide B, Kaehler KC, Loquai C, Mohr P, Gutzmer R, Dummer R, Gabriel S, Wu CJ, Schadendorf D, Garraway LA (2015) Genomic correlates of response to CTLA-4 blockade in metastatic melanoma. Science 350(6257):207–211. doi:10.1126/science.aad0095
82. Rizvi NA, Hellmann MD, Snyder A, Kvistborg P, Makarov V, Havel JJ, Lee W, Yuan J, Wong P, Ho TS, Miller ML, Rekhtman N, Moreira AL, Ibrahim F, Bruggeman C, Gasmi B, Zappasodi R, Maeda Y, Sander C, Garon EB, Merghoub T, Wolchok JD, Schumacher TN, Chan TA (2015) Cancer immunology. Mutational landscape determines sensitivity to PD-1 blockade in non-small cell lung cancer. Science 348(6230):124–128. doi:10.1126/science.aaa1348
83. Moloney FJ, Comber H, O'Lorcain P, O'Kelly P, Conlon PJ, Murphy GM (2006) A population-based study of skin cancer incidence and prevalence in renal transplant recipients. Br J Dermatol 154(3):498–504. doi:10.1111/j.1365-2133.2005.07021.x
84. Topalian SL, Taube JM, Anders RA, Pardoll DM (2016) Mechanism-driven biomarkers to guide immune checkpoint blockade in cancer therapy. Nat Rev Cancer 16(5):275–287. doi:10.1038/nrc.2016.36
85. Liu XS, Mardis ER (2017) Applications of immunogenomics to cancer. Cell 168(4):600–612. doi:10.1016/j.cell.2017.01.014
86. Naito Y, Saito K, Shiiba K, Ohuchi A, Saigenji K, Nagura H, Ohtani H (1998) CD8+ T cells infiltrated within cancer cell nests as a prognostic factor in human colorectal cancer. Cancer Res 58(16):3491–3494
87. Zhang L, Conejo-Garcia JR, Katsaros D, Gimotty PA, Massobrio M, Regnani G, Makrigiannakis A, Gray H, Schlienger K, Liebman MN, Rubin SC, Coukos G (2003)

Intratumoral T cells, recurrence, and survival in epithelial ovarian cancer. N Engl J Med 348(3):203–213. doi:10.1056/NEJMoa020177
88. Yarchoan M, Johnson BA 3rd, Lutz ER, Laheru DA, Jaffee EM (2017) Targeting neoantigens to augment antitumour immunity. Nat Rev Cancer 17(4):209–222. doi:10.1038/nrc.2016.154
89. Hyman DM, Taylor BS, Baselga J (2017) Implementing genome-driven oncology. Cell 168(4):584–599. doi:10.1016/j.cell.2016.12.015
90. Hundal J, Carreno BM, Petti AA, Linette GP, Griffith OL, Mardis ER, Griffith M (2016) pVAC-Seq: a genome-guided in silico approach to identifying tumor neoantigens. Genome Med 8(1):11. doi:10.1186/s13073-016-0264-5
91. Yadav M, Jhunjhunwala S, Phung QT, Lupardus P, Tanguay J, Bumbaca S, Franci C, Cheung TK, Fritsche J, Weinschenk T, Modrusan Z, Mellman I, Lill JR, Delamarre L (2014) Predicting immunogenic tumour mutations by combining mass spectrometry and exome sequencing. Nature 515(7528):572–576. doi:10.1038/nature14001
92. Gros A, Parkhurst MR, Tran E, Pasetto A, Robbins PF, Ilyas S, Prickett TD, Gartner JJ, Crystal JS, Roberts IM, Trebska-McGowan K, Wunderlich JR, Yang JC, Rosenberg SA (2016) Prospective identification of neoantigen-specific lymphocytes in the peripheral blood of melanoma patients. Nat Med 22(4):433–438. doi:10.1038/nm.4051
93. Newman AM, Liu CL, Green MR, Gentles AJ, Feng W, Xu Y, Hoang CD, Diehn M, Alizadeh AA (2015) Robust enumeration of cell subsets from tissue expression profiles. Nat Methods 12(5):453–457. doi:10.1038/nmeth.3337
94. Aran D, Butte AJ (2016) Digitally deconvolving the tumor microenvironment. Genome Biol 17(1):175. doi:10.1186/s13059-016-1036-7
95. Hackl H, Charoentong P, Finotello F, Trajanoski Z (2016) Computational genomics tools for dissecting tumour-immune cell interactions. Nat Rev Genet 17(8):441–458. doi:10.1038/nrg.2016.67
96. Doering TA, Crawford A, Angelosanto JM, Paley MA, Ziegler CG, Wherry EJ (2012) Network analysis reveals centrally connected genes and pathways involved in CD8+ T cell exhaustion versus memory. Immunity 37(6):1130–1144. doi:10.1016/j.immuni.2012.08.021
97. Paley MA, Kroy DC, Odorizzi PM, Johnnidis JB, Dolfi DV, Barnett BE, Bikoff EK, Robertson EJ, Lauer GM, Reiner SL, Wherry EJ (2012) Progenitor and terminal subsets of CD8+ T cells cooperate to contain chronic viral infection. Science 338(6111):1220–1225. doi:10.1126/science.1229620
98. Wherry EJ, Ha SJ, Kaech SM, Haining WN, Sarkar S, Kalia V, Subramaniam S, Blattman JN, Barber DL, Ahmed R (2007) Molecular signature of CD8+ T cell exhaustion during chronic viral infection. Immunity 27(4):670–684. doi:10.1016/j.immuni.2007.09.006
99. Chiou VL, Burotto M (2015) Pseudoprogression and immune-related response in solid tumors. J Clin Oncol 33(31):3541–3543. doi:10.1200/JCO.2015.61.6870
100. Seymour L, Bogaerts J, Perrone A, Ford R, Schwartz LH, Mandrekar S, Lin NU, Litiere S, Dancey J, Chen A, Hodi FS, Therasse P, Hoekstra OS, Shankar LK, Wolchok JD, Ballinger M, Caramella C, de Vries EG, Recist Working Group (2017) iRECIST: guidelines for response criteria for use in trials testing immunotherapeutics. Lancet Oncol 18(3):e143–e152. doi:10.1016/S1470-2045(17)30074-8
101. McGranahan N, Swanton C (2017) Clonal heterogeneity and tumor evolution: past, present, and the future. Cell 168(4):613–628. doi:10.1016/j.cell.2017.01.018
102. Tavare R, Escuin-Ordinas H, Mok S, McCracken MN, Zettlitz KA, Salazar FB, Witte ON, Ribas A, Wu AM (2016) An effective immuno-PET imaging method to monitor CD8-dependent responses to immunotherapy. Cancer Res 76(1):73–82. doi:10.1158/0008-5472.CAN-15-1707
103. Kohrt HE, Tumeh PC, Benson D, Bhardwaj N, Brody J, Formenti S, Fox BA, Galon J, June CH, Kalos M, Kirsch I, Kleen T, Kroemer G, Lanier L, Levy R, Lyerly HK, Maecker H, Marabelle A, Melenhorst J, Miller J, Melero I, Odunsi K, Palucka K, Peoples G, Ribas A, Robins H, Robinson W, Serafini T, Sondel P, Vivier E, Weber J, Wolchok J, Zitvogel L, Disis ML, Cheever MA, Cancer Immunotherapy Trials N (2016) Immunodynamics: a cancer

immunotherapy trials network review of immune monitoring in immuno-oncology clinical trials. J Immunother Cancer 4:15. doi:10.1186/s40425-016-0118-0
104. Masucci GV, Cesano A, Hawtin R, Janetzki S, Zhang J, Kirsch I, Dobbin KK, Alvarez J, Robbins PB, Selvan SR, Streicher HZ, Butterfield LH, Thurin M (2016) Validation of biomarkers to predict response to immunotherapy in cancer: volume I – pre-analytical and analytical validation. J Immunother Cancer 4:76. doi:10.1186/s40425-016-0178-1
105. Schwaederle M, Husain H, Fanta PT, Piccioni DE, Kesari S, Schwab RB, Patel SP, Harismendy O, Ikeda M, Parker BA, Kurzrock R (2016) Use of liquid biopsies in clinical oncology: pilot experience in 168 patients. Clin Cancer Res doi:10.1158/1078-0432.CCR-16-0318
106. Das R, Verma R, Sznol M, Boddupalli CS, Gettinger SN, Kluger H, Callahan M, Wolchok JD, Halaban R, Dhodapkar MV, Dhodapkar KM (2015) Combination therapy with anti-CTLA-4 and anti-PD-1 leads to distinct immunologic changes in vivo. J Immunol 194(3):950–959. doi:10.4049/jimmunol.1401686
107. Weide B, Di Giacomo AM, Fonsatti E, Zitvogel L (2015) Immunologic correlates in the course of treatment with immunomodulating antibodies. Semin Oncol 42(3):448–458. doi:10.1053/j.seminoncol.2015.02.016
108. Maude SL, Barrett D, Teachey DT, Grupp SA (2014) Managing cytokine release syndrome associated with novel T cell-engaging therapies. Cancer J 20(2):119–122. doi:10.1097/PPO.0000000000000035
109. Wang S, Charbonnier LM, Noval Rivas M, Georgiev P, Li N, Gerber G, Bry L, Chatila TA (2015) MyD88 adaptor-dependent microbial sensing by regulatory T cells promotes mucosal tolerance and enforces commensalism. Immunity 43(2):289–303. doi:10.1016/j.immuni.2015.06.014
110. Telesford KM, Yan W, Ochoa-Reparaz J, Pant A, Kircher C, Christy MA, Begum-Haque S, Kasper DL, Kasper LH (2015) A commensal symbiotic factor derived from Bacteroides fragilis promotes human CD39(+)Foxp3(+) T cells and Treg function. Gut Microbes 6(4):234–242. doi:10.1080/19490976.2015.1056973
111. Sivan A, Corrales L, Hubert N, Williams JB, Aquino-Michaels K, Earley ZM, Benyamin FW, Lei YM, Jabri B, Alegre ML, Chang EB, Gajewski TF (2015) Commensal Bifidobacterium promotes antitumor immunity and facilitates anti-PD-L1 efficacy. Science 350(6264):1084–1089. doi:10.1126/science.aac4255
112. Hegde PS, Karanikas V, Evers S (2016) The where, the when, and the how of immune monitoring for cancer immunotherapies in the era of checkpoint inhibition. Clin Cancer Res 22(8):1865–1874. doi:10.1158/1078-0432.CCR-15-1507
113. Wan JC, Massie C, Garcia-Corbacho J, Mouliere F, Brenton JD, Caldas C, Pacey S, Baird R, Rosenfeld N (2017) Liquid biopsies come of age: towards implementation of circulating tumour DNA. Nat Rev Cancer 17(4):223–238. doi:10.1038/nrc.2017.7
114. Ott PA, Hodi FS, Kaufman HL, Wigginton JM, Wolchok JD (2017) Combination immunotherapy: a road map. J Immunother Cancer 5:16. doi:10.1186/s40425-017-0218-5
115. Postow MA, Callahan MK, Wolchok JD (2015) Immune checkpoint blockade in cancer therapy. J Clin Oncol 33(17):1974–1982. doi:10.1200/JCO.2014.59.4358
116. Lim WA, June CH (2017) The principles of engineering immune cells to treat cancer. Cell 168(4):724–740. doi:10.1016/j.cell.2017.01.016
117. Galluzzi L, Buque A, Kepp O, Zitvogel L, Kroemer G (2015) Immunological effects of conventional chemotherapy and targeted anticancer agents. Cancer Cell 28(6):690–714. doi:10.1016/j.ccell.2015.10.012
118. Schadt EE, Bjorkegren JL (2012) NEW: network-enabled wisdom in biology, medicine, and health care. Sci Transl Med 4(115):115rv111. doi:10.1126/scitranslmed.3002132
119. Demaria S, Coleman CN, Formenti SC (2016) Radiotherapy: changing the game in immunotherapy. Trends Cancer 2(6):286–294. doi:10.1016/j.trecan.2016.05.002
120. Kline J, Brown IE, Zha YY, Blank C, Strickler J, Wouters H, Zhang L, Gajewski TF (2008) Homeostatic proliferation plus regulatory T-cell depletion promotes potent rejection of B16 melanoma. Clin Cancer Res 14(10):3156–3167. doi:10.1158/1078-0432.CCR-07-4696

121. Ebert PJ, Cheung J, Yang Y, McNamara E, Hong R, Moskalenko M, Gould SE, Maecker H, Irving BA, Kim JM, Belvin M, Mellman I (2016) MAP kinase inhibition promotes T cell and anti-tumor activity in combination with PD-L1 checkpoint blockade. Immunity 44(3):609–621. doi:10.1016/j.immuni.2016.01.024
122. Beers SA, Glennie MJ, White AL (2016) Influence of immunoglobulin isotype on therapeutic antibody function. Blood 127(9):1097–1101. doi:10.1182/blood-2015-09-625343
123. Zitvogel L, Galluzzi L, Viaud S, Vetizou M, Daillere R, Merad M, Kroemer G (2015) Cancer and the gut microbiota: an unexpected link. Sci Transl Med 7(271):271ps271. doi:10.1126/scitranslmed.3010473
124. Vetizou M, Pitt JM, Daillere R, Lepage P, Waldschmitt N, Flament C, Rusakiewicz S, Routy B, Roberti MP, Duong CP, Poirier-Colame V, Roux A, Becharef S, Formenti S, Golden E, Cording S, Eberl G, Schlitzer A, Ginhoux F, Mani S, Yamazaki T, Jacquelot N, Enot DP, Berard M, Nigou J, Opolon P, Eggermont A, Woerther PL, Chachaty E, Chaput N, Robert C, Mateus C, Kroemer G, Raoult D, Boneca IG, Carbonnel F, Chamaillard M, Zitvogel L (2015) Anticancer immunotherapy by CTLA-4 blockade relies on the gut microbiota. Science 350(6264):1079–1084. doi:10.1126/science.aad1329
125. Melero I, Berman DM, Aznar MA, Korman AJ, Perez Gracia JL, Haanen J (2015) Evolving synergistic combinations of targeted immunotherapies to combat cancer. Nat Rev Cancer 15(8):457–472. doi:10.1038/nrc3973
126. Roh W, Chen PL, Reuben A, Spencer CN, Prieto PA, Miller JP, Gopalakrishnan V, Wang F, Cooper ZA, Reddy SM, Gumbs C, Little L, Chang Q, Chen WS, Wani K, De Macedo MP, Chen E, Austin-Breneman JL, Jiang H, Roszik J, Tetzlaff MT, Davies MA, Gershenwald JE, Tawbi H, Lazar AJ, Hwu P, Hwu WJ, Diab A, Glitza IC, Patel SP, Woodman SE, Amaria RN, Prieto VG, Hu J, Sharma P, Allison JP, Chin L, Zhang J, Wargo JA, Futreal PA (2017) Integrated molecular analysis of tumor biopsies on sequential CTLA-4 and PD-1 blockade reveals markers of response and resistance. Sci Transl Med 9 (379). doi:10.1126/scitranslmed.aah3560
127. Sharma P, Hu-Lieskovan S, Wargo JA, Ribas A (2017) Primary, adaptive, and acquired resistance to cancer immunotherapy. Cell 168(4):707–723. doi:10.1016/j.cell.2017.01.017
128. Vesely MD, Kershaw MH, Schreiber RD, Smyth MJ (2011) Natural innate and adaptive immunity to cancer. Annu Rev Immunol 29:235–271. doi:10.1146/annurev-immunol-031210-101324
129. Morrissey KM, Yuraszeck TM, Li CC, Zhang Y, Kasichayanula S (2016) Immunotherapy and novel combinations in oncology: current landscape, challenges, and opportunities. Clin Transl Sci 9(2):89–104. doi:10.1111/cts.12391
130. Spranger S, Gajewski T (2013) Rational combinations of immunotherapeutics that target discrete pathways. J Immunother Cancer 1:16. doi:10.1186/2051-1426-1-16
131. Liu L, Mayes PA, Eastman S, Shi H, Yadavilli S, Zhang T, Yang J, Seestaller-Wehr L, Zhang SY, Hopson C, Tsvetkov L, Jing J, Zhang S, Smothers J, Hoos A (2015) The BRAF and MEK inhibitors dabrafenib and trametinib: effects on immune function and in combination with immunomodulatory antibodies targeting PD-1, PD-L1, and CTLA-4. Clin Cancer Res 21(7):1639–1651. doi:10.1158/1078-0432.CCR-14-2339
132. Khalil DN, Smith EL, Brentjens RJ, Wolchok JD (2016) The future of cancer treatment: immunomodulation, CARs and combination immunotherapy. Nat Rev Clin Oncol 13(5):273–290. doi:10.1038/nrclinonc.2016.25

Chapter 2
Pharmacokinetics and Pharmacodynamics of Immunotherapy

Lisa H. Lam, Swan D. Lin, and Ji Sun

Abstract Over the last decade, there have been exciting advances in the development of monoclonal antibodies (mAbs), adoptive cellular therapies, vaccines, and viruses in eliciting immune responses against tumor cells with promising results in patients. This chapter highlights some of the immunotherapies that are in late-stage development or have received regulatory approval and summarizes their mechanisms of action, pharmacokinetics (PK), and pharmacodynamics (PD). This chapter summarizes the PK and PD of single-agent immunotherapies from publicly available sources through 2016. Advances in the field of immunotherapy have revolutionized oncology practice. The field is rapidly changing, and at any given time, there are hundreds of ongoing clinical trials with immunotherapies as single agents or in various combinations with another immunotherapy, targeted therapy, radiation therapy, or chemotherapy. Available data from new studies may provide additional insight for clinical PK and PD for immunotherapies in new patient populations.

Keywords Cellular therapy (CT) products • CGT products • Gene therapy (GT) products • Pharmacology • Pharmacokinetics • Pharmacodynamics • Oncology • Cancer immunotherapy • Immune checkpoint inhibitors

---

L.H. Lam, PharmD
Genentech, Inc., 1 DNA Way, South San Francisco, CA 94080, USA
e-mail: lam.lisa@gene.com

S.D. Lin, PharmD
Skaggs School of Pharmacy & Pharmaceutical Sciences, University of California, San Diego, 9500 Gilman Drive, La Jolla, CA 92093, USA
e-mail: sdlin@ucsd.edu

J. Sun, PharmD, PhD (✉)
Moores Cancer Center, University of California, San Diego, 3855 Health Sciences Drive, La Jolla, CA 92037, USA
e-mail: j2sun@ad.ucsd.edu

S.P. Patel, R. Kurzrock (eds.), *Early Phase Cancer Immunotherapy*, Current Cancer Research, DOI 10.1007/978-3-319-63757-0_2

2.1 Introduction

Immunology and oncology are two fields that have long been linked together when it was first reported that an injection of an inactive bacteria into sarcoma cells could lead to shrinkage of the tumor [1]. Immunotherapy is an approach to treating cancer by activating the patients' own immune defenses to fight malignant cells. Immunotherapy has wide-ranging potential and has been studied and used in a variety of solid and hematologic tumors [2]. Initial use of cancer immunotherapy was through harnessing the downstream effects of cytokines with the use of immune-modulating agents such as interleukin-2 (IL-2) and interferons (IFN) with limited success. Over the last decade, there have been exciting advances in the development of monoclonal antibodies (mAbs), adoptive cellular therapies, vaccines, and viruses in eliciting immune responses against tumor cells with promising results in patients (Fig. 2.1).

The human monomeric immunoglobulin (Ig) antibody structure is comprised of two light chains (two classes: κ and λ) and two heavy chains (five classes: μ, δ, γ, α, ε). There are five different human Ig subtypes comprised of different combinations of light and heavy chain classes (IgA, IgD, IgE, IgG, and IgM). Each Ig isotype is further divided into subclasses, such as IgG1, IgG2, IgG3, and IgG4 for the IgG isotype [3]. Each antibody has a fragment antigen-binding (Fab) and fragment constant (Fc) region [4]. Furthermore, each subclass differs in sequence, structure, and binding properties to cellular Fc receptors (FcR), which facilitate communication between Ig antibodies and the immune system. Each of the isotypes, IgM, IgG, IgA, and IgE, have receptors that bind exclusively to antibodies of that isotype: FcμR, FcγR, FcαR, and FcεR, respectively [3].

The pharmacokinetic (PK) properties of mAbs differ from those of small chemical molecules. Parenteral administration is the most typical route of administration for mAbs because of their instability in the gastrointestinal tract and poor membrane permeability. Elimination occurs primarily through peptide and amino acid catabolism. The pharmacological effect of mAbs depends on the type of target, including whether it is soluble or membrane bound [4].

This chapter highlights some of the immunotherapies that are in late-stage development or have received regulatory approval and summarizes their mechanisms of action, PK and pharmacodynamics (PD). This chapter summarizes the PK and PD of single-agent immunotherapies from publicly available sources through 2016 (Table 2.1). Advances in the field of immunotherapy have revolutionized oncology practice. The field is rapidly changing and at any given time there are hundreds of ongoing clinical trials with immunotherapies as single agents or in various combinations with another immunotherapy, targeted therapy, radiation therapy, or chemotherapy. Available data from new studies may provide additional insight for clinical PK and PD for immunotherapies in new patient populations.

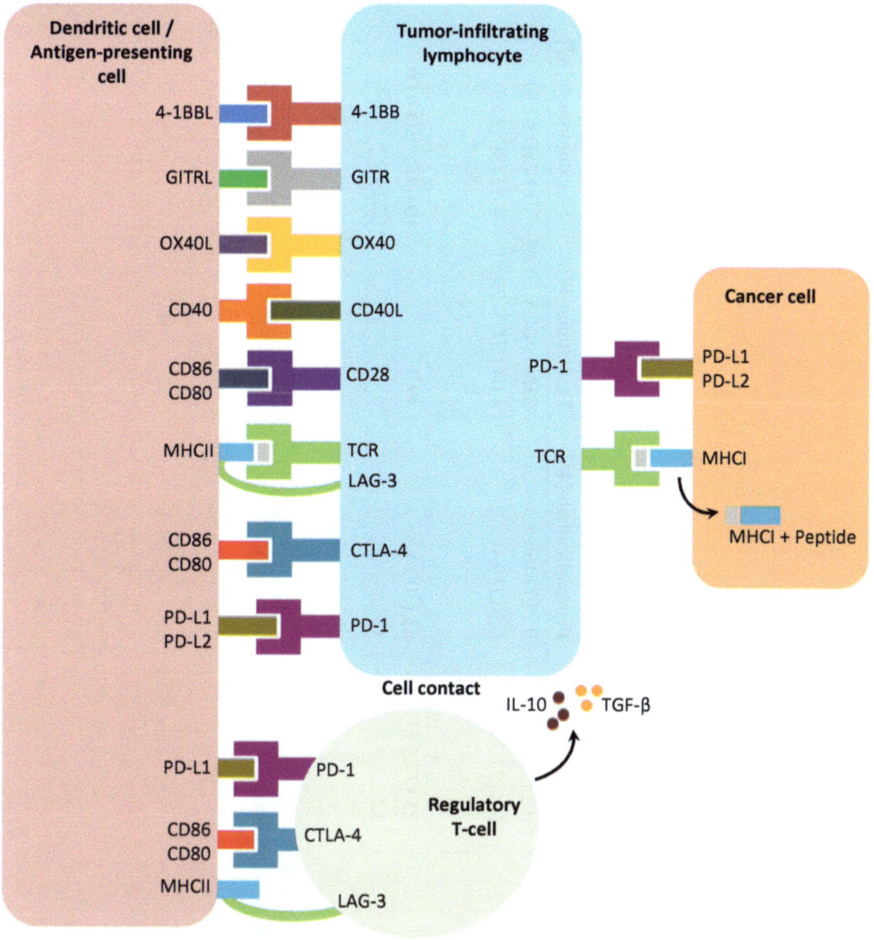

Fig. 2.1 An overview of the major targets and mechanisms of action of immunotherapies in oncology. In tumor microenvironments, T-cell antitumor activity is suppressed by immune inhibitory cell surface proteins expressed on tumor cells (such as programmed cell death ligands PD-L1 and PD-L2) or cytokines (such as transforming growth factor beta [TGF-β] and interleukin [IL]-10). Regulatory T cells also play a role in downregulating the immune system in tumor microenvironments through binding of cell surface receptors (including cytotoxic T lymphocyte-associated antigen 4 [CTLA-4] and programmed death-1 [PD-1]) to inhibitory ligands. Immune checkpoint inhibitors directed against CTLA-4, PD-1, and PD-L1 can augment release of immune stimulating cytokines and activate T-cell mediated antitumor activity. Immunostimulatory monoclonal antibodies have also been developed to target cell surface receptors on tumor-infiltrating lymphocytes (TILs) to activate stimulatory receptors and increase antitumor immunity. Targets for immunostimulatory agents include 4-1BB, glucocorticoid-induced tumor necrosis factor (TNF)-like receptor (GITR), and OX40, among others (Figure adapted from Khalil [2])

Table 2.1 Summary of population PK parameters (single agent) for approved immunotherapy

	Ipilimumab [12, 14]	Atezolizumab [54, 55]	Nivolumab [37]	Pembrolizumab [46]	Elotuzumab [76]	Blinatumomab [82]
Clearance (L/day)	0.4 (%CV 38)	0.2	0.2 (53.9%)	0.212 (46%)	0.086 (%CV 31.6)	70.1 (SD 67.9)
Volume of distribution at steady state (L)	4.16 (%CV 15.8)	6.9	6.8 (27.3%)	6.1 (21%)	4.04 (%CV 20.3)	4.52 (SD 2.89)
Half-life (days)	15.4 (%CV 34)	27	25 (77.5%)	23 (30%)	49.3	0.0875 (SD 0.06)
Time to reach steady state (weeks)	9	6 to 9	12	19	8	0.14

Note: Reported numbers are population PK parameter estimates
Abbreviations: *%CV* percent coefficient of variation, *SD* standard deviation

2.2 Immune Checkpoint Inhibitors

One mechanism by which immunotherapy works in cancer therapy is through the blockage of negative regulatory receptors and inhibitory checkpoints in the tumor microenvironment [5]. Antitumor T cells are naturally active against tumor antigens in most cancers; however, T cells may be rendered ineffective in the tumor microenvironment due to immune checkpoints, which are the collective immune resistance mechanisms that result in immune escape by the tumor [6]. Therefore, blocking of immune checkpoints results in enhancement of antitumor T-cell activity and shifts the balance from immune resistance to immune destruction of the tumor. Several classes of mAb checkpoint inhibitors have been developed, including anti-CTLA-4, anti-PD-1 and anti-PD-L1 antibodies.

2.2.1 Anti-CTLA-4 Antibodies

CTLA-4, also known as CD152, is a negative immune regulatory receptor expressed on surface of T cells, which play an important role in central anticancer adaptive immune response. Activation of CTLA-4 through binding to its ligands, CD80 and CD86, results in downregulation of T-cell activity against tumor cells. Blocking of CD80 and CD86 to CTLA-4 receptor can restore the immune function of T cells. Following blockage of CTLA-4, immune stimulating cytokines, such as IL-2 and IFN-γ, are released, resulting in T-cell activation and increased antitumor immunity [2, 7]. In recent years, antibody therapeutics targeted against CTLA-4 have been developed and tested in a number of cancers, most notably in metastatic or refractory melanoma, non-small cell lung cancer (NSCLC), and renal cell carcinoma (RCC). Although immune activation through central T-cell blockage of CTLA-4 is critical in eliciting antitumor response, greater T-cell activation may also lead to autoimmunity, as evidenced in patients who develop immune-related adverse events (irAEs) [8]. The most common irAEs are diarrhea, colitis, hepatitis, skin toxicities (such as rash or pruritis), and endocrinopathies (such as thyroid or pituitary dysfunction). Of note, relative to the anti-CTLA-4 antibodies, the anti-PD-1 antibodies have a different toxicity profile to ipilimumab with fewer high grade events [9, 10].

2.2.1.1 General ADME/Preclinical Pharmacokinetics

Ipilimumab and tremelimumab are two mAbs targeting CTLA-4. As with most mAb therapeutics, the administration of these drugs is through the parenteral, intravenous (IV) route. In general, anti-CTLA-4 antibodies are well distributed in the vascular system. The metabolism and elimination of large molecule therapeutics are well characterized through catabolic processes with little involvement from renal or hepatic organ systems.

Both ipilimumab and tremelimumab are directed against human CTLA-4 receptors; thus animal studies in various nonprimate species are limited. Preclinical PK studies for ipilimumab and tremelimumab were conducted in cynomolgus monkeys because both antibodies are cross reactive with cynomolgus monkeys with similar binding affinity to human CTLA4. After IV administration in cynomolgus monkeys, plasma clearance (CL) was low and the mean half-lives of anti-CTLA-4s were long, ranging from 8.5 to 14 days for ipilimumab and 9.1 to 11 days for tremelimumab [11, 12].

2.2.1.2 Ipilimumab

Ipilimumab is the first therapeutic antibody targeting human CTLA-4 and is approved in over 47 countries for the treatment of patients with unresectable or metastatic melanoma as monotherapy or in combination with nivolumab and as adjuvant treatment of patients with cutaneous melanoma [13].

Description and Human Dosing

Ipilimumab is a fully human mAb of IgG1-κ class consisting of four polypeptide chains with a molecular weight of 148 kDa. Ipilimumab has two identical heavy chains consisting of 447 amino acids each linked through interchain disulfide bonds to two identical κ light chains of 215 amino acids each. The approved dose for treatment of metastatic or refractory melanoma is 3 mg/kg administered IV every 3 weeks (Q3W) for a total of four doses. For the treatment of adjuvant melanoma, the dose is 10 mg/kg IV Q3W for four doses followed by 10 mg/kg every 12 weeks for up to 3 years [12, 14]. The dose selection of 3 mg/kg and 10 mg/kg was based on a phase 2 dose-ranging study that showed improved overall response rates with increasing doses from 0.3 to 10 mg/kg, but increased rates of Grade 3 and 4 adverse events in the highest dose group of 10 mg/kg [15].

Human Pharmacokinetics

In clinical trials, ipilimumab has been studied in advanced melanoma patients at doses ranging from 0.3 to 10 mg/kg IV Q3W for four doses. Ipilimumab exhibits linear PK with steady-state concentrations reached by the third dose of the Q3W regimen and mean half-life of approximately 15 days. The mean CL after 10 mg/kg IV administration was 18.3 mL/h and mean steady-state volume of distribution (V_{ss}), was 5.75 L [12].

Population Pharmacokinetics

The population PK model for ipilimumab was developed using PK data from patients with advanced melanoma from three phase 2 studies (CA184-007, CA184-008, and CA184-002; $N = 420$) and was validated with PK data from the

CA184-004 phase 2 study (*N* = 79). Ipilimumab PK data were well described by a linear two-compartment model with zero-order infusion and first-order elimination. From population PK analysis, the PK of ipilimumab was determined to be linear and dose proportional in the dose range of 0.3–10 mg/kg. The model parameters are time independent and comparable to those estimated by noncompartmental analyses from clinical studies. With multiple dosing, systemic accumulation was less than 1.5 fold. Steady-state levels of ipilimumab were reached by the third dose with a mean minimum concentration (C_{min}) of 19.4 mcg/mL at the 3 mg/kg dose level or 58.1 mcg/mL at the 10 mg/kg dose level. The mean value of CL, V_{ss} and half-life were estimated at 16.8 mL/h, 7.47 L, and 15.4 days, respectively [12, 16].

Body weight was identified as a significant covariate for central volume (V_c) and CL. The CL of ipilimumab increased with higher body weight, supporting the weight-based dosing. There was no significant increase in exposure with increasing body weight on an mg/kg basis. The steady-state C_{min} was relatively uniform over the body weight range of 40–140 kg in the model. Baseline lactate dehydrogenase (LDH) level was also identified as a significant covariate for CL. Steady-state exposure (area under the curve [AUC]) tends to decrease with increasing LDH, but this is likely not clinically significant based on existing safety and efficacy data [12, 16]. Incorporation of body weight and log-transformed LDH into the final population PK model explained approximately 24% and 52% of the base model variability of CL and V_c, respectively [16].

Exposure-Response Relationships

The PD response of anti-CLTA-4 antibodies in reducing tumor immunosuppression can be evaluated by activation of circulating T cells and immune cytokines. In both preclinical ex vivo studies and human clinical trials, elevated IL-2 and absolute lymphocyte counts were observed following administration of an anti-CTLA-4 antibody [14]. In melanoma patients with low baseline absolute lymphocyte counts, those treated with ipilimumab demonstrated longer overall survival (OS) compared to patients not treated with ipilimumab.

Data from 498 PK-evaluable patients from studies CA184-004, CA184-007, and CA184-002 were used for exposure-response (E-R) analyses for ipilimumab. Increasing steady-state C_{min} was associated with increased OS with both 3 mg/kg and 10 mg/kg doses. OS at the median steady-state C_{min} or ipilimumab at 0.3 mg/kg was estimated to be 0.85- and 0.58-fold lower relative to that at the median $C_{min,ss}$ for the 3 and 10 mg/kg doses, respectively. A stepwise Cox proportional hazard model identified C_{min} as a significant independent predictor of OS and predicted that for a 10 mcg/mL increase in exposure, the hazard ratio would decrease by 10%. In terms of safety, grade 2 and higher immune-related AEs (irAEs) were also associated with increased ipilimumab steady-state C_{min}. The model predicted that at median C_{min} of 3 and 10 mg/kg doses, Grade 2 and higher irAEs were approximately 33% and 51%, respectively, whereas Grade 3 and higher irAEs were approximately 13% and 24%, respectively [14, 16].

2.2.1.3 Tremelimumab

Tremelimumab is another anti-CTLA-4 antibody that is currently in development as monotherapy and in combination with other targeted therapies or immunotherapies for a number of advanced malignancies [17].

Description and Human Dosing

Tremelimumab is a humanized mAb of IgG2 class expressed and purified from NS0 murine myeloma cell lines. It has an overall molecular weight of approximately 149 kDa including oligosaccharides. The clinical dose of tremelimumab in phase three trials is 15 mg/kg administered as a continuous IV infusion every 90 days for a total of four doses [17].

Human Pharmacokinetics

Tremelimumab administered following a single IV infusion in clinical patients exhibited a biphasic PK profile. Mean systemic exposure increased in a dose-proportional manner for doses ranging from 1 to 15 mg/kg. The estimate of CL, V_{ss}, and terminal-phase half-life are consistent with those of natural IgG2 antibodies at 0.132 mL/h/kg, 81.2 mL/kg, and 22.1 days, respectively [11, 18, 19].

Population Pharmacokinetics

Population PK analysis of tremelimumab was performed on combined data from phase 1 through 3 studies in a total of 654 metastatic melanoma patients [20]. The base model was best described by a two-compartment model with log-transformed concentrations. The population estimate for CL and volume of the central compartment (V_c) were 0.26 L/day and 3.97 L, respectively. CL was faster in males, patients with higher values of creatinine CL (CrCl), patients with higher values of endogenous Ig, and patients with relatively poor baseline prognostic factors. Central V was higher in males and patients with higher body weight. In the final PK model, the covariates were sex, ECOG performance status, CrCl, endogenous IgG, LDH, and C-reactive protein (CRP) on CL and body weight and sex on V_c [20]. CRP on CL may have the most clinically important effect. There is 100% certainty that the CL would be greater than 120% of the value for an individual with a median CRP in patients with CRP levels greater than 16.5 times the upper normal limit.

Exposure-Response Relationships

Based on the population PK model for tremelimumab, slower CL was associated with longer median OS. The median OS for 147 patients in the fast CL group was 9.6 months compared to 15.8 months for the 146 patients in the slow CL group. The hazard ratio for death was 0.54 ($p < 0.001$). Prognostic covariates favoring longer survival in the slower clearance group included ECOG performance status, disease metastatic stages, and endogenous levels of LDH and CRP [20].

2.2.2 *Anti-PD-1 and PD-L1 Antibodies*

PD-1 is an inhibitory receptor involved in immune checkpoint signaling and is highly expressed on the surface of tumor-infiltrating lymphocytes (TILs), including cytotoxic T cells, B cells, and macrophages [2, 21]. The ligands for the PD-1 receptor, PD-L1 and PD-L2, are expressed on malignant tumor cells and antigen-presenting cells [2, 22, 23]. Binding of PD-L1/PD-L2 on a tumor cell with the PD-1 receptor on TILs results in decreased T-cell activation, proliferation, and cytokine production, ultimately contributing to inhibition of active T-cell immune surveillance of tumors [24]. Upregulation of PD-1 ligands occurs in some tumors and can contribute to inhibition of active T-cell immune surveillance [25]. MAbs act as checkpoint inhibitors by blocking inhibitory receptors for T cells, such as blocking the interaction between PD-1 and PD-L1/PD-L2. This blockage stimulates T-cell function by reactivating the function of pre-existing tumor-specific cytotoxic T cells in the tumor microenvironment [7, 26–28]. Nivolumab, pembrolizumab, and MEDI-0680 (AMP-514) are mAbs directed toward PD-1 that have shown activity in various types of cancers. Atezolizumab, durvalumab, avelumab, and BMS-936559 are mAbs directed toward PD-L1 that have shown activity in various types of cancers [29, 30]. This section mainly focuses on the publicly available data on nivolumab, pembrolizumab, and atezolizumab, which have received regulatory approval in various countries for multiple oncology indications.

2.2.2.1 Nivolumab

Nivolumab is a fully human, IgG4 κ isotype mAb that binds PD-1 (dissociation rate constant, $K_D = 3.06$ nM) [31]. Nivolumab consists of four polypeptide chains and contains an engineered hinge region mutation (S228P) designed to prevent the exchange of IgG4 molecules [25]. The IgG4 isotype reduces binding to Fc receptors and minimizes cellular and complement-mediated cytolytic functions [26].

Description and Human Dosing

The initial dose chosen for phase 1 studies of 0.3 mg/kg is over 200-fold lower than the dose level suggested by the "no observable adverse effect level" considerations from preclinical toxicology studies [25]. In the dose-escalation/dose-expansion study in patients with melanoma, NSCLC, or other solid tumors (MDX1106-03; $N = 306$) with doses from 0.1 to 10 mg/kg every 2 weeks (Q2W), the maximum tolerable dose was not reached [32]. In the MDX1106-03 study, the trough concentration of the first dose was >16 mcg/mL for the 3 mg/kg Q2W dose, which was >160 times of the binding EC50 of 0.1 mcg/mL [31, 33].

The 3 mg/kg Q2W was selected as the clinical dose based on the safety and efficacy in the MDX1106-03 study, which included patients with melanoma and NSCLC [25, 33, 34]. In addition, data from in vitro, preclinical, and the clinical analysis of E-R in CheckMate-037 and CheckMate-063 support the dose selection. Therefore, the 3 mg/kg Q2W dose was considered appropriate for late-stage clinical development across tumor types, including melanoma and NSCLC [33–36]. However, based on E-R analyses for nivolumab, a flat 240 mg dose replaced the weight-based dosing regimen as described below.

Population Pharmacokinetics

Based on the data from three phase 1, three phase 2, and five phase 3 clinical studies in 1895 patients with solid tumors treated with nivolumab, the PK profile of nivolumab was characterized by noncompartment analysis and population PK analysis. The population PK analysis demonstrated that the PK of nivolumab is linear in the dose range of 0.1–20 mg/kg with time-varying CL. CL is independent of dose within the dose range of 0.1–20 mg/kg. It is hypothesized that the decrease in nivolumab CL over the course of treatment may be associated with improvement in disease status and the corresponding decrease in the rate of cancer-related cachexia.

Based on the population PK model for single-agent nivolumab dosed 0.1–20 mg/kg as single or multiple doses Q2W or Q3W, nivolumab V_{ss} is 6.8 L, CL is 8.2 mL/h, terminal $t_{1/2}$ were estimated to be 25 days, and steady state was achieved by 12 weeks of 3 mg/kg Q2W repeated dosing, with an accumulation index (AI) estimated to be approximately 3.7-fold [33, 34, 37].

Nivolumab population PK was described with a two-compartment model with zero-order IV infusion and first-order elimination. The effects of various covariates on nivolumab PK were assessed. Nivolumab CL and V increase with body weight. The final model included the effects of baseline performance status, baseline body weight, and baseline estimated glomerular filtration rate (eGFR), sex, and race on CL, and effects of baseline body weight and sex on volume of distribution in the central compartment. Sex, performance status, baseline eGFR, age, race, baseline lactate dehydrogenase, mild hepatic impairment, tumor type, tumor burden, and PD-L1 expression had a significant but not clinically relevant (<20%) effect on nivolumab CL [33, 34, 38].

Exposure-Response Relationships

No exposure-efficacy relationship has been identified for nivolumab in melanoma or NSCLC patients based on the primary endpoint of overall response rate (ORR) in MDX1106-03, CheckMate-037, and CheckMate-063. In the MDX1106-03 dose-escalation and dose-expansion study, in patients with malignant melanoma, a flat exposure-ORR relationship was identified over the dose range of 0.1–10 mg/kg [33]. Similarly, for NSCLC patients in MDX1106-03, a flat E-R for ORR was identified over the dose range of 3 to 10 mg/kg, with ORR of 3% (n = 33), 24.3% (n = 37), and 20.3% (n = 59) for doses of 1, 3, and 10 mg/kg doses Q2W, respectively [34].

Data from MDX1106-03, CheckMate-037, and CheckMate-063 were used to characterize the relationship between average concentration at steady state (average C_{ss}) and the time to first Grade 3 or higher drug-related AEs or AEs leading to discontinuation. In general, there appeared to be no exposure-safety relationship between exposure (as measured by average C_{ss}) and time to first Grade 3+ drug-related AEs, AEs leading to discontinuation, and all grade 3 + AEs for nivolumab at 3 mg/kg Q2W based on the currently available clinical safety data.

On September 13, 2016, the Food and Drug Administration (FDA) modified the dosage regimen for nivolumab from 3 mg/kg Q2W to a flat dose of 240 mg Q2W for RCC, metastatic melanoma, and NSCLC. A flat dose of 240 mg was selected based on equivalence to the approved 3 mg/kg dose at the median body weight of approximately 80 kg in patients with solid tumors. Demographic data from patients with RCC (n = 603), melanoma (n = 826), or NSCLC (n = 648) across nine CheckMate studies were included in the pooled data set. Based on model-predicted simulations, the overall exposure at the 240 mg Q2W flat dose is similar (less than 6% difference) to 3 mg/kg Q2W. The predicted OS benefit and risk of AEs leading to discontinuation or death were similar across tumor types for both dosing regimens. Subgroup safety analyses did not demonstrate a clinically meaningful relationship between nivolumab exposure or BW and frequency or severity of AEs. Similarly, there was no clinically meaningful relationship between nivolumab exposure or body weight and frequency or severity of AEs [37, 39, 40].

2.2.2.2 Pembrolizumab

Pembrolizumab is a humanized IgG4 κ isotype mAb that binds to PD-1 with high affinity (K_D = 29 pM), antagonizing the interaction of PD-1 with PD-L1 and PD-L2, with a half maximal inhibitory concentration (IC50) between 0.1 and 0.3 nM [41, 42]. It was generated by grafting the variable region sequences of a mouse anti-human PD-1 antibody onto a human IgG4 κ isotype framework containing a stabilizing S228P Fc mutation [24].

Description and Human Dosing

KEYNOTE-001 was an open-label phase 1 dose-escalation and dose-expansion study in multiple tumor types. In the dose-escalation portion of KEYNOTE-001 (Part A, n = 10), pembrolizumab was dosed at 1, 3, and 10 mg/kg on days 1 and 28 and Q2W thereafter; maximum tolerated dose was not reached [24]. In Part A1 (n = 7), patients were administered pembrolizumab 10 mg/kg Q2W, which was a predetermined maximum administered dose. In Part A2 (n = 13), 13 patients were randomly assigned to one of three parallel, 3-week, intrapatient dose-escalation schedules (dose range 0.005–10 mg/kg), followed by treatment with 2 or 10 mg/kg Q3W.

The clinical dose of 2 mg/kg Q2W was supported by translational PK/PD analyses based on clinical IL-2 biomarker data and preclinical data in mice, which relied on interspecies extrapolation. These two PK/PD analysis methods converged on a similar dose regimen of 1–2 mg/kg Q3W as the lowest dose with high optimal likelihood of maximizing clinical efficacy. The potential for lesser efficacy was predicted at doses below 1 mg/kg. Thus, a dosage regimen of 2 mg/kg Q3W was proposed for the pivotal cohorts of the KEYNOTE-001 trial, along with the previously planned higher dose of 10 mg/kg Q2W to inform the dose selection for registration [43].

Population Pharmacokinetics

The original melanoma filing submission of pembrolizumab relied on the data from a single clinical study, KEYNOTE-001. Therefore, the focus of clinical pharmacology characterization was on model-based approaches that could leverage sparse PK, safety, and efficacy data. For the original melanoma filing, the PK profile of pembrolizumab was described using population PK analysis based on data collected from 476 patients enrolled in Parts A, B1, B2, C, and D of the KEYNOTE-001 study. Part A had intensive PK sampling and Parts B1, B2, C, and D had sparse sampling. In this initial population PK analysis (n = 476), none of the covariates tested appeared to have a clinically meaningful effect on pembrolizumab CL (no covariate changed clearance by more than 30%). Body weight-based dosing was deemed acceptable based on the exposure variation.

The most recently published population PK analysis for pembrolizumab used data from 2841 patients with various cancers who received pembrolizumab doses of 1–10 mg/kg Q2W or 2–10 mg/kg Q3W. Pembrolizumab PK were described adequately by a two-compartment model with linear CL; nonlinearity was observed at doses well below 1 mg/kg [44]. CL was found to depend on body weight allometrically. Sex, eGFR, albumin, tumor burden, and prior ipilimumab treatment had statistically significant effects on pembrolizumab CL. Sex, albumin, and prior ipilimumab treatment had statistically significant effects on pembrolizumab central volume. However, these covariates lacked clinical significance [45]. Clearance was found to be lower by 17% in female patients ($P < 0.0001$), translating into a 20% increase in AUC in female subjects ($N = 900$), which is small in relation to the exposure margins and, therefore, did not have clinical relevance. Because therapeutic antibodies are too large to pass through the glomerular membrane of the kidney, renal insufficiency was not expected to significantly impact pembrolizumab exposure, therefore, eGFR was not considered a clinically significant covariate. Relative to an ECOG performance status of 1, an ECOG performance status of 0 was associated with a 7.3% increase in CL. Similarly, cancer type (14.5% increase for patients with NSCLC) and ipilimumab status (13.9% increase in clearance for patients pre-treated with ipilimumab) had a statistically significant effect on clearance. At the 90th percentile of baseline tumor burden distribution, clearance was increased by 8.79% relative to a typical subject, translating to a 9.17% reduction in AUC. However, because of the limited volume of distribution for pembrolizumab, the total level of pembrolizumab outside the blood is expected to be low. Tumor volume represents only a fraction of total body volume, therefore, tumors have a limited potential to contribute to total body CL of pembrolizumab [45].

Pembrolizumab CL at steady state was estimated as 212 mL/day, volume of distribution at steady state is 6.1 L, and $t_{1/2}$ is 23 days. Steady-state concentrations were reached by 19 weeks of repeated Q3W dosing and the systemic accumulation was 2.2-fold. The PK of pembrolizumab is dose proportional in the dose range of 2–10 mg/kg Q3W [46]. The latest and most mature version of the population PK model will be continuously refined with more data with the expanding pembrolizumab clinical programs [43].

Exposure-Response Relationships

Data for E-R analyses for clinical activity (n = 365) and E-R analyses for adverse events (n = 409) were collected from Parts B1, B2, and D [47]. There was a flat E-R relationship between steady-state exposure and ORR for patients in Part B2 of KEYNOTE-001 (n = 173), which supports the 2 mg/kg dosing as opposed to the 10 mg/kg dosing regimen. In addition, the mean time to response was 15 weeks for the 2 mg/kg arm compared to 12 weeks for the 10 mg/kg arm, with median duration of response not reached for either arm; the proportion of nonprogressing patients was the same for each arm (90%). The E-R relationship for safety in terms of both adverse events of grade 3–5 or serious AE and adverse events of special interest of pembrolizumab is flat across the exposure range observed with doses ranging from 1 to 10 mg/kg [47].

In an integrated population PK analysis using efficacy and safety data from the final NSCLC expansion cohort of KEYNOTE-001, in which patients received either pembrolizumab 2 mg/kg Q3W, 10 mg/kg Q3W, or 10 mg/kg Q2W, the final model showed a flat E-R relationship for efficacy and safety [42].

For all melanoma submissions to date (November 2016), OS data were not sufficiently mature to establish robust E-R relationships. Therefore, exposure-efficacy evaluations supporting pembrolizumab dose selection centered on tumor size kinetics. The E-R relationship for tumor size (sum of longest dimension of tumor lesions) and pembrolizumab exposure in melanoma (n = 897) and NSCLC (n = 496) patients showed a flat E-R relationship for tumor size response across the 2 mg/kg Q3W to 10 mg/kg Q2W dosage range, indicating that a near-maximal response was achieved at 2 mg/kg Q3W. This approach will also be extended across other solid tumors [43, 48].

Using a population PK model developed with data from KEYNOTE-001, KEYNOTE-002, and KEYNOTE-006, simulations indicate that the fixed 200 mg Q3W dose of pembrolizumab would provide exposure similar to weight-based dosing regimens used in previous pembrolizumab studies. Therefore, both dosing regimens of 200 mg and 2 mg/kg are appropriate for pembrolizumab, as both provide similar exposure distributions, with no advantage to either dosing approach [49, 50]. The FDA has approved the fixed 200 mg Q3W dosing regimen in NSCLC and head and neck squamous cell carcinoma [46].

2.2.2.3 Atezolizumab

Atezolizumab is an Fc-engineered, humanized, nonglycosylated IgG1 κ isotype mAb that directly binds to PD-L1 (K_D = 0.4 nM) and blocks interactions with the PD-1 (IC50 82.8 pM) and B7.1/CD80 (IC50 48.5 pM) receptors [51, 52]. It is composed of two light chains consisting of 214 amino acid residues and two heavy chains consisting of 448 amino acid residues [53, 54]. The Fc region was engineered with a modification to eliminate antibody-dependent cell-mediated cytotoxicity (ADCC) at clinical doses, preventing depletion of activated T cells [52]. Atezolizumab is currently FDA approved for treatment of NSCLC and urothelial carcinoma [54].

Description and Human Dosing

The dose-escalation portion of the phase 1 PCD4989g study included atezolizumab doses ranging from 0.01 to 20 mg/kg Q3W and included patients receiving 1200 mg Q3W, which is the fixed dose equivalent of 15 mg/kg [55]. A maximum tolerated dose was not achieved and no dose-limiting toxicities were observed at any dose level. The 15 mg/kg Q3W dose level was sufficient to maintain a trough concentration of 6 mcg/mL [56, 57]. In the dose-expansion portion of the study, atezolizumab was dosed by weight at 15 mg/kg, as well as a fixed, nonweight-based dose of 1200 mg Q3W. In the phase 1 JO28944 study, atezolizumab was dosed at either 10 or 20 mg/kg Q3W [53, 55]. The current FDA-approved dose for atezolizumab is 1200 mg Q3W [54].

Population Pharmacokinetics

A population PK analysis using a two-compartment linear model with first-order elimination from the central compartment described serum atezolizumab PK in the dose range of 1–20 mg/kg, including the fixed dose 1200 mg Q3W. This model was built based on pooled PK data from 472 cancer patients in the PCD4989g (N = 466) and JO28944 (N = 6) studies and was validated using PK data from the phase 2 IMvigor 210 study (GO29293) in patients with metastatic urothelial bladder cancer [55]. Atezolizumab patient exposure increased dose proportionally over the dose range of 1–20 mg/kg, including the fixed dose 1200 mg Q3W. At atezolizumab doses <1.0 mg/kg, atezolizumab exposure was less than dose proportional [54]. The population PK model predicted V_{ss} is 6.9 L, CL is 0.2 L/day, $t_{1/2}$ was estimated to be 27 days, and steady state was achieved after 6–9 weeks of repeated dosing, with an AI estimated to be approximately 1.91-fold for exposure (AUC) [53, 54].

Patients with body weight lower than 54 kg would have up to a 32% increase in steady-state AUC (AUC_{ss}) than the typical patient. However, the population PK analysis did not show any other clinically meaningful differences in atezolizumab exposure (less than 28% change in exposure from the typical patient) following a fixed dose (1200 mg Q3W) or a dose adjusted for weight (15 mg/kg Q3W) [55]. Because of the lack of safety concern in addition to an assessment of the PK characteristics of atezolizumab (target serum concentration of 6 mcg/mL), a 1200 mg fixed dosage (equivalent to an average body weight-based dose of 15 mg/kg) Q3W was adopted for later clinical trials. No covariate was identified to have a clinically relevant effect on atezolizumab PK. In the population PK analysis, a typical patient is a male without positive postbaseline antidrug antibody (ADA), weighing 77 kg, with an albumin level of 40 g/L, and a tumor burden of 63 mm. Patients with metastatic urothelial carcinoma did not show any trend of having different PK parameters than patients with other tumor types [53].

Exposure-Response Relationships

PK data from 306 patients receiving atezolizumab 1200 mg Q3W as second-line or greater treatment in cohort 2 of the IMvigor 210 study was used to establish the E-R relationship for ORR. A univariate analysis using a logistic model showed that there is no correlation between ORR and trough concentration of atezolizumab in the first cycle. In addition, analysis of the E-R relationship for progression-free survival (PFS) showed no clear differences in PFS among the atezolizumab exposure quartiles. The difference in atezolizumab exposure when evaluated at extreme values of weight compared to the typical patient following administration of the flat dose of 1200 mg Q3W would not be expected to be clinically meaningful or require dose adjustment by body size. These results suggest no improved efficacy would be expected with atezolizumab doses higher than 1200 mg Q3W. Additionally, the E-R relationship is flat for all three IC score groups (IC0, IC1, and IC2/3). Based on multivariate analysis, the statistically significant covariates identified for ORR were higher baseline ECOG score or greater number of metastatic sites, which are associated with lower probability to respond, whereas higher IC score is associated with higher probability to respond.

PK data from both cohorts of IMvigor 210 (423 out of 429 patients) in combination with PK data from PCD4989g (90 out of 92 patients) were used to establish the E-R relationship for safety. There appeared to be no significant exposure-safety relationship between adverse events and exposure within the range following atezolizumab administration of 1200 mg Q3W. The relationship between the AUC_{ss} and incidence of AEs appears to be flat [53].

2.2.2.4 Durvalumab

Durvalumab (MEDI4736) is a selective, high-affinity, engineered human IgG1 κ isotype mAb that blocks PD-L1 binding to PD-1 (IC50 0.1 nM) and B7.1/CD80 (IC50 0.04 nM). Durvalumab does not bind to PD-L2, which plays a role in controlling inflammation in normal lung tissue. An engineered triple mutation in the Fc antibody domain is designed to reduce ADCC and complement-dependent cytotoxicity. Durvalumab is currently in development as monotherapy and in combination with other targeted therapies or immunotherapies for a number of advanced malignancies [58, 59].

Description and Human Dosing

In the CD-ON-MEDI4736-1108 phase 1 dose-escalation and dose-expansion study, PK data were collected from 292 PK-evaluable patients following 0.1, 0.3, 1.0, 3.0, and 10 mg/kg Q2W and 15 mg/kg Q3W doses of durvalumab (1954 serum concentrations). Durvalumab PK was best described using a two-compartment population PK model with both linear and nonlinear (target-mediated) CL. Durvalumab exhibited nonlinear (dose-dependent) PK. No covariates were identified to have a clinically relevant impact on PK parameters. The population estimate for linear CL was 0.25 L/day, V in the central compartment was 3.3 L, and concentration at half maximal elimination (K_M) was 0.4 mcg/L. Greater than 99% target saturation (soluble and membrane bound) is expected at durvalumab concentrations ≥40 mcg/mL. PK simulations indicate that following 10 mg/kg Q2W, over 90% patients are expected to maintain PK exposure ≥40 mcg/mL throughout the dosing interval. Based on preclinical/clinical PK, PD, and safety data, a dose of 10 mg/kg Q2W was selected for the dose-expansion phase of the study and for further clinical development in phase 2 and 3 studies [60, 61].

2.2.2.5 Avelumab

Avelumab (MSB0010718C) is a fully human IgG1 mAb targeting PD-L1, which can mediate ADCC of tumor cells [62, 63]. Avelumab is currently in development as monotherapy and in combination with other targeted therapies or immunotherapies for several advanced malignancies [64–66].

Description and Human Dosing

In a phase 1 trial in patients with advanced solid tumors, dose-escalation and dose-expansion trial (3 + 3 design) was performed four dose levels of 1, 3, 10, or 20 mg/kg Q2W. PK parameters were evaluated on 53 patients in the dose-escalation portion and 600 patients in the dose-expansion portion. The mean half-life of avelumab at 10 mg/kg was 102 h, mean Cmax was 301 mcg/mL, and mean C_{min} was 22 mcg/mL. The PK profile was linear over the dose range and the population PK model was best described by a two-compartment model. One immune-related dose-limiting toxicity was reported at the 20 mg/kg dose level. Target occupancy was >95% over the biweekly dosing interval at 10 mg/kg, therefore, the 10 mg/kg dose was selected for dose expansion and further clinical trials [65, 66].

2.3 Immunostimulatory Antibody Therapies

Although immune checkpoint inhibitors can indirectly enhance antitumor T-cell activity, newer antibody therapeutics have been developed that can directly stimulate and elicit an immune response against malignant cells. High dose IL-2 is well known to promote cytotoxic T-cell and natural killer (NK) cell cytolytic activity and IFN alpha 2-b stimulates IL-12 secretion that also promotes T-cell activity. These traditional immunomodulating cytokines have now largely fallen out of favor in cancer immunotherapy due to the development of more efficacious immunostimulatory therapies.

The mechanism of action for immunostimulatory antibodies can vary based on the costimulatory receptor targeted. Currently, several antibody therapeutics are underdevelopment, including antibody targets for OX40 (CD134), 4-1BB (CD137 or TNFRSF9), GITR (CD357), and several others [7]. OX40 is expressed on CD4+ and CD8+ T cells and can be activated through binding to its ligand, OX40L from antigen-presenting cells (APCs). MEDI-6469 is an agonist antibody of OX40 currently under development in phase 1 clinical trials in patients with advanced solid tumors [67]. 4-1BB is another costimulatory receptor that is expressed on activated T cells, activated NK cells and constitutively on dendritic and regulatory T cells. When 4-1BBB is activated by its natural ligand, 4-1BBL, it promotes activity of T cells, dendritic cells, monocytes, and neutrophils. Two agonist antibodies for 4-1BB are currently under development, including urelumab and utomilumab (PF-05082566) [68–70]. In clinical studies with 4-1BB antibody agonists, high-dose regimens resulted in severe liver toxicities. Currently, lower doses of urelumab and utomilumab are being studied in monotherapy and combination therapy for a number of solid malignancies [71, 72]. GITR is another costimulatory target. GITR expression increases after stimulation of CD4+ and CD8+ T cells resulting in increased proliferation and effector function. GITR may also play a role in reverse suppression by regulatory T cells and leucocyte adhesion. Currently several GITR targeted antibodies are being studied in phase 1 clinical trials in advanced melanoma or other advanced solid tumors [73, 74]. Although agonist antibodies for OX40, 4-1BB, and GITR are currently under development in solid tumor malignancies, elotuzumab and blinatumomab are two other immunostimulatory antibodies with different targets and mechanisms of actions that have been FDA approved for hematologic malignancies. Elotuzumab and blinatumomab PK and PD will be described in more detail in this section.

2.3.1 *Elotuzumab*

Elotuzumab is a mAb directed against signaling lymphocyte activation molecule family 7 (SLAMF7) that is FDA approved for use in combination therapy with lenalidomide and dexamethasone in second-line treatment of patients with multiple myeloma. The immunostimulatory effect of elotuzumab is a result of direct activation of NK cells through signaling of SLAMF7. Additionally, elotuzumab can also elicit indirect tumor cell death via traditional ADCC. Elotuzumab mediates dose-dependent, ADCC against SLAMF7 expressing multiple myeloma cells. Elotuzumab binds to SLAMF7, which is a glycoprotein expressed on NK cells and myeloma cells, resulting in their direct activation. Elotuzumab bound to myeloma cells further activates NK cells via a cluster of differentiation 16 (CD16) mediated pathway, thereby enabling selective killing of myeloma cells with minimal effects on normal tissue cells [75, 76].

Elotuzumab is a 148 kDa humanized recombinant IgG1 mAb consisting of the complementarity determining regions of the mouse antibody, MuLuc63, grafted onto human IgG1 heavy and κ light chain framework regions. The recommended dose for elotuzumab in multiple myeloma is 10 mg/kg IV every week for the first two cycles followed by every 2 weeks thereafter [77].

2.3.1.1 General ADME/Preclinical Pharmacokinetics

Preclinical studies of elotuzumab consist of primarily in vitro safety assessments and in vivo biological activity assessment of elotuzumab target selectivity and toxicity. Based on nonclinical studies, SLAMF7 is expressed by >95% of multiple myeloma cells and its expression is independent of cytogenetic abnormalities. In xenographed mice with human myeloma, elotuzumab was found to inhibit tumor growth and the effect was enhanced in further xenographed models with coadministration with bortezomib and lenalidomide. PK properties have not been characterized in animal studies for elotuzumab due to its lack of cross reactivity to other species [77].

2.3.1.2 Human Pharmacokinetics

Several clinical trials were conducted in multiple myeloma patients using elotuzomab as a single agent and in combination. One single agent and two combination dose-escalation studies were conducted to assess the dose-response characteristics and dose-limiting toxicities of elotuzumab. Following a single IV administration of elotuzumab, the maximum drug concentration increased in a dose-proportional manner across the dose range of 0.5–20 mg/kg. AUC increased greater than proportionally with dose (nonlinear), indicative of target-mediated clearance. Geometric mean clearance of elotuzumab ranged from 15.5 to 69.3 mL/h and decreased with an increase in dose, suggesting a saturation of target-mediated CL. Elotuzumab V was approximately 3–6 L, which is similar to serum volume [75, 77]. Following administration of elotuzumab every 7 days for the first 2 cycles and every 14 days for all subsequent cycles in combination with lenalidomide and dexamethasone, the steady-state C_{min} concentrations associated with the 10 and 20 mg/kg doses were above the anticipated therapeutic trough concentration of 70 mcg/mL [77, 78].

2.3.1.3 Population Pharmacokinetics

Population PK analyses for elotuzumab were conducted using data from four clinical studies, including the pivotal phase 3 trial in combination with lenolidamide and dexamethasone in multiple myeloma patients [79]. The analysis included a total of 6958 elotuzumab serum concentration values from 375 patients. Elotuzumab PK was best characterized by a two-compartment model with zero-order IV infusion, parallel linear and Michaelis-Menten elimination from the central compartment, and additional target-mediated elimination from the peripheral compartment [80].

Baseline body weight influenced the linear component of clearance, the distributional clearance, and volume of distribution of elotuzumab. Both CL and V_c increased with weight; weight-based dosing generated uniform exposures across the range of weights and minimized interindividual variability of elotuzumab exposure. M (myeloma) protein, a measure of myeloma disease burden, was also identified as a major covariate of elotuzumab clearance. There was also a correlation seen between high baseline M-protein and lower exposure. Coadministration of lenalidomide/dexamethasone was estimated to reduce elotuzumab CL by 35%. The target-mediated CL increased with increasing serum M-protein at baseline. There was almost a three-fold increase in target-mediated CL in patients with baseline serum M-protein of 8 g/dL compared with patients with a value of 0 g/dL. Furthermore, steady-state AUC was 45% lower for patients win the top quartile of serum M-protein values compared to patients in the lowest quartile. As M-protein is secreted by tumor cells, elevated serum M-protein reflects higher tumor burden, and higher target-mediated elimination at higher levels of serum M-protein is consistent with target-mediated elimination of elotuzumab by binding to tumor cells. All other covariates tested had an effect <20% on model parameters and are unlikely to have clinically meaningful effects [76, 80].

2.3.1.4 Exposure-Response Relationships

The E-R analysis for PFS was conducted using data from multiple myeloma patients for elotuzumab. E-R analyses and the target-mediated clearance of the drug suggest that patients with lower exposure of the drug may benefit from an increased dose. This was supported by evaluating baseline disease burden using M-protein, β2-microglobulin, and LDH. There was no difference in median PFS between patients with elotuzumab average C_{ss} in the lowest quartile of elotuzumab exposure (average C_{ss} < 209 mcg/mL) and patients on active control of lenalidomide and dexamethasone, after controlling for potential confounding factors such as high M-protein, higher β2-microglobulin, ECOG score, and higher LDH levels. Patients with elotuzumab concentrations in the higher three quartiles of exposure showed treatment benefit with longer PFS compared to active control. Further analysis of patients with high tumor burden (high baseline M-protein) and lower exposure are needed to conclude dose optimization in this population [76].

2.3.2 *Blinatumomab*

Other immunostimulatory agents activate costimulatory targets to activate adaptive antitumor immunity or directly stimulate NK cells, such as elotuzumab. In contrast, blinatumomab utilizes a cell directed therapy with through binding of two targets. The therapeutic action of blinatumomab is a result of activation and redirection of cytotoxic T lymphocytes to malignant cells. Blinatumomab is a bispecific CD19-directed CD3 T-cell engager (BiTE) indicated for the treatment of Philadelphia chromosome-negative relapsed or refractory B-cell precursor acute lymphoblastic leukemia (ALL). Blinatumomab binds to CD19, an antigen expressed on the surface of B cells, and CD3 expressed on the surface of T cells. It activates and engages T cells through formation of the CD3 T-cell receptor complex and directs the cytotoxic T lymphocyte to CD19-positive benign and malignant B cells. In in vitro studies, blinatumomab binding to CD3-positive T cells and CD19-positive target B cells resulted in the release of cytokines, including IL-2, TNF-α, and IFN-γ, which aid in the activation of T cells [81].

Blinatumomab is a recombinant nonglycosylated protein (504 amino acids, 55 kDa) that was developed by genetic engineering from two distinct murine mAbs directed against CD19 and CD3. The amino terminus of blinatumomab contains the CD3-binding region, whereas the carboxy terminus contains the CD19-binding region. A single cycle of treatment consists of 28 days of continuous blinatumomab IV infusion, followed by a 2-week treatment-free interval. Dosing is weight based and begins at 9 mcg/day on days 1–7 and 28 mcg/day on subsequent days and cycles for patients greater than or equal to 45 kg. For patients under 45 kg, dosing begins at 5 mcg/m^2/day on days 1–7 and increases to 15 mcg/m^2/day on subsequent days and cycles [82].

2.3.2.1 General ADME/Preclinical Pharmacokinetics

Blinatumomab binds with similar potency to human and chimpanzee B and T cells and animal studies have been conducted in nonprimate and primate species. Following single or multiple doses through IV, subcutaneous (SC) or intraperitoneal (IP) administration, blinatumomab exposure increased dose dependently. Blinatumomab exhibited a fast elimination with a half-life of 1.8 h in chimpanzees. There was no apparent drug accumulation following multiple dosing [83].

2.3.2.2 Human Pharmacokinetics

In humans, blinatumomab PK appear linear over a dose range of 5–90 mcg/m^2/day following continuous IV infusion in patients with ALL and non-Hodgkin's lymphoma (NHL) [81]. Steady state was achieved within 1 day of continuous IV infusion and remained stable over time during the infusion period and mean C_{ss} values increased dose proportionally. At the clinical doses of 9 mcg/day and 28 mcg/day for the treatment of relapsed/refractory ALL, the mean (standard deviation; SD) C_{ss} was 211 (258) pg/mL and 621 (502) pg/mL, respectively [82]. Unlike other antibody therapeutics, the mean elimination half-life of blinatumomab is short, at approximately 2.1 h and the estimated mean systemic CL was 2.92 L/h. Like other therapeutic antibodies, mean V is close to serum V at 4.52 L [83, 84].

2.3.2.3 Population Pharmacokinetics

A population PK model for blinatumomab was developed from four adult clinical trials with a total of 322 subjects and 2587 serum samples. A one-compartment linear model with a mixture model to identify two subpopulations with different CL was used. The model described the time course of blinatumomab concentrations after continuous IV infusion of different doses in several hematological malignancies. The geometric mean of V was 3.40 L. For 90% of the population, the geometric mean for CL was 1.36 L/h, but 10% of the population had typical CL of 5.49 L/h. Renal function was identified as a significant factor on CL with 50% reduction in CrCL associated with a 20% reduction in systemic CL. The reason for the 10% population with a four-fold higher systemic CL is unknown. Other tested covariates, including body size, age, sex, and creatinine CL, did not have clinically meaningful effects on blinatumomab exposure. The effect of race on PK could not be evaluated as >90% of study subjects were Caucasians [83].

2.3.2.4 Exposure-Response Relationships

The pharmacodynamics of blinatumomab can be characterized by T-cell activation and initial redistribution, reduction in peripheral B-cells, and transient cytokine elevation. Following continuous infusion with blinatumomab, peripheral T-cell counts initially declined within the first 6 h due to the initial redistribution from periphery to tissues. Baseline or above baseline levels were recovered and seen during subsequent 2–7 days of treatment. Redistribution of NK cells and monocytes exhibited kinetics similar to those observed for T cells. B-cell counts in the periphery decreased rapidly and become undetectable during treatment at doses ≥5 mcg/m^2/day (or 9 mcg/day) in most patients. No recovery of B-cell counts was observed during the 14-day drug free period between cycles. Transient increases in cytokines were observed 2 days after blinatumomab administration. The elevated cytokines returned to baseline levels within 24–48 h during the first infusion period. The magnitude of cytokine elevation trended with the dose level received. In subsequent cycles, the cytokine elevation occurred in fewer patients and with lesser intensity compared to the initial 48 h of the first treatment cycle [83].

The E-R relationship for blinatumomab was studied using data from the pivotal phase 2 clinical trial, MT103-211 in relapsed/refractory ALL patients. Patients received 28 mcg/day infusion of blinatumomab and steady-state concentrations were measured. As a result of the analysis, there was an increase in remission rate in correlation to an increase in exposures. Baseline characteristics and disease risk factors were major confounders to this analysis. It was found that patients with lower exposure who exhibited lower remission rate were also patients with higher blast cells and CD19-positive B cells but lower CD3-postive T cells. Thus, it is difficult to differentiate the true contribution of exposure on efficacy due to variability in baseline disease severity and B- and T-cell counts [83].

2.4 Immunogenicity

As with any antibody drug therapy, there is a potential for patients to develop ADAs. The likelihood of developing antidrug antibodies with humanized antibodies such as the checkpoint inhibitors and elotuzumab is low [77]. In clinical trials, 1.1% of patients treated with ipilimumab had measurable anti-ipilimumab antibodies, although no patients tested positive for neutralizing antibodies [14]. In phase 1 through 3 studies with tremelimumab evaluating immunogenicity, the incidence of developing ADA was <6% overall [11].

Among 1086 nivolumab-treated patients, 138 patients (12.7%) were ADA positive, only three (0.3%) of whom were persistently positive for ADA (positive at two consecutive time points at least 8 weeks apart), and nine (0.8%) were positive for neutralizing antibodies (NAbs) at one time point. The presence of ADAs was not associated with hypersensitivity, infusion reactions, or loss of efficacy and had minimal impact on nivolumab CL. Additionally, the presence of NAbs was not associated with loss of efficacy [85]. In the 153 patients treated with pembrolizumab with the dosage regimen of 2 mg/kg Q3W, 97 of them had a concentration of pembrolizumab in the last postdose sample below the drug tolerance level of the antiproduct antibody assay. None of these 97 patients tested positive for treatment-emergent anti-pembrolizumab antibodies [47]. The ADA incidence to atezolizumab was 31.7%, 16.7%, and 41.9% in the studies PCD4989g, JO28944, and IMvigor 210, respectively. Overall, ADA positivity did not seem to impact efficacy or safety of atezolizumab. The incidence of adverse events of special interest (AESI) for atezolizumab was similar irrespective of postbaseline ADAs status [53, 55].

Of 390 patients across four clinical studies who were treated with elotuzumab and evaluable for the presence of antiproduct antibodies, 72 patients (18.5%) tested positive for treatment-emergent antiproduct antibodies by an electrochemiluminescent assay. In 63 (88%) of these 72 patients, antiproduct antibodies occurred within the first 2 months of the initiation of treatment. Antiproduct antibodies resolved by 2–4 months in 49 (78%) of these 63 patients. Neutralizing antibodies were detected in 19 of 299 patients in the randomized trial in multiple myeloma [76–78].

Less information regarding immunogenicity of durvalumab, avelumab, and blinatumomab is available. As of February 2015, eight of 388 patients treated with durvalumab were ADA positive [61]. In clinical studies, <1% of treated patients produced anti-blinotumomab antibodies [82]. Of 79 patients treated with avelumab in a phase 3 trial, three patients were ADA positive [64]. To date, no infusion related reactions occurred in patients who tested positive for antidrug antibodies and no effect was seen on HLA status and immunogenicity.

2.5 Studies in Special Populations

In general, the use and evaluation of cancer immunotherapy in special populations is limited. To date, there are no published studies for cancer immunotherapy antibodies in patients with hepatic or renal impairment. However, the impact of varying degrees of hepatic or renal impairment on PK parameters was assessed in population PK analyses. Patients with moderate to severe hepatic impairment were generally not included in the clinical trials of mAbs [76, 77, 82, 83].

Studies in other special populations, such as pregnant women are also lacking, as most trials excluded pregnant or lactating women. It is well known that antibodies may be transferred from the mother to the infants through breastfeeding; therefore, breastfeeding while on treatment with checkpoint inhibitors or immunostimulatory antibodies is generally not recommended [14, 37, 46, 54, 77, 82]. Limited information regarding pregnancy and lactation is available from animal studies.

See Table 2.2 for a summary of FDA-approved immunotherapy dosing recommendations in special populations.

2.6 Adoptive Cellular Therapy

2.6.1 Description and Human Dosing

Advances in the use of adoptive cellular therapy to treat cancer have yielded unprecedented results in hematological malignancies and are being tested in solid tumors. The purpose of adoptive cellular therapy is to elicit a robust immune-mediated antitumor response. Adoptive cellular therapy is based on ex vivo manipulation of homologous or heterologous T cells through selection and expansion of TILs, gene transfer of a synthetic T-cell receptors, or insertion of a chimeric antigen receptor (CAR) into T cells. This section mainly discusses the PK/PD of CAR T cells.

CAR T cells are engineered to express synthetic receptors that direct T cells to specific antigens for tumor elimination [86]. CARs consist of an intracellular signaling domain of a T-cell receptor linked by a spacer with an extracellular antigen-recognition domain (single chain fragment of variable region), which permits recognition of a specific antigen by a T cell. This stimulates T-cell proliferation,

Table 2.2 Summary of FDA-approved immunotherapy use in specific populations

	Renal impairment	Hepatic impairment	Pregnancy or lactation	Geriatrics	Pediatrics
Ipilimumab [14]	No dose adjustment	No dose adjustment is needed for patients with mild hepatic impairment (total bilirubin [TB] >1.0–1.5 times ULN or AST > ULN). Ipilimumab has not been studied in patients with moderate (TB >1.5–3.0 times ULN and any AST) or severe (TB >3 times ULN and any AST) hepatic impairment	It is not known whether ipilimumab is secreted in human milk. In monkeys, ipilimumab was present in milk Advise women to discontinue nursing during treatment with ipilimumab and for 3 months following the final dose Human IgG1 is known to cross the placental barrier and ipilimumab is an IgG1; therefore, ipilimumab has the potential to be transmitted from the mother to the developing fetus. There is insufficient human data for ipilimumab exposure in pregnant women Preclinical studies in pregnant cynomolgus monkeys found higher incidences of abortion, stillbirths, premature deliveries, and infant mortality after administration of ipilimumab. Fetal harm from ipilimumab was also found to occur in a dose related manner	No overall differences in safety or efficacy were reported between the elderly patients (≥65 years) and younger patients (<65 years)	Safety and effectiveness of ipilimumab have not been established in pediatric patients
Blinatumomab [82]	No starting dose adjustment for mild or moderate renal impairment. No formal studies have been conducted in patients with severe renal impairment (CLcr <30 mL/min) or patients on hemodialysis for blinatumomab [83]	No formal PK studies using blinatumomab have been conducted in patients with hepatic impairment	There is no information regarding the presence of blinatumomab in human milk, the effects on the breastfed infant, or the effects on milk production. Advise patients not to breastfeed during and for at least 48 h after treatment with blinatumomab Due to the potential for B-cell lymphocytopenia in infants following exposure to blinatumomab in utero, the infant's B lymphocytes should be monitored before the initiation of live virus vaccination	No overall differences in safety or effectiveness were observed between these patients and younger patients. Elderly patients experienced a higher rate of neurological toxicities, including cognitive disorder, encephalopathy, confusion, and serious infections	No differences in efficacy were observed between the different age subgroups. The adverse reactions in blinatumomab-treated pediatric patients were similar in type to those seen in adult patients. The steady-state concentrations of blinatumomab were comparable in adult and pediatric patients at the equivalent dose levels based on BSA-based regimens

Elotuzumab [76]	Clinically significant differences were not observed in the PK of elotuzumab based on renal impairment ranging from mild to severe (CLcr 15 to 89 mL/min) renal impairment or end-stage renal disease (CLcr <15 mL/min) with or without hemodialysis	Clinically significant differences were not observed in the PK of elotuzumab based on mild (NCI-CTEP) hepatic impairment. The PK of elotuzumab in patients with moderate to severe hepatic impairment is unknown	There are no studies with elotuzumab with pregnant women to inform any drug associated risks. Animal reproduction studies have not been conducted with elotuzumab. There is no information on the presence of elotuzumab in human milk, the effect on the breastfed infant, or the effect on milk production. Breastfeeding is not recommended	No overall differences in efficacy or safety were observed between patients ≥65 years and patients <65 years	Safety and effectiveness have not been established in pediatric patients
Atezolizumab [54]	Based on a population PK analysis, no dose adjustment of atezolizumab is recommended for patients with renal impairment	Based on a population PK analysis, no dose adjustment of atezolizumab is recommended for patients with mild hepatic impairment. Atezolizumab has not been studied in patients with moderate or severe hepatic impairment	Animal reproduction studies have not been conducted with atezolizumab to evaluate its effect on reproduction and fetal development. There are no available data on the use of atezolizumab in pregnant women	No overall differences in safety or efficacy were observed between patients ≥65 years of age and younger patients	The safety and effectiveness of atezolizumab have not been established in pediatric patients
Nivolumab [37]	No dose adjustment	No dose adjustment in patients with mild hepatic impairment. Nivolumab has not been studied in patients with moderate or severe hepatic impairment	In animal reproduction studies, administration of nivolumab to cynomolgus monkeys from the onset of organogenesis through delivery resulted in increased abortion and premature infant death. Human IgG4 is known to cross the placental barrier and nivolumab is an IgG4; therefore, nivolumab has the potential to be transmitted from the mother to the developing fetus. It is not known whether nivolumab is present in human milk. Advise women to discontinue breastfeeding during treatment with nivolumab	No overall differences in safety or effectiveness were reported between elderly patients and younger patients	The safety and effectiveness of nivolumab have not been established in pediatric patients
Pembrolizumab [46]	There was no clinically important effect on the CL of pembrolizumab based on renal impairment (eGFR ≥15 mL/min/1.73 m^2)	There was no clinically important effect on the CL of pembrolizumab based on mild hepatic impairment. There is insufficient information to determine whether there are clinically important differences in the CL of pembrolizumab in patients with moderate or severe hepatic impairment	There are no available human data informing the risk of embryo-fetal toxicity. Animal reproduction studies have not been conducted with pembrolizumab to evaluate its effect on reproduction and fetal development. It is not known whether pembrolizumab is excreted in human milk. Instruct women to discontinue nursing during treatment with pembrolizumab and for 4 months after the final dose	No overall differences in safety or effectiveness were observed between elderly patients and younger patients	The safety and effectiveness of pembrolizumab have not been established in pediatric patients

Abbreviations: *CL* clearance, *CLcr* creatinine clearance, *eGFR* estimated glomerular filtration rate. *NCI-CTEP* National Cancer Institute Cancer Therapy Evaluation Program cytolysis, and cytokine secretion to eliminate the target T cell. The patient's own T cells or those from an allogenic donor are isolated via leukapheresis, activated, and genetically modified with CARs to generate CAR T cells, which are then infused into the patient. This approach carries low risk for graft versus host disease [87–89]. Targets for CAR T extracellular antigen-binding domain include CD19, CD20, CD22, CD33, ROR1, Ig κ isotype, B-cell maturation antigen, CD138, CD123, and Lewis Y antigen for hematological malignancies and prostate-specific membrane antigen, fibroblast activation protein alpha, CEA, CD171, GD2, glypican-3, HER2, IL-13R alpha for solid tumors [2, 89]. CAR T cells can identify unprocessed antigens without the expression of major histocompatibility antigens, including proteins, carbohydrate and lipids, thus increasing the range of potential targets [89]. Once infused and the CAR T cells engage with tumor associated antigens, intracellular activation domains and costimulatory domains initiate CAR T-cell proliferation, activation, release of proinflammatory cytokines, and cytolysis of target tumor cells. Four generations of CAR T cells have been developed and are being tested in more than 100 clinical trials to treat hematological and solid malignancies [87, 88].

First-generation CAR T cells contain one signaling domain, whereas second, third, and fourth generations contain additional one, two, or three, costimulatory domains, respectively [88]. First-generation CAR T cells have only one intracellular activation signal (CD3-ζ) [90–92]. To achieve immediate expansion and long term persistence of therapeutic T cells, costimulatory signaling domains are combined with the primary signaling domains. Second-generation CARs have an additional costimulatory signal (CD28 or 4-1BB) [93, 94]. Third generation of CARs have two additional costimulatory signals (CD28 and 4-1BB) [95, 96]. Fourth generation of CARs (armored CAR or TRUCK CAR) are genetically engineered to produce proinflammatory cytokines (IL-12) or immunostimulatory molecules such as 4-1BBL or CD40L [97–100]. To sustain long term cell persistence and corresponding efficacy, procedures have been established that include different gene transfer techniques (retroviral or lentiviral), supplementation with IL-2, IL-7, IL-15, IL-21 for better ex vivo expansion [101] and preconditioning of the host with nonmyeloablative chemotherapy (cyclophosphamide and fludarabine) [102, 103] (Fig. 2.2).

Several distinguishing factors affect the clinical outcomes of CAR T cells, including CAR composition, ex vivo expansion techniques, cytokine support, formulation variation (cell origin (autologous/allogeneic), cell type, cell design, pharmacological properties, excipients, preservation method and packaging), dose calculation, administration method (systemic infusion vs. local administration) and usage of preconditioning chemotherapy. Thus, it is difficult to generalize the therapeutic class' PK and PD behavior. This section outlines the PK/PD of second-generation anti-CD19 CAR T cells.

One of the first successes of CAR T cells is the treatment of relapsed and/or refractory pediatric and adult B-ALL using CD19-targeted CAR T cells. Up to now, over 40 trials are targeting CD19 to treat hematologic malignancies, including NHL, chronic lymphocytic leukemia, and ALL [87, 104–107].

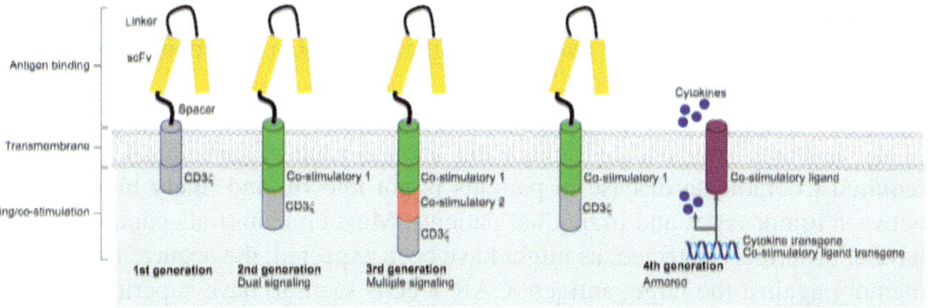

Fig. 2.2 An overview of the basic structure of four generations of CARs. The basic CAR structure (first generation) includes an extracellular domain, a transmembrane domain, and an intracellular domain. The extracellular domain includes an antigen-binding region of both heavy and light chains of a monoclonal antibody that is usually derived from a single-chain variable fragment (scFv). The intracellular domain generally includes a cell-signaling component derived from the endogenous T-cell receptor that can overcome immunosuppression associated with the tumor microenvironment. Subsequent generations of CARs have added one (second generation) or more (third and fourth generations) costimulatory signaling components on the intracellular domain to improve T-cell activation and promote antitumor immunity. Costimulatory signaling components may include: CD28, 4-1BB, or OX40, among others. Fourth-generation CAR T cells (armored CAR T cells) combine an earlier generation CAR with the addition of various genes, including cytokine and costimulatory ligand transgenes (Figure adapted from Khalil et al. [2] and Batlevi et al. [129])

2.6.2 *Pharmacokinetics*

T cells engineered with a "second-generation" CAR with combined 4-1BB-CD3ξ signaling underwent extensive amplification upon administration to the patients, eliminated high tumor burdens and persisted for at least 3 years, with retention of antitumor activity. With respect to the eliminated tumor mass, it was calculated that one CAR T cell is capable of killing as many as 1000 leukemic cells [87].

In an open-label phase 1 dose-escalation study of CD19-CAR T cells in children and young adults with ALL or NHL ($N = 21$), peak circulating blood CAR T-cell numbers were measured by flow cytometry or quantitative polymerase chain reaction (qPCR). Patients received either 1×10^6 or 3×10^6 CAR-transduced T cells/kg. The expansion cohort was treated at the maximum tolerated dose of 1×10^6 cells/kg. Of 17 ALL patients with available cerebrospinal fluid (CSF) specimens, 11 had detectable CAR T cells in CSF. Eighteen of 21 patients had detectable circulating CAR T cells by flow cytometry. Peak expansion occurred within 14 days.

In a study of 15 patients with advanced B-cell malignancies, patients received fludarabine followed by a single infusion of anti-CD19 CAR T cells. The number of CAR T cells infused ranged from 1×10^6 to 5×10^6 cells/kg. The peak levels of CAR T cells were detected in the blood at a peak levels ranging from 9 to 777 cells/mcL, with peak levels between 7 and 17 days after infusion, then decreased rapidly [105]. The CAR T cells were detected in blood of patients for up to 181 days after infusion [105]. A few clinical trials have shown that CAR T-cell persistence can be increased by lymphodepleting conditioning chemotherapy that include cyclophosphamide and fludarabine. This also led to enhanced clinical response rate and toxicity [88].

CAR T-cell persistence is likely an important factor in determining the efficacy of the antitumor response, although the optimal time of survival of CAR T cells required to eradicate disease in patients is not known, and likely highly variable between tumor types and individual patients. Most clinical trials conducted to date have not routinely detected, as might have been expected, the occurrence of lifelong memory against the target antigen. CAR T cells seem to have superior persistence in pediatric patients and 4-1BB has been shown to be a superior costimulatory signal to increase persistence [108]. Because CAR T cells are able to expand exponentially in vivo post-infusion in response to antigen stimulus, the number of CAR T cells following expansion is expected to vary between individuals.

2.6.3 Pharmacodynamics

In a phase 1 dose-escalation study of CD19-CAR T cells in children and young adults with ALL or NHL, peak circulating blood CAR T-cell numbers were higher in patients obtaining lymphoma responses of complete response or partial response compared to patients obtaining responses of stable disease or progressive disease [94].

Biomarker analyses are typically performed on blood and tumor samples to evaluate predictive and PD markers for anti-CD19 CAR T cells, such as induction of cytokine and chemokine production. Preliminary data from earlier trials demonstrate that infusion of anti-CD19 CAR T cells in subjects with B-cell malignancies results in increased cytokine concentration in peripheral blood, with the concomitant expected aplasia of normal B cells. PD parameter levels followed a similar pattern (rapid increase immediately after product infusion followed by a return to baseline levels) as observed for the anti-CD19 CAR T cells themselves. Exploratory analyses may explore biomarkers for cytokine and chemokine production, such as immune homeostatic cytokines IL-2 and IL-15; inflammatory cytokines IL-6, IL-1, SAA, GM-CSF, CRP, and TNF-alpha; immune-modulating cytokines IL-5, IL-10, and IFN-r; chemokines IP-10, IL-8, MCP-1, MIP-1 beta, and Eotaxin; and immune effector molecules Granzyme A, B, perforin, and sFasL.

2.6.4 Discussion and Future Direction

Due to the unique immunobiology of CAR T cells, the relationships between dose, efficacy, and toxicity may not follow relationships expected from noncell therapeutics. Though dose-escalation schemes are still employed for these agents in phase 1 safety and dose finding trials, caution should be taken when using PK/PD results to guide the selection of dosage and infusion frequency.

Though there are not yet any FDA-approved cellular and gene therapies (CGT) on the market, the FDA has provided detailed recommendations regarding the design of early phase clinical trials of these products [109]. CGT products are different from traditional small molecule therapeutic agents with distinct features such as extended persistence and biological activities even after one administration, and tendency to induce immunogenicity. Additionally, it may not feasible to perform traditional preclinical PK studies, as extrapolation from animal dose to a clinical dose may not be reliable or informative. Very importantly, CGT products are affected by the manufacturing process. These autologous and allogeneic cell products are manufactured for individual subjects and therefore there may be significant individual variability attributed to characteristics of the donor or recipient. The cell viability and potency of CGT products may decline rapidly following time of formulation, therefore cryopreservation should be considered if these cells are not administered shortly after manufacturing.

To design early phase clinical trials for CGT products, considerations should be given to address the unique features discussed above. Though half-log increments can be used for dose escalation, single dose administration should also be explored because CGT products can persist in vivo for extended period. For CGT products with less tolerance risk, larger cohort size (as opposed to the traditional 3 + 3 design) may be needed to ensure the safety before dose escalation.

Investigational pharmacy services supporting clinical research institutions have been at a unique position to handle patient-derived CGT products such as CAR T cells. Each batch is manufactured separately and each lot sis tracked (product accountability). The source (allogeneic and autologous donors) typically receive a treatment prior to harvest of cells. Recipients also receive myeloablative chemotherapy conditioning before the CGT engraftment administration. Due to the uncertainty of the severity and frequency of adverse reactions of CGT products, extended safety monitoring, subject follow-up and symptom controls with pharmaceuticals justified the involvement of research pharmacists' role in this new type of multi-modality therapeutics.

2.7 Oncolytic Viruses

2.7.1 Description and Human Dosing

Talimogene laherparepvec (T-vec, Imlygic) is oncolytic immunotherapy based on a modified herpes simplex virus type-1 (HSV-1) that is designed to selectively replicate in tumor tissue and to stimulate a systemic antitumor immune response [110–113]. Other oncolytic viruses in clinical development include vaccinia virus JX-594 (Pexa-vec, pexastimogene devacirepvec) for hepatocellular carcinoma, adenovirus CG0070 for bladder cancer, reovirus Reolysin (pelareorep) for head and neck cancer, and G47Δ, a third-generation oncolytic HSV-1, for glioblastoma. This review mainly focuses on talimogene laherparepvec which has received regulatory approval in the US and Europe for melanoma [114].

In talimogene laherparepvec, the HSV-1 viral genes ICP34.5 and ICP47 have been deleted and replaced by the coding sequence to produce human granulocyte macrophage colony stimulating factor (GM-CSF) [113]. ICP47 blocks antigen presentation by major histocompatibility complex molecules of infected cells. ICP34.5 is known as the "neurovirulence factor" that promotes viral replication in normal cells with an intact anti-viral response. In normal cells, deletion of ICP34.5 renders HSV-1 unable to replicate. However, because cancer cells are in defect of the shut-off response, ICP34.5-deficient HSV-1 can still replicate in cancer cells [114–120].

Intralesional administration of talimogene laherparepvec results in oncolysis of cells within injected tumors. Iterative viral replication within permissive tumor tissue results in lytic cell destruction and local release of progeny virus and tumor cell antigens. GM-CSF, the product of the viral transgene, is also produced locally to recruit and stimulate cellular immune responses and antigen-presenting cells which, in addition to relevant tumor-derived antigens, are required for the initiation of a systemic antitumor immune response. Overall, this strategy is expected to result in the destruction of injected tumors via oncolysis and also uninjected sites of disease (including micrometastases) via a systemic antitumor immune response [121].

In the single dose group of a phase 1 clinical trial of 30 patients with solid tumors (breast, head and neck, colorectal, melanoma), patients were exposed to a single dose of 10^6, 10^7, or 10^8 plaque-forming units (PFU)/mL [122]. In the multidose group, seronegative patients were given an initial dose of 10^6 PFU/mL 3 weeks before escalation to higher viral concentrations up to 10^8 PFU/mL, which was then repeated every 2 weeks. Approximately one third of patients were seronegative for HSV with all seroconverting 3–4 weeks after the first dose. No dose-limiting toxicities were observed when the initial dose was 10^6 PFU/mL. Therefore, this dose was selected as the starting dose, followed 3 weeks later by a higher dose of 10^8 PFU/mL, which is then dosed q2w until maximum clinical response, toxicity or confirmed disease progression. This regimen was adopted for subsequent clinical development [123].

In the OPTiM phase 3 randomized trial in patients with unresected stage IIIB–IV melanoma, 436 patients were randomly assigned in a 2:1 ratio to intralesional T-Vec or subcutaneous GM-CSF treatment arms [124]. T-Vec was administered at a concentration of 10^8 PFU/mL injected into 1 or more skin or subcutaneous tumors on Days 1 and 15 of each 28-day cycle for up to 12 months, whereas GM-CSF was administered at a dose of 125 mcg/m^2/day subcutaneously for 14 consecutive days followed by 14 days of rest, in 28-day treatment cycles for up to 12 months.

The FDA-approved recommended starting dose is up to a maximum of 4 mL at a concentration of 10^6 (1 million) PFU/mL. Subsequent doses should be administered up to 4 mL at a concentration of 10^8 (100 million) PFU/mL [125].

2.7.2 Pharmacokinetics

Typical human PK studies are not relevant for the oncolytic virus talimogene laherparepvec. The pharmacology of talimogene laherparepvec is defined by the analysis of the biodistribution in the blood and urine and live virus shedding at time points post-injection [126].

Talimogene laherparepvec is administered by intralesional injection. The Amgen 20 120 324 study evaluates the biodistribution and shedding of tamilogene laherparepvec in melanoma patients who received intralesional talimogene laherparepvec at a dose and schedule similar to the current FDA-approved dose. In the initial 20 patients analyzed, talimogene laherparepvec DNA was present in the blood in 85% of patients, and in the urine of 20% of patients during the study. Peak levels of tamilogene laherparepvec DNA were detected in urine on the day of treatment. Most of the positive samples were from blood or urine samples collected at time points within the first 24 h after the injection of talimogene laherparepvec. Viral DNA was generally observed to clear from the blood prior to the next injection. Infectious talimogene laherparepvec virus was detected at the injection site of three patients (15%) at a single time point each, all within the first week after the initial injection. Additionally, the exterior of the occlusive dressings was positive for talimogene laherparepvec DNA, but not for infectious virus, in 70% of patients during the study. The number of patients with measurable DNA on the exterior of the occlusive dressings declined over time with no measurable DNA by the third treatment in the 13 patients tested [127].

2.7.3 Pharmacodynamics: Immune Profiling and Tumor Immunogenicity

To date, there has been no reported E-R correlation between antibody titers and therapeutic responses or adverse events [123].

In an analysis of 11 patients treated at the Rush University Medical Center site for the Amgen study 002/003, samples from injected and uninjected melanoma lesions from 11 subjects enrolled were analyzed for the changes in populations of effector (CD8 + perforin+), regulatory (CD4 + FoxP3+), and suppressor T cells (CD8 + FoxP3+), as well as for the generation of melanoma-derived antigen-specific T lymphocytes after talimogene laherparepvec administration; these samples were compared to melanoma tumor samples from untreated individuals. Results from this study demonstrated that treatment with talimogene laherparepvec increased the appearance of CD4+ and CD8+ T lymphocytes with both memory (CD45RO) and activation markers (CD25 and HLA-DR) in injected lesions. In addition, the treatment resulted in generation of CD8+ T cells capable of recognizing melanoma-derived peptides, such as MART-1, in peripheral blood and in regressing uninjected tumors, consistent with the priming of systemic immunity against defined melanoma antigens. Additionally, it was found that treatment with talimogene laherparepvec resulted in decreased levels of regulatory and suppressor T cells compared to uninjected melanoma lesions, suggesting local and systemic changes in otherwise inhibitory tumor microenvironment were initiated by administration of talimogene laherparepvec. Based on these results, it is evident that treatment with talimogene laherparepvec results in the generation of anti-melanoma immune response, both locally and systemically [128].

2.8 Conclusion

This chapter highlighted the mechanisms of action, PK and PD of some of the more recently approved cancer immunotherapies. For the monoclonal antibody-based therapeutics, population PK estimates of CL and V were consistent across most of the agents discussed here. V is typically around the volume of plasma, indicating high distribution in the central compartment with minimal tissue distribution. Elimination of monoclonal antibodies occurs through catabolic degradation with minimal hepatic and renal contributions. Half-lives are generally long, on the order of days versus hours with small molecule drugs.

The PK for cellular therapies and viruses are difficult to characterize. Dosing of adoptive cellular therapy and viruses are dependent on yield and the PK is related to T-cell lifespan postadministration. Typical PK parameters for small molecules and antibody therapeutics generally cannot be used to describe the PK for cellular therapies or viruses.

Although the focus of this chapter was on checkpoint inhibitors, adoptive cellular therapy, and oncolytic viruses, many more exciting therapies are currently under development. These agents under development utilize diverse mechanisms of action to modulate antitumor immunity. In particular, immunostimulatory agents with novel costimulatory targets, cellular therapy, oncolytic viruses and vaccines, and even immunomodulating small molecules are on the horizon. It is anticipated that these innovative developments, along with personalization of clinical use of cancer immunotherapy, will improve efficacy and safety in patients with various cancer types.

References

1. Coley WB (1991) The treatment of malignant tumors by repeated inoculations of erysipelas. With a report of ten original cases. 1893. Clin Orthop Relat Res 262:3–11
2. Khalil DN, Smith EL, Brentjens RJ, Wolchok JD (2016) The future of cancer treatment: immunomodulation, CARs and combination immunotherapy. Nat Rev Clin Oncol 13(5):273–290. doi:10.1038/nrclinonc.2016.25. Epub 2016 Mar 15. PMID: 26977780
3. Brezski RJ, Georgiou G (2016) Immunoglobulin isotype knowledge and application to Fc engineering. Curr Opin Immunol 40:62–69

4. Dostalek M, Gardner I, Gurbaxani BM, Rose RH, Chetty M (2013) Pharmacokinetics, pharmacodynamics and physiologically-based pharmacokinetic modelling of monoclonal antibodies. Clin Pharmacokinet 52(2):83–124
5. Pardoll DM (2012) The blockade of immune checkpoints in cancer immunotherapy. Nat Rev Cancer 12(4):252–264
6. Chen DS, Mellman I (2013) Oncology meets immunology: the cancer-immunity cycle. Immunity 39(1):1–10
7. Sathyanarayanan V, Neelapu SS (2015) Cancer immunotherapy: strategies for personalization and combinatorial approaches. Mol Oncol 9(10):2043–2053
8. Bertrand A, Kostine M, Barnetche T, Truchetet ME, Schaeverbeke T (2015) Immune related adverse events associated with anti-CTLA-4 antibodies: systematic review and meta-analysis. BMC Med 13:211
9. Spain L, Diem S, Larkin J (2016) Management of toxicities of immune checkpoint inhibitors. Cancer Treat Rev 44:51–60
10. Bourke JM, O'Sullivan M, Khattak MA (2016) Management of adverse events related to new cancer immunotherapy (immune checkpoint inhibitors). Med J Aust 205(9):418–424
11. Tarhini AA (2013) Tremelimumab: a review of development to date in solid tumors. Immunotherapy 5(3):215–229
12. Center for Drug Evaluation and Research (2016) Yervoy (ipilimumab) Clinical Pharmacology Biopharmaceutics Review(s). Application number 125377Orig1s000. Available at: http://www.accessdata.fda.gov/drugsatfda_docs/nda/2011/125377Orig1s000ClinPharmR.pdf. Accessed 12 Nov 2016
13. Camacho LH (2015) CTLA-4 blockade with ipilimumab: biology, safety, efficacy, and future considerations. Cancer Med 4(5):661–672
14. Yervoy (ipilimumab) Prescribing Information (2015) Princeton: Bristol-Myers Squibb Co.; October 2015. Available at: http://packageinserts.bms.com/pi/pi_yervoy.pdf. Accessed 14 Nov 2016
15. Wolchok JD, Neyns B, Linette G et al (2010) Ipilimumab monotherapy in patients with pretreated advanced melanoma: a randomised, double-blind, multicentre, phase 2, dose-ranging study. Lancet Oncol 11(2):155–164
16. Feng Y, Masson E, Dai D et al (2014) Model-based clinical pharmacology profiling of ipilimumab in patients with advanced melanoma. Br J Clin Pharmacol 78(1):106–117
17. Comin-Anduix B, Escuin-Ordinas H, Ibarrondo FJ (2016) Tremelimumab: research and clinical development. Onco Targets Ther 9:1767–1776
18. Ribas A, Chesney JA, Gordon MS et al (2012) Safety profile and pharmacokinetic analyses of the anti-CTLA4 antibody tremelimumab administered as a one hour infusion. J Transl Med 10:236
19. Ribas A, Camacho LH, Lopez-Berestein G et al (2005) Antitumor activity in melanoma and anti-self responses in a phase I trial with the anti-cytotoxic T lymphocyte-associated antigen 4 monoclonal antibody CP-675,206. J Clin Oncol 23(35):8968–8977
20. Wang E, Kang D, Bae KS et al (2014) Population pharmacokinetic and pharmacodynamic analysis of tremelimumab in patients with metastatic melanoma. J Clin Pharmacol 54(10):1108–1116
21. Pardoll D (2015) Cancer and the immune system: basic concepts and targets for intervention. Semin Oncol 42(4):523–538
22. Patel SP, Kurzrock R (2015) PD-L1 expression as a predictive biomarker in cancer immunotherapy. Mol Cancer Ther 14(4):847–856
23. Goodman A, Patel SP, Kurzrock R (2016) PD-1-PD-L1 immune-checkpoint blockade in B-cell lymphomas. Nat Rev Clin Oncol 14:203–220
24. Patnaik A, Kang SP, Rasco D et al (2015) Phase I study of pembrolizumab (MK-3475; Anti-PD-1 monoclonal antibody) in patients with advanced solid tumors. Clin Cancer Res 21(19):4286–4293
25. Farolfi A, Schepisi G, Conteduca V et al (2016) Pharmacokinetics, pharmacodynamics and clinical efficacy of nivolumab in the treatment of metastatic renal cell carcinoma. Expert Opin Drug Metab Toxicol 12(9):1089–1096

26. Wong RM, Scotland RR, Lau RL et al (2007) Programmed death-1 blockade enhances expansion and functional capacity of human melanoma antigen-specific CTLs. Int Immunol 19(10):1223–1234
27. Iwai Y, Ishida M, Tanaka Y et al (2002) Involvement of PD-L1 on tumor cells in the escape from host immune system and tumor immunotherapy by PD-L1 blockade. Proc Natl Acad Sci U S A 99(19):12293–12297
28. Blank C, Mackensen A (2007) Contribution of the PD-L1/PD-1 pathway to T-cell exhaustion: an update on implications for chronic infections and tumor evasion. Cancer Immunol Immunother 56(5):739–745
29. Lu J, Lee-Gabel L, Nadeau MC, Ferencz TM, Soefje SA (2015) Clinical evaluation of compounds targeting PD-1/PD-L1 pathway for cancer immunotherapy. J Oncol Pharm Pract 21(6):451–467
30. Homet Moreno B, Ribas A (2015) Anti-programmed cell death protein-1/ligand-1 therapy in different cancers. Br J Cancer 112(9):1421–1427
31. Center for Drug Evaluation and Research (2016) Opdivo (nivolumab) Pharmacology Review(s). Application number. Available at: http://www.accessdata.fda.gov/drugsatfda_docs/nda/2014/125554Orig1s000PharmR.pdf. Accessed 12 Nov 2016
32. Topalian SL, Hodi FS, Brahmer JR et al (2012) Safety, activity, and immune correlates of anti-PD-1 antibody in cancer. N Engl J Med 366(26):2443–2454
33. Center for Drug Evaluation and Research (2016) Opdivo (nivolumab) Clinical Pharmacology Biopharmaceutics Review(s). Application number 125554Orig1s000. Available at: http://www.accessdata.fda.gov/drugsatfda_docs/nda/2014/125554Orig1s000ClinPharmR.pdf. Accessed 12 Nov 2016
34. Center for Drug Evaluation and Research (2016) Opdivo (nivolumab) Clinical Pharmacology Biopharmaceutics Review(s). Application number 125527Orig1s000. Available at: http://www.accessdata.fda.gov/drugsatfda_docs/nda/2015/125527Orig1s000ClinPharmR.pdf. Accessed 12 Nov 2016
35. Weber JS, D'Angelo SP, Minor D et al (2015) Nivolumab versus chemotherapy in patients with advanced melanoma who progressed after anti-CTLA-4 treatment (CheckMate 037): a randomised, controlled, open-label, phase 3 trial. Lancet Oncol 16(4):375–384
36. Rizvi NA, Mazieres J, Planchard D et al (2015) Activity and safety of nivolumab, an anti-PD-1 immune checkpoint inhibitor, for patients with advanced, refractory squamous non-small-cell lung cancer (CheckMate 063): a phase 2, single-arm trial. Lancet Oncol 16(3):257–265
37. Opdivo (nivolumab) Prescribing Information (2016) Princeton: Bristol-Myers Squibb Co; November 2016. Available at: http://packageinserts.bms.com/pi/pi_opdivo.pdf. Accessed 14 Nov 2016
38. Bajaj G, Wang X, Agrawal S et al (2016) Model-Based Population Pharmacokinetic Analysis of Nivolumab in Patients With Solid Tumors. CPT Pharmacometrics Syst Pharmacol 6:58–66
39. U.S. Food and Drug Administration (2016) Modification of the Dosage Regimen for Nivolumab. Published online September 2016. Available at: http://www.fda.gov/Drugs/InformationOnDrugs/ApprovedDrugs/ucm520871.htm. Accessed 14 November 2016
40. Zhao X, Suryawanshi S, Hruska M, et al (2016) Assessment of nivolumab (NIVO) benefit-risk profile from a 240 mg flat dose versus a 3 mg/kg dosing regimen in patients with solid tumor. Presented at the European Society for Medical Oncology Congress 2016, Copenhagen, Denmark, 7–11 October 2016
41. Center for Drug Evaluation and Research (2016) Keytruda (pembrolizumab) Pharmacology Review(s). Application number 125514Orig1s000. Available at: http://www.accessdata.fda.gov/drugsatfda_docs/nda/2014/125514Orig1s000PharmR.pdf. Accessed 13 Nov 2016
42. Chatterjee M, Turner DC, Felip E et al (2016) Systematic evaluation of pembrolizumab dosing in patients with advanced non-small-cell lung cancer. Ann Oncol 27(7):1291–1298
43. de Greef R, Elassaiss-Schaap J, Chatterjee M et al (2016) Pembrolizumab: role of modeling and simulation in bringing a novel immunotherapy to patients with melanoma. CPT Pharmacometrics Syst Pharmacol 6:5–7

44. Elassaiss-Schaap J, Rossenu S, Lindauer A et al (2016) Using model-based "Learn and confirm" to reveal the pharmacokinetics-pharmacodynamics relationship of pembrolizumab in the KEYNOTE-001 trial. CPT Pharmacometrics Syst Pharmacol 6:21–28
45. Ahamadi M, Freshwater T, Prohn M et al (2016) Model-based characterization of the pharmacokinetics of pembrolizumab: a humanized anti-PD-1 monoclonal antibody in advanced solid tumors. CPT Pharmacometrics Syst Pharmacol 6:49–57
46. Keytruda (pembrolizumab) Prescribing Information (2016) Whitehouse Station: Merck & Co, Inc.; October 2016. Available at: http://www.merck.com/product/usa/pi_circulars/k/keytruda/keytruda_pi.pdf. Accessed 6 Nov 2016
47. Center for Drug Evaluation and Research (2016) Keytruda (pembrolizumab) Clinical Pharmacology and Biopharmaceutics Review(s). Application number 125514Orig1s000. Available at: http://www.accessdata.fda.gov/drugsatfda_docs/nda/2014/125514Orig1s000ClinPharmR.pdf. Accessed 13 Nov 2016
48. Chatterjee M, Turner DC, Ahamadi M, et al (2015) Model-based analysis of the relationship between pembolizumab exposure and efficacy in patients with melanoma and NSCLC: across indication comparison. Presented at the Annual Meeting of the Population Approach Group in Europe, Hersonissos, Greece, 2–5 June 2015
49. Freshwater T, Stone J, de Greef R, et al (2015) Assessment of pembrolizumab (MK-3475) dosing strategy based on population pharmacokinetics and exposure-response models. Presented at the 6th American Conference on Pharmacometrics, Arlington, 3–7 October 2015
50. Reck M, Rodriguez-Abreu D, Robinson AG et al (2016) Pembrolizumab versus chemotherapy for PD-L1-positive non-small-cell lung cancer. N Engl J Med 375:1823–1833
51. Center for Drug Evaluation and Research (2016) Tecentriq (atezolizumab) Clinical Pharmacology Review(s). Application number 761034Orig1s000. Available at: http://www.accessdata.fda.gov/drugsatfda_docs/nda/2016/761034Orig1s000PharmR.pdf. Accessed 14 Nov 2016
52. Herbst RS, Soria JC, Kowanetz M et al (2014) Predictive correlates of response to the anti-PD-L1 antibody MPDL3280A in cancer patients. Nature 515(7528):563–567
53. Center for Drug Evaluation and Research (2016) Tecentriq (atezolizumab) Clinical Pharmacology and Biopharmaceutics Review(s). Application number 761034Orig1s000. Available at: http://www.accessdata.fda.gov/drugsatfda_docs/nda/2016/761034Orig1s000ClinPharmR.pdf. Accessed 12 Nov 2016
54. Tecentriq (atezolizumab) Prescribing Information (2016) South San Francisco: Genentech, Inc; October 2016. Available at: https://www.gene.com/download/pdf/tecentriq_prescribing.pdf. Accessed 5 Nov 2016
55. Stroh M, Winter H, Marchand M et al (2016) The clinical pharmacokinetics and pharmacodynamics of atezolizumab in metastatic urothelial carcinoma. Clin Pharmacol Ther 102:305–312
56. Powles T, Eder JP, Fine GD et al (2014) MPDL3280A (anti-PD-L1) treatment leads to clinical activity in metastatic bladder cancer. Nature 515(7528):558–562
57. Mizugaki H, Yamamoto N, Murakami H et al (2016) Phase I dose-finding study of monotherapy with atezolizumab, an engineered immunoglobulin monoclonal antibody targeting PD-L1, in Japanese patients with advanced solid tumors. Investig New Drugs 34(5):596–603
58. Massard C, Gordon MS, Sharma S et al (2016) Safety and efficacy of durvalumab (MEDI4736), an anti-programmed cell death ligand-1 immune checkpoint inhibitor, in patients with advanced urothelial bladder cancer. J Clin Oncol 34(26):3119–3125
59. Planchard D, Yokoi T, McCleod MJ et al (2016) A phase III study of durvalumab (MEDI4736) with or without tremelimumab for previously treated patients with advanced NSCLC: rationale and protocol design of the ARCTIC study. Clin Lung Cancer 17(3):232–236 e231
60. Song X, Pak M, Chavez C, et al (2015) Population pharmacokinetics of MEDI4736, a fully human antiprogrammed death ligand 1 (PD-L1) monoclonal antibody, in patients with advanced solid tumors. Presented at the European Cancer Congress 2015, Vienna, Austria, 25–29 September 2015

61. Song X, Pak M, Liang M, et al (2015) Pharmacokinetics and pharmacodynamics of MEDI4736, a fully human anti-programmed death ligand 1 (PD-L1) monoclonal antibody, in patients with advanced solid tumors. Abstract submitted to the 2015 Americal Society of Clinical Oncology Annual Meeting, Chicago, 29 May–2 June 2015
62. Grenga I, Donahue RN, Lepone LM, Richards J, Schlom J (2016) A fully human IgG1 anti-PD-L1 MAb in an in vitro assay enhances antigen-specific T-cell responses. Clin Transl Immunology 5(5):e83
63. Boyerinas B, Jochems C, Fantini M et al (2015) Antibody-dependent cellular cytotoxicity activity of a novel anti-PD-L1 antibody avelumab (MSB0010718C) on human tumor cells. Cancer Immunol Res 3(10):1148–1157
64. Kaufman HL, Russell J, Hamid O et al (2016) Avelumab in patients with chemotherapy-refractory metastatic Merkel cell carcinoma: a multicentre, single-group, open-label, phase 2 trial. Lancet Oncol 17(10):1374–1385
65. Heery CR, O'Sullivan Coyne GH, Marte JL, et al (2015) Pharmacokinetic profile and receptor occupancy of avelumab (MSB0010718C), an anti-PD-L1 monoclonal antibody, in a phase I, open-label, dose escalation trial in patients with advanced solid tumors. Presented at the 2015 Americal Society of Clinical Oncology Annual Meeting, Chicago, 29 May–2 June 2015
66. Arkenau H-T, Kelly K, Patel MR, et al (2015) Phase I JAVELIN solid tumor trial of avelumab (MSB0010718C), an anti-PD-L1 antibody: Safety and pharmacokinetics. Presented at the European Society for Medical Oncology Symposium on Immuno-Oncology 2015, Lausanne, Switzerland, 20–21 November 2015
67. MedImmune LLC (2016) A Phase 1 Study of MEDI0562 in Adult Subjects With Selected Advanced Solid Tumors. In: ClinicalTrials.gov [Internet]. Bethesda (MD): National Library of Medicine (US). 2000- [cited 2016 Nov 11]. Available from: https://clinicaltrials.gov/ct2/show/NCT02318394 NLM Identifier: NCT02318394
68. Segal NH, Logan TF, Hodi FS et al (2016) Results From an Integrated Safety Analysis of Urelumab, an Agonist Anti-CD137 Monoclonal Antibody. Clin Cancer Res 23:1929–1936
69. Pfizer, Inc and Merck Sharp & Dohme Corp (2016) A Study Of 4-1BB Agonist PF-05082566 Plus PD-1 Inhibitor MK-3475 In Patients With Solid Tumors (B1641003/KEYNOTE-0036). In: ClinicalTrials.gov [Internet]. Bethesda (MD): National Library of Medicine (US). 2000- [cited 2016 Nov 11]. Available from: https://clinicaltrials.gov/ct2/show/NCT02179918 NLM Identifier: NCT02179918
70. Pfizer, Inc and Kyowa Hakko Kirin Company, Ltd (2016) A Study of PF-05082566 In Combination With Mogamulizumab In Patients With Advanced Solid Tumors. In: ClinicalTrials.gov [Internet]. Bethesda (MD): National Library of Medicine (US). 2000- [cited 2016 Nov 11]. Available from: https://clinicaltrials.gov/ct2/show/NCT02444793 NLM Identifier: NCT02444793
71. Chester C, Ambulkar S, Kohrt HE (2016) 4-1BB agonism: adding the accelerator to cancer immunotherapy. Cancer Immunol Immunother 65(10):1243–1248
72. Makkouk A, Chester C, Kohrt HE (2016) Rationale for anti-CD137 cancer immunotherapy. Eur J Cancer 54:112–119
73. GITR, Inc. and Cancer Research Institute (2016) Trial of TRX518 (Anti-GITR mAb) in Stage III or IV Malignant Melanoma or Other Solid Tumors (TRX518–001). In: ClinicalTrials.gov [Internet]. Bethesda (MD): National Library of Medicine (US). 2000- [cited 2016 Nov 11]. Available from: https://clinicaltrials.gov/ct2/show/NCT01239134 NLM Identifier: NCT01239134
74. Knee DA, Hewes B, Brogdon JL (2016) Rationale for anti-GITR cancer immunotherapy. Eur J Cancer 67:1–10
75. Zonder JA, Mohrbacher AF, Singhal S et al (2012) A phase 1, multicenter, open-label, dose escalation study of elotuzumab in patients with advanced multiple myeloma. Blood 120(3):552–559
76. Center for Drug Evaluation and Research (2016) Empliciti (elotuzumab) Clinical Pharmacology and Biopharmaceutics Review(s). Application number 761035Orig1s000. Available at: http://www.accessdata.fda.gov/drugsatfda_docs/nda/2015/761035Orig1s000ClinPharmR.pdf. Accessed 11 Nov 2016

77. Empliciti (elotuzumab) Prescribing Information (2016) Princeton: Bristol-Myers Squibb Co.; November 2015. Available at: http://packageinserts.bms.com/pi/pi_empliciti.pdf. Accessed 11 Nov 2016
78. Berdeja J, Jagannath S, Zonder J et al (2016) Pharmacokinetics and safety of elotuzumab combined with lenalidomide and dexamethasone in patients with multiple myeloma and various levels of renal impairment: results of a phase Ib study. Clin Lymphoma Myeloma Leuk 16(3):129–138
79. Lonial S, Dimopoulos M, Palumbo A et al (2015) Elotuzumab therapy for relapsed or refractory multiple myeloma. N Engl J Med 373(7):621–631
80. Gibiansky L, Passey C, Roy A, Bello A, Gupta M (2016) Model-based pharmacokinetic analysis of elotuzumab in patients with relapsed/refractory multiple myeloma. J Pharmacokinet Pharmacodyn 43(3):243–257
81. Zhu M, Wu B, Brandl C et al (2016) Blinatumomab, a bispecific T-cell engager (BiTE((R))) for CD-19 targeted cancer immunotherapy: clinical pharmacology and its implications. Clin Pharmacokinet 55(10):1271–1288
82. Blincyto (blinatumomab) Prescribing Information (2016) Thousand Oaks: Amgen Inc.; September 2016. Available at: http://pi.amgen.com/united_states/blincyto/blincyto_pi_hcp_english.pdf. Accessed 11 Nov 2016
83. Center for Drug Evaluation and Research (2016) Blincyto (blinatumomab) Clinical Pharmacology Biopharmaceutics Review(s). Application number 125557Orig1s000. Available at: http://www.accessdata.fda.gov/drugsatfda_docs/nda/2014/125557Orig1s000ClinPharmR.pdf. Accessed 11 Nov 2016
84. Goebeler ME, Knop S, Viardot A et al (2016) Bispecific T-cell engager (BiTE) antibody construct blinatumomab for the treatment of patients with relapsed/refractory non-hodgkin Lymphoma: final results from a phase I study. J Clin Oncol 34(10):1104–1111
85. Agrawal S, Statkevich P, Bajaj G et al (2016) Evaluation of Immunogenicity of Nivolumab Monotherapy and Its Clinical Relevance in Patients With Metastatic Solid Tumors. J Clin Pharmacol 26:202–204
86. Newick K, O'Brien S, Moon E, Albelda SM (2016) CAR T Cell Therapy for Solid Tumors. Annu Rev Med 68:139–152
87. Holzinger A, Barden M, Abken H (2016) The growing world of CAR T cell trials: a systematic review. Cancer Immunol Immunother 65(12):1433–1450
88. Jackson HJ, Rafiq S, Brentjens RJ (2016) Driving CAR T-cells forward. Nat Rev Clin Oncol 13(6):370–383
89. Allegra A, Innao V, Gerace D, Vaddinelli D, Musolino C (2016) Adoptive immunotherapy for hematological malignancies: current status and new insights in chimeric antigen receptor T cells. Blood Cells Mol Dis 62:49–63
90. Jensen MC, Popplewell L, Cooper LJ et al (2010) Antitransgene rejection responses contribute to attenuated persistence of adoptively transferred CD20/CD19-specific chimeric antigen receptor redirected T cells in humans. Biol Blood Marrow Transplant 16(9):1245–1256
91. Lamers CH, Sleijfer S, van Steenbergen S et al (2013) Treatment of metastatic renal cell carcinoma with CAIX CAR-engineered T cells: clinical evaluation and management of on-target toxicity. Mol Ther 21(4):904–912
92. Till BG, Jensen MC, Wang J et al (2008) Adoptive immunotherapy for indolent non-Hodgkin lymphoma and mantle cell lymphoma using genetically modified autologous CD20-specific T cells. Blood 112(6):2261–2271
93. Savoldo B, Ramos CA, Liu E et al (2011) CD28 costimulation improves expansion and persistence of chimeric antigen receptor-modified T cells in lymphoma patients. J Clin Invest 121(5):1822–1826
94. Lee DW, Kochenderfer JN, Stetler-Stevenson M et al (2015) T cells expressing CD19 chimeric antigen receptors for acute lymphoblastic leukaemia in children and young adults: a phase 1 dose-escalation trial. Lancet 385(9967):517–528
95. Carpenito C, Milone MC, Hassan R et al (2009) Control of large, established tumor xenografts with genetically retargeted human T cells containing CD28 and CD137 domains. Proc Natl Acad Sci U S A 106(9):3360–3365

96. Zhong XS, Matsushita M, Plotkin J, Riviere I, Sadelain M (2010) Chimeric antigen receptors combining 4-1BB and CD28 signaling domains augment PI3kinase/AKT/Bcl-XL activation and CD8+ T cell-mediated tumor eradication. Mol Ther 18(2):413–420
97. Chmielewski M, Kopecky C, Hombach AA, Abken H (2011) IL-12 release by engineered T cells expressing chimeric antigen receptors can effectively Muster an antigen-independent macrophage response on tumor cells that have shut down tumor antigen expression. Cancer Res 71(17):5697–5706
98. Kerkar SP, Goldszmid RS, Muranski P et al (2011) IL-12 triggers a programmatic change in dysfunctional myeloid-derived cells within mouse tumors. J Clin Invest 121(12):4746–4757
99. Pegram HJ, Lee JC, Hayman EG et al (2012) Tumor-targeted T cells modified to secrete IL-12 eradicate systemic tumors without need for prior conditioning. Blood 119(18):4133–4141
100. Zhang L, Morgan RA, Beane JD et al (2015) Tumor-infiltrating lymphocytes genetically engineered with an inducible gene encoding interleukin-12 for the immunotherapy of metastatic melanoma. Clin Cancer Res 21(10):2278–2288
101. Xu Y, Zhang M, Ramos CA et al (2014) Closely related T-memory stem cells correlate with in vivo expansion of CAR.CD19-T cells and are preserved by IL-7 and IL-15. Blood 123(24):3750–3759
102. Riddell SR, Sommermeyer D, Berger C et al (2014) Adoptive therapy with chimeric antigen receptor-modified T cells of defined subset composition. Cancer J 20(2):141–144
103. Turtle CJ, Berger C, Sommermeyer D, et al. (2015) Immunotherapy with CD19-specific chimeric antigen receptor (CAR)-modified T cells of defined subset composition. Presented at the 2015 Annual Society of Clinical Oncology Annual Meeting, Chicago, 29 May–2 June 2015
104. Brentjens RJ, Riviere I, Park JH et al (2011) Safety and persistence of adoptively transferred autologous CD19-targeted T cells in patients with relapsed or chemotherapy refractory B-cell leukemias. Blood 118(18):4817–4828
105. Kochenderfer JN, Dudley ME, Feldman SA et al (2012) B-cell depletion and remissions of malignancy along with cytokine-associated toxicity in a clinical trial of anti-CD19 chimeric-antigen-receptor-transduced T cells. Blood 119(12):2709–2720
106. Porter DL, Hwang WT, Frey NV et al (2015) Chimeric antigen receptor T cells persist and induce sustained remissions in relapsed refractory chronic lymphocytic leukemia. Sci Transl Med 7(303):303ra139
107. Kochenderfer JN, Dudley ME, Kassim SH et al (2015) Chemotherapy-refractory diffuse large B-cell lymphoma and indolent B-cell malignancies can be effectively treated with autologous T cells expressing an anti-CD19 chimeric antigen receptor. J Clin Oncol 33(6):540–549
108. Croft M (2003) Co-stimulatory members of the TNFR family: keys to effective T-cell immunity? Nat Rev Immunol 3(8):609–620
109. Center for Biologics Evaluation and Research. Guidance for Industry: Considerations for the Design of Early-Phase Clinical Trials of Cellular and Gene Therapy Products. June 2015. Available at: http://www.fda.gov/downloads/Biologi.../UCM359073.pdf. Accessed 30 Dec 2016
110. Liu BL, Robinson M, Han ZQ et al (2003) ICP34.5 deleted herpes simplex virus with enhanced oncolytic, immune stimulating, and anti-tumour properties. Gene Ther 10(4):292–303
111. Mineta T, Rabkin SD, Yazaki T, Hunter WD, Martuza RL (1995) Attenuated multi-mutated herpes simplex virus-1 for the treatment of malignant gliomas. Nat Med 1(9):938–943
112. Spivack JG, Fareed MU, Valyi-Nagy T et al (1995) Replication, establishment of latent infection, expression of the latency-associated transcripts and explant reactivation of herpes simplex virus type 1 gamma 34.5 mutants in a mouse eye model. J Gen Virol 76(Pt 2):321–332
113. Andtbacka RH, Ross M, Puzanov I et al (2016) Patterns of clinical response with talimogene laherparepvec (T-VEC) in patients with melanoma treated in the OPTiM phase III clinical trial. Ann Surg Oncol 23(13):4169–4177
114. Fukuhara H, Ino Y, Todo T (2016) Oncolytic virus therapy: a new era of cancer treatment at dawn. Cancer Sci 107(10):1373–1379

115. Mohr I, Sternberg D, Ward S et al (2001) A herpes simplex virus type 1 gamma34.5 second-site suppressor mutant that exhibits enhanced growth in cultured glioblastoma cells is severely attenuated in animals. J Virol 75(11):5189–5196
116. Poppers J, Mulvey M, Khoo D, Mohr I (2000) Inhibition of PKR activation by the proline-rich RNA binding domain of the herpes simplex virus type 1 Us11 protein. J Virol 74(23):11215–11221
117. He B, Chou J, Brandimarti R et al (1997) Suppression of the phenotype of gamma(1)34.5-herpes simplex virus 1: failure of activated RNA-dependent protein kinase to shut off protein synthesis is associated with a deletion in the domain of the alpha47 gene. J Virol 71(8):6049–6054
118. MacKie RM, Stewart B, Brown SM (2001) Intralesional injection of herpes simplex virus 1716 in metastatic melanoma. Lancet 357(9255):525–526
119. Markert JM, Medlock MD, Rabkin SD et al (2000) Conditionally replicating herpes simplex virus mutant, G207 for the treatment of malignant glioma: results of a phase I trial. Gene Ther 7(10):867–874
120. Sundaresan P, Hunter WD, Martuza RL, Rabkin SD (2000) Attenuated, replication-competent herpes simplex virus type 1 mutant G207: safety evaluation in mice. J Virol 74(8):3832–3841
121. Advani SJ, Weichselbaum RR, Whitley RJ, Roizman B (2002) Friendly fire: redirecting herpes simplex virus-1 for therapeutic applications. Clin Microbiol Infect 8(9):551–563
122. Hu JC, Coffin RS, Davis CJ et al (2006) A phase I study of OncoVEXGM-CSF, a second-generation oncolytic herpes simplex virus expressing granulocyte macrophage colony-stimulating factor. Clin Cancer Res 12(22):6737–6747
123. Rehman H, Silk AW, Kane MP, Kaufman HL (2016) Into the clinic: Talimogene laherparepvec (T-VEC), a first-in-class intratumoral oncolytic viral therapy. J Immunother Cancer 4:53
124. Andtbacka RH, Kaufman HL, Collichio F et al (2015) Talimogene Laherparepvec Improves Durable Response Rate in Patients With Advanced Melanoma. J Clin Oncol 33(25):2780–2788
125. Imlygic (talimogene laherparepvec) Prescribing Information. Thousand Oaks: Amgen Inc.; October 2015. Available at: http://pi.amgen.com/united_states/imlygic/imlygic_pi.pdf. Accessed 21 November 2016
126. Center for Biologics Evaluation and Research. Imlygic (talimogene laherparepvec, T-VEC, OncoVEX). Clinical Review. Submission tracking number 125518. Available at: http://www.fda.gov/downloads/BiologicsBloodVaccines/CellularGeneTherapyProducts/ApprovedProducts/UCM474612.pdf. Accessed 20 Nov 2016
127. Center for Biologics Evaluation and Research. Imlygic (talimogene laherparepvec, T-VEC, OncoVEX). Clinical Pharmacology and Toxicology Review. Submission tracking number 125518. Accessed 20 Nov 2016. Available at: http://www.fda.gov/downloads/BiologicsBloodVaccines/CellularGeneTherapyProducts/ApprovedProducts/UCM474613.pdf
128. Kaufman HL, Kim DW, DeRaffele G et al (2010) Local and distant immunity induced by intralesional vaccination with an oncolytic herpes virus encoding GM-CSF in patients with stage IIIc and IV melanoma. Ann Surg Oncol 17(3):718–730
129. Batlevi CL, Matsuki E, Brentjens RJ, Younes A. Novel immunotherapies in lymphoid malignancies. Nat Rev Clin Oncol. 2016;13(1):25-40. doi:10.1038/nrclinonc.2015.187. Epub 2015 Nov 3. PMID: 26525683

Chapter 3
Immunotherapeutic Biomarkers and Selection Strategies

Young Kwang Chae, Timothy J. Taxter, Ludimila L. Cavalcante, and Francis J. Giles

Abstract Immunotherapy has been one of the recent major breakthroughs in cancer therapy. The basic mechanism of immunotherapy agents is to facilitate the immune system to view cancer cells as a foreign presence. The recent success demonstrated by immune checkpoint inhibition in melanoma has launched a boom in immune checkpoint inhibitor trials in several different histologies, but these unfortunately have not shown the same outcome as melanoma. There still exists a significant gap to bridge in therapeutic improvement of these therapies, with patient selection still a major unresolved issue.

Advancements in preclinical modeling and tumor and immune cell sequencing technology have had a significant impact on the types of immune-related biomarkers that can be evaluated. These advancements are both a blessing and challenge for clinicians attempting to make sense of rapidly changing landscape of immunotherapy. This is both true in community practice using immunotherapy treatment for their patients and for academic clinicians involved in designing and conducting immunotherapy clinical trials who are essential in developing correlative studies to evaluate potential biomarkers. Here in this chapter, we aim to discuss the immunotherapeutic biomarkers and the overall selection strategies.

Keywords Predictive biomarkers • Immunotherapy • PD-L1 • Tumor mutational burden

Y.K. Chae (✉) • L.L. Cavalcante • F.J. Giles
Division of Hematology Oncology, Department of Medicine, Northwestern University Feinberg School of Medicine, Chicago, IL, USA
e-mail: young.chae@northwestern.edu; ludimila.cavalcante@northwestern.edu; francis.giles@northwestern.edu

T.J. Taxter
Department of Pathology, Northwestern University Feinberg School of Medicine, Chicago, IL, USA
e-mail: timothy.taxter@northwestern.edu

S.P. Patel, R. Kurzrock (eds.), *Early Phase Cancer Immunotherapy*,
Current Cancer Research, DOI 10.1007/978-3-319-63757-0_3

3.1 Introduction

Immunotherapies in their short existence have already revolutionized the treatment of some forms of cancer with non-small cell lung cancer being at the forefront of success stories. On the surface, their different mechanisms of action seem relatively simple. Whether its checkpoint inhibitors leading to T-cell activation or tumor vaccines priming immunity in a similar fashion as infectious disease vaccines, the unifying concept is clear; facilitate the immune system to view cancer cells as a foreign presence. The translation of that concept into reality, however, is far from clear. The recent success demonstrated by immune checkpoint inhibition in melanoma has launched a boom in immune checkpoint inhibitor trials in several different histologies, but these unfortunately have not shown the same response rates as melanoma and renal cell carcinoma. Altogether, these response rates average only about 20% [1], leaving a significant gap to bridge in therapeutic improvement of these therapies, with patient selection still a major unresolved issue.

Just as targeted therapies are affected by histologic variations in molecular pathways, immunotherapeutic efficacy is determined by numerous variables intrinsic to a patient's tumor and the exquisite heterogeneity of the immune system. Understanding this complexity has been an evolving process. The conceptual frameworks put forth by Schreiber et al. introducing "cancer immune surveillance" and then later "cancer immunoediting" highlight this ongoing investigation into how the immune system interacts with cancer cells and how it can be modulated by immunotherapeutics. A key component in this process has been improved experimental models. Specifically, advancements in mouse models, which had hampered immunology research for much of the twentieth century, are allowing for a more in-depth understanding of tumor immunology. In the clinical realm, advancements in sequencing technology have had a significant impact on the types of immune-related biomarkers that can be evaluated. These advancements are both a blessing and challenge for clinicians attempting to make sense of rapidly changing landscape of immunotherapy. This is both true in community practice and for clinicians involved in immunotherapy clinical trial development who are essential in developing correlative studies to evaluate potential biomarkers. Here in this chapter, we aim to discuss the immunotherapeutic biomarkers and selection strategies.

3.2 Biomarkers: Definition and Clinical Utility

Biomarkers have a variety of clinical uses in oncology, ranging anywhere from screening for malignancies, estimating risk of developing cancer, determining prognosis of disease, predicting or monitoring response to therapy and monitoring for disease recurrence [2]. According to the National Cancer Institute (NCI), a biomarker is "a biological molecule found in blood, other body fluids, or tissues that is a sign of a normal or abnormal process, or of a condition or disease," such as cancer [3]. These can include proteins such as an enzyme or receptor, nucleic acid, antibodies, peptides, or even gene expression and proteomic signatures, among a very wide gamut of categories. Biomarkers can be found in easily accessible sites such as the peripheral blood or other fluids (e.g., urine, sputum, stool, etc.) or can be derived invasively from biopsied tissue or aspirated fluid (e.g., pleural, abdominal, etc.). Genetic biomarkers can be inherited, in which case they would be detectable in germ line DNA isolated from peripheral blood, sputum, or buccal cells, or they can be somatic, and identified as mutations in DNA derived directly from the tumor.

Prognostic biomarkers help patients with an oncologic diagnosis to determine the likelihood of disease recurrence, regardless of treatment. This speaks of the natural history of the disease as it pertains to that individual. Traditionally, the tumor's clinicopathologic features were considered the determinants of prognosis, but more recently, new technologies like gene expression signatures are being developed based on individual tumor assessment [4, 5]. As an example, circulating tumor cells were found to be prognostic of overall survival (OS) in several tumor types, including breast, colorectal, and prostate cancers, among others [6–8].

Predictive biomarkers are used as modifiers of response to specific therapies and useful in determining which treatments have the likelihood of being most effective. For instance, in colorectal tumors, somatic mutations in the KRAS protein are associated with a poor response to antiepithelial growth factor receptor (EGFR) therapies such as panitumumab and cetuximab [9]. Another example would be the presence of HER2 overexpression or amplification in breast or gastric tumors which predict response for anti-HER2 therapies like trastuzumab [10–12].

As mentioned above, the advent of immune checkpoint inhibitor therapies has drastically changed the therapeutic scenario of solid tumor oncology and even of some hematologic malignancies, but defining which patients derive the most benefit from these treatments is of crucial importance and currently under active investigation. Therefore, defining the appropriate predictive biomarkers will be the key to the advancement of these therapies in the future. In this chapter, we will focus on predictive biomarkers currently under investigation for the evaluation of response to immunotherapies; these include immune cell markers (such as PD-L1, CTLA-4, tumor-infiltrating lymphocytes (TILs), and T-cell receptor sequencing), immune transcriptomic profiling, mismatch repair (MMR) status, tumor mutational burden, neoantigen expression, germline biomarkers, and finally host-related biomarkers. We will analyze the advantages and limitations of each of these biomarker modalities and their applications in clinical context and ultimately propose a potential paradigm toward personalized cancer immunotherapy in the future.

3.3 Immune Cell Markers

3.3.1 PD-L1

3.3.1.1 PD-L1 Expression

The immune anticancer response is regulated by an array of molecules and steps ultimately leading to effective killing of cancer cells in what is now termed the "cancer-immunity cycle" [13]. This can be achieved in part by the regulation of

T-cell activation, which requires two signals. The first is through the T-cell receptor (TCR), by recognition of antigens presented via the major histocompatibility complex (MHC) on antigen-presenting cells (APCs). The second is through the binding of costimulatory and coinhibitory molecules expressed on T cells and APCs [14, 15]. PD-L1 expression has been identified in a variety of cell types, including benign tissue cells such as hepatocytes, endothelial, pancreatic, and muscle cells, as well as peripheral blood cells like B cells, dendritic cells, T cells, macrophages, and mast cells [16]. PD-L2 is another ligand for PD-1 and can be found in dendritic cells, macrophages, and mast cells [17].

PD-L1 has also been identified in 20–50% of human cancers, with a wide variability reported for any given solid tumor histology [18]. The PD-1-PD-L1/PD-L2 interaction between T cell and tumor cell/APC, respectively, has been recognized as a negative immune modulating interaction causing T-cell inhibition and consequently leading to shutting down of the immune response and cancer survival [18]. In other words, PD-1, a molecule on the T cell, is involved in diminishing T-cell activation of cells expressing PD-L1 and PD-L2 (the tumor and APCs), leading to T-cell immunologic tolerance [19].

This discovery has led to the development of several cancer immunotherapy agents targeting the PD-1-PD-L1/PD-L2 interaction, with anti-PD-1 and anti-PD-L1 monoclonal antibodies demonstrating overall response rates ranging from 13 to 38% as single agents, but with unprecedented duration of responses in a broad range of tumor types, and now leading the way in transforming cancer treatment paradigms in several solid tumors [1]. These agents include the anti-PD-1 antibodies nivolumab and pembrolizumab, both IgG4 antibodies which have been FDA approved in the treatment of several cancer histologies, and more recently the anti-PD-L1 agents atezolizumab, durvalumab, and avelumab [18, 20–56]. With a similar side effect profile, as well as overall response rates recently found to be comparable among these therapies, along with our knowledge of the benefit to a limited subset of patients and elevated cost of these treatments, the selection of candidate subjects most likely to benefit from these immune checkpoint therapies is crucial [57].

3.3.1.2 PD-L1 Assays

PD-L1 expression in tumor cells has emerged as an important diagnostic marker and currently is used to guide therapy decisions with several agents. PD-L1 expression is measured using a combination of specific PD-L1 detection antibodies and immunohistochemistry (IHC) [58]. Unfortunately, there is considerable variability in testing, with each drug manufacturer developing their own assay which differs in PD-L1 detection antibodies, cutoff values for PD-L1 positivity, tissue preparation, and other processing differences. In addition, some stain strictly tumor membrane, while others incorporate both membrane and immune cells to form complex scoring systems, making the task of comparing data across histologies and even clinical trials a daunting one [18, 22, 24, 30, 35, 45, 50, 59]. Table 3.1 lists the currently available assays stratified by immune checkpoint agent.

Table 3.1 Diagnostic partners with their respective agents [18, 20–56]

Drug	Nivolumab (anti-PD-1) BMS	Pembrolizumab (anti-PD-1) Merck	Atezolizumab (anti-PD-L1) Roche/Genentech	Durvalumab (anti-PD-L1) AstraZeneca	Avelumab (anti-PD-L1) Pfizer/Merck Serono
Diagnostic partner	Dako	Dako	Ventana	Ventana	Dako
Clones	28–8	22-C3	SP142	SP263	73–10
Companion vs. complementary	Complementary (not required)	Companion for NSCLC (required) Complementary in other histologies (not required)	Complementary (not required)	Not FDA approved yet	Not FDA approved yet
Cells scored/ Compartment	Tumor cell membrane (and stroma)	Tumor cell membrane	Tumor cells Immune cells	Tumor cell membrane	Tumor cells Immune cells
Tissue	Archival	Fresh or archival tissue	Archival/fresh	Archival/fresh	Unknown
Cut-point for (+)	PD-L1 (+) >1% Strong (+) >5%	PD-L1 (+) >1% Strong (+) >50%	TC/IC 3 (+) TC/IC 2 (+) TC/IC 1 (+) TC/IC 0 (−)	PD-L1 (+) ≥ 25%	PD-L1 (+) ≥1% or 5% Merkel cell vs Javelin trials

This inconsistency in PD-L1 testing methods has contributed significantly to the wide variability in results demonstrated throughout clinical trials with immunotherapy drugs to date [18, 20–56] and rendered the clinical utility of PD-L1 as a predictive marker a subject of much debate. Currently, PD-L1 testing has been approved by the FDA as either a complementary assay, not affecting the decision to start treatment (applicable to nivolumab, atezolizumab, and pembrolizumab in NSCLC histologies), or as a companion diagnostic assay, whereby a negative result would preclude patients from receiving therapy (i.e., pembrolizumab in NSCLC). In the case of NSCLC, when considering therapy with pembrolizumab, PD-L1 testing by the approved companion assay is required prior to starting therapy. Of note, the cutoffs used for positivity of the Dako 22C3 assay have undergone several adjustments since the initial FDA approval of pembrolizumab in October 2015, with an initial cutoff of >50% for positivity, and just recently modified to ≥1% PD-L1 expression of tumor cells [28, 34] (Table 3.1).

Clinical Applications: Trial Data of PD-L1 Expression in Several Tumor Histologies

Determining predictive biomarkers for immunotherapy treatment has become increasingly pressing, as the decision to give immune checkpoint drugs, the choice between single agent or combination immune checkpoint inhibition and timing of therapy (1st line vs. ≥2 lines), needs to be balanced with considerations on known overall limited response rates (~20% across histologies) [1] with single agent, the significantly higher risk of severe autoimmune adverse events from combination therapy, and financial burden from this therapy vs. an alternative treatment, respectively.

Current data indicates that overexpression of PD-L1 on the tumor surface correlates with better responses to anti-PD-1 therapies; however, notable responses have been observed in tumors with low levels of PD-L1 expression, making the predictive value of this biomarker clinically challenging [60]. We will present the current clinical data on the validity of PD-L1 testing as a predictive marker of response in FDA-approved histologies of melanoma, lung cancer, bladder cancer, renal cell carcinoma (RCC), Hodgkin lymphoma, and head and neck cancers.

Specific details on PD-L1 testing in different histologies and ORR in clinical trials are described in Table 3.2 [55]. A cutoff of 5% for expression of PD-L1 in tumor cells was used to define positivity and performed in 42 of the 296 patients enrolled on this trial. After 1 year of follow-up, 9 of 25, or 36% of PD-L1 positive patients, showed objective responses to treatment, while none of the 17 patients with PD-L1-negative disease responded to therapy.

Clinical Trial Data of PD-L1 Expression as a Predictive Marker in FDA-Approved Histologies

The number of clinical trials testing immune checkpoint inhibitors in oncology has rapidly expanded in the last couple of years, with several histologies now receiving FDA approval for routine clinical use of these agents. Moreover, the current trend is to move these therapies earlier in the sequence of regimens, with numerous studies currently testing different approaches thus making the need for a predictive biomarker essential in these treatment decisions. We will discuss here the PD-L1 biomarker data available in advanced phase studies of the currently FDA approved histologies, these being melanoma, NSCLC, RCC, Hodgkin lymphoma, bladder cancer, and head and neck cancer.

3.3.1.3 PD-L1 Expression in Melanoma

Melanoma is known for its highly immunogenic qualities and was the first histology to have immune checkpoint inhibitors FDA approved for wide use. The first drug was the anti-CTLA-4 inhibitor ipilimumab, followed by the anti-PD-1 inhibitors nivolumab and pembrolizumab and more recently the combination of nivolumab and ipilimumab

There are a plethora of phase III trials demonstrating the benefit of nivolumab as monotherapy and in combination with ipilimumab, compared to chemotherapy for the treatment of melanoma [56, 61–63]. PD-L1 cutoffs have not yet been established for melanoma patients, and current phase III data have not been definitive in demonstrating a clear benefit for any specific threshold. For instance, CheckMate 037 and 066 both looked at nivolumab vs. chemotherapy, in the second- and first-line settings, respectively, both demonstrating survival benefits for the nivolumab-treated patients compared to chemotherapy, regardless of PD-L1 status, with a threshold of ≥5% for positivity [56, 63]. In the groundbreaking phase III study of ipilimumab and nivolumab combination compared to nivolumab or ipilimumab alone, CheckMate 067, which interestingly at cutoffs of either ≥1 or ≥5%, did not show significant differences in PFS in PD-L1-positive patients receiving nivolumab vs. the combination, although there were differences in response rates (72.1% vs. 57.5% for the combination vs. nivolumab alone for PD-L1 positive (≥5%) patients and 21.3% for ipilimumab [61]. However, for those patients negative for PD-L1 (<5%), both response rates and PFS were improved with the combination vs. single agent nivolumab and even more pronounced than ipilimumab. These important results suggested that the combination of nivolumab and ipilimumab could be more beneficial for those patients with PD-L1 negative melanomas, although clear cutoffs remain a subject of debate.

In KEYNOTE-006, pembrolizumab monotherapy was compared to ipilimumab regardless of PD-L1 status, although 80% had PD-L1-positive tumors (≥1%) [64]. Both a significantly higher response rate and PFS were noted for pembrolizumab compared to ipilimumab, across all groups, regardless of PD-L1 status. However, the number of PD-L1-negative patients was relatively small and confidence intervals were large for that group. ORR were reported at 33.7% for pembrolizumab given every 2 weeks (P <0.001 vs. ipilimumab), 32.9% for pembrolizumab every 3 weeks (P <0.001), and 11.9% for ipilimumab [64]. A later analysis of the trial showed the best benefit of pembrolizumab in PD-L1+ and treatment naïve patients than their previously treated counterparts [27]. There was also a relationship between increasing PD-L1 expression and improved outcomes when PD-L1 was

Table 3.2 Pivotal clinical trials in FDA-approved histologies with respective PD-L1 data

Histology	Therapeutic agent & antibody	Study	Phase of clinical trial	% expressing PD-L1 and cutoffs (%)	ORR	Median PFS	Median OS	References
Melanoma								
	Nivolumab (Dako 28–8)							
	Nivo vs. chemo after ipi failure	CheckMate 037	Phase III	52% (<5%)	20.3% (95% CI, 11.3–32.2) vs. 13% for nivo vs. chemo	NR	NR	[56]
				46% (≥5%)	43.6% (30.3–57.7) vs. 9.1% (2.8–33.6)	NR	NR	
	Nivo/ipi vs. ipi	CheckMate 069	Phase II	35% (<5%)	55% (95% CI, 42–69) for nivo/ipi	50% (95% CI, 36–63) for nivo/ipi vs. ipi at 12 mo	75% (95% CI, 61–84) for nivo/ipi vs. ipi at 12 mo	[198]
				15% (≥5%)	58% (95% CI 37–78)	48% (27–66) at 12 mo	71% (48–85) at 12 mo	
				22% (<1%)	46% (95% CI, 29–63)	45% (27–61) at 12 mo	71% (52–83) at 12 mo	
				28% (≥1%)	64% (49–78)	53% (37–66) at 12 mo	76% (60–86) at 12 mo	
	Nivo vs. dacarbazine	CheckMate 066	Phase III *(1st line)*	64.5% (<5%)	NR	NR	NE vs. 10.2mo (95% CI,7.6–11.8) for nivo vs. dacarbazine	[63]
				35.6% (≥ 5%)	NR	NR	NE vs. 12.4 mo (9.2-NE)	

	Nivo vs. nivo/ ipi vs. ipi	CheckMate 067	Phase III	(<5%)	54.8% (47.8–61.6) for nivo + ipi, 41.3% (34.6–48.4) for nivo, 17.8% (12.8–23.8) for Ipi	11.2 mo for nivo + ipi, HR = 0.42 for nivo + ipi vs. ipi; 5.3 mo for nivo, HR = 0.60 for nivo vs. ipi; 2.8 mo for ipi	NR	[61]
				(≥ 5%)	72.1% (59.9–82.3), 57.5% (45.9–68.5), 21.3% (12.7–32.3)	14 mo for nivo + ipi HR = 0.40 for nivo + ipi vs. ipi; 14 mo for nivo HR = 0.40 for nivo vs. ipi; 3.9 mo for ipi	NR	
	Pembrolizumab (Dako 22-C3)							
	Pembro (q2 wks vs. q3 wks) vs. ipilimumab	KEYNOTE-006	Phase III	(<1%)	NR	HR = 0.67 (95% CI, 0.41–1.11) for pembro q2 wks; HR = 0.76 (0.47–1.24) for q3 wks	HR = 0.91 (95% CI, 0.49–1.69) for pembro q2 wks; HR = 1.02 (0.56–1.85) for q3 wks	[64]
				(≥ 1%) 80.6% in q2 wks, 79.8% in q3 wks, 80.9% in ipi	NR	HR = 0.53 (95% CI, 0.41–0.67) for pembro q2wks; HR = 0.52 (0.40–0.66) for pembro q3 wks	HR = 0.55 (95% CI 0.40–0.76) for pembro q2wks; HR = 0.58 (0.42–0.79) for pembro q3 wks	
	Pembrolizumab	KEYNOTE-001	Phase I	NR	NR	NR	NR	[44]
NSCLC								
	Nivolumab (Dako 28–8)							

(continued)

Table 3.2 (continued)

Histology	Therapeutic agent & antibody	Study	Phase of clinical trial	% expressing PD-L1 and cutoffs (%)	ORR	Median PFS	Median OS	References
	Nivo vs. docetaxel	CheckMate 017	Phase III (squamous)	47% (≥1%)	17% vs. 17%	HR, 0.70; 95% CI, 0.53–0.94; vs. HR, 1.19; 95% CI, 0.88–1.61	HR, 0.59; 95% CI, 0.43–0.82; vs. 0.90; 95% CI, 0.66–1.24	[26]
				31% (≥5%)	21% vs. 15%	HR, 0.54; 95% CI, 0.39–0.76; vs. HR, 1.31; 95% CI, 1.01–1.71	HR, 0.43; 95% CI, 0.30–0.63; vs. HR, 1.01; 95% CI, 0.77–1.34	
				27% (≥10%)	19% vs. 16%	HR, 0.52; 95% CI, 0.37–0.75; vs. HR, 1.24; 95% CI, 0.96–1.61	HR, 0.4; 95% CI, 0.26–0.59; vs. HR, 1.0; 95% CI, 0.76–1.31	
	Nivo vs. docetaxel	CheckMate 057	Phase III (non-squamous)	53% (≥1%)	31% vs. 9%	NR	NR	[25]
				41% (≥5%)	36% vs. 10%	NR	NR	
				37% (≥10%)	37% vs. 11%	NR	NR	
	Nivo vs. docetaxel	CheckMate 026	Phase III *(1st line)*	78% (≥5%)	NR	4.2 vs 5.9 mo; HR = 1.15, 95% CI 0.91–1.45; $p = 0.25$) for nivo vs. docetaxel	14.4 vs. 13.2 mo for nivo vs. docetaxel (HR = 1.02, 95% CI 0.80–1.30)	[53]
	Pembrolizumab (Dako 22-C3)							
	Pembrolizumab	KEYNOTE-001	Phase Ib (squamous and non-squamous)	23% (PS <1%)	11% vs. NR	NR	NR	[32]

				38% (PS ≥1% to <50%)	17% vs. NR	NR	NR	
				34% (PS ≥50%)	45% vs. NR	6.3 mo (95% CI, 2.9–12.5) vs. NR	NRe (95% CI, 9.3-NRe) vs. NR	
	Pembro vs. docetaxel	KEYNOTE-010	Phase II/III (squamous and non-squamous)	43% (PS ≥50%)	30% vs. NR	NR	2 mg/kg: 14.9 mo (95% CI, 10.4–NRe); 10 mg/kg: 17.3 mo (95% CI, 11.8-NRe) vs. NR	[34]
	Pembro vs. 1st line chemo	KEYNOTE-024	Phase III *(1st line)*	100% (PS ≥ 50%)	44.8% vs. 27.8% for pembro vs. chemo	10.3 mo (95% CI, 6.7 –NR) vs. 6 mo (95% CI, 4.2 to 6.2) for pembro vs. chemo	80.2% vs. 72.4% at 6 mo, $p = 0.005$ for pembro vs. chemo	[42]
	Atezolizumab (Ventana SP 142)							
	Atezolizumab	FIR	Phase II (squamous and non-squamous)	100% (TC 3 or IC 3, cohort 1)	29% vs. NA	43% with 12 wk (95% CI, 6–80%) vs. NA	NR	[54]
				100% (TC 3 or IC 3, Cohort 2)	17% vs. NA	49% with 12 wk (95% CI, 30–69%) vs. NA	NR	
				100% (TC 3 or IC 3, Cohort 3)	17% vs. NA	NR	NR	

(continued)

Table 3.2 (continued)

Histology	Therapeutic agent & antibody	Study	Phase of clinical trial	% expressing PD-L1 and cutoffs (%)	ORR	Median PFS	Median OS	References
	Atezolizumab vs. docetaxel	POPLAR	Phase II (squamous and non-squamous)	65% (TC 1/2/3 or IC 1/2/3)	18% vs. 8%	2.8 mo (NS) vs. NA	15.5 mo (significant) vs. NA	[30]
				35% (TC 2/3 or IC 2/3)	22% vs. 13%	3.4 mo (NS) vs. NA	15.1 mo (significant) vs. NA	
				17% (TC 3 or IC 3)	38% vs. 12%	7.8 mo (NS) vs. NA	15.5 mo (NS) vs. NA	
	Atezolizumab vs. docetaxel	OAK	Phase III	45% (TC 0 and IC 0)	7.8 vs 10.6% (atezo vs. docetaxel)	2.6 mo (1.7–2.9) vs. 4.0 mo (3.1–4.2) for atezo vs. docetaxel	12.6 vs. 8.9 mo; HR 0.75 (0.59–0.96) for atezo vs. docetaxel	[45]
				54% (TC 1/2/3 or IC 1/2/3)	17.8 vs. 16%	2.8 mo (2.6–4.0) vs. 4.1 mo (2.9–4.3)	15.7 vs 10.3 mo; HR 0.74 (0.58–0.93)	
				31% (TC 2/3 or IC 2/3)	22.5 vs. 12.5%	4.1 mo (2.8 vs 5.3) vs. 3.6 mo (2.8–4.2)	16.3 vs 10.8 mo; HR 0.67 (0.49–0.90)	
				16% (TC 3 or IC 3)	30.6 vs. 10.8%	4.2 mo (2.9–7) vs. 3.3 mo (2.7–4.2)	20.5 vs. 8.9 mo; HR 0.41 (0.27–0.64)	
	Atezolizumab	BIRCH	Phase II *(1st line)*	100% (TC 3 or IC 3, Cohort 1)	26% vs. NA	48% with 6 mo (95% CI, 35–61%) vs. NA	79% with 6 mo (95% CI, 69–89%) vs. NA	[24]
				100% (TC 3 or IC 3, Cohort 2)	24% vs. NA	34% with 6 mo (95% CI, 26–43%) vs. NA	80% with 6 mo (95% CI, 72–87%) vs. NA	

				100% (TC 3 or IC 3, Cohort 3)	27% vs. NA	39% with 6 mo (95% CI, 30–48%) vs. NA	75% with 6 mo (95% CI, 67–83%) vs. NA	
	Durvalumab (Ventana SP 263)							
	Durvalumab	ATLANTIC	Phase II	30% (<25%)	7.5% (95% CI, 3.1–14.5)	1.9 mo (1.8–1.9)	34.5% at 12 mo (25–44.1)	[31]
				47% (≥25%)	16.4% (95% CI, 10.8–23.5)	3.3 mo (1.9–3.7)	48% at 12 mo (39.3–55.5)	
				22% (≥90%)	30.9% (95% CI, 20.2–43.3)	2.4 mo (1.8–5.5)	51% at 12 mo (36.9–63.2)	
Renal cell carcinoma								
	Nivolumab (Dako 28–8)							
	Nivo vs. Everolimus	CheckMate 025	Phase III	76% (<1%)	NR	NR	27.4 mo (21.4-NE) vs. 21.2 mo (17.7–26.2) for nivo vs. everolimus	[38]
				24% (≥1%)	NR	NR	21.8 mo (16.5–28.1) vs. 18.8 mo (11.9–19.9)	
				11% (≥5%)	NR	NR	21.9 mo (14-NE) vs. 18.1 (10.3- NE)	
Bladder cancer								
	Atezolizumab (Ventana SP 142)	IMvigor210	Phase II	32% (IC 0)	21% (95% CI, 9–36)	NR	19.1 mo (9.8-NE) for combined IC 0/1 group	[50]

(continued)

Table 3.2 (continued)

Histology	Therapeutic agent & antibody	Study	Phase of clinical trial	% expressing PD-L1 and cutoffs (%)	ORR	Median PFS	Median OS	References
				40% (IC 1)	21% (95% CI, 10–35)	NR	NR	
				67% (IC 1/2/3)	24% (95% CI, 15–35)	NR	NR	
				27% (IC 2/3)	28% (95% CI, 14–47)	NR	12.3 mo (6.0-NE) for IC 2/3	
	Nivolumab (Dako 28–8)	CheckMate 032	Phase I/II	54% (<1%)	26.2% (13.9–42·0)	2.8 mo (95% CI, 1.4–6.5)	9.9 mo (95% CI, 7- NE)	[52]
				32% (≥1%)	24% (9.4–45.1)	5.5 mo (95% CI 1.4–11.2)	16.2 mo (95% CI 7.6 – NE)	
				18% (≥5%)	NR	NR	NR	
	Pembrolizumab (Dako 22-C3)	KEYNOTE-045	Phase III	70% (Ps <10%)	NR	NR	NR	[23]
	Pembro vs. chemo			30% (Ps ≥10%)	21.6% (95% CI, 12.9–32.7) vs. 6.7% (2.5 to 13.9) for pembro vs. chemo	HR = 0.89 (95% CI, 0.61–1.28) $p = 0.24$	HR = 0.57 (95% CI, 0.37–0.88) $p = 0.0048$	
Hodgkin lymphoma								
	Nivolumab (PD-L1 by FISH)		Phase I	Of 50% evaluable pts., all were PD-L1 + by FISH	87% ORR; 17% CR	86% at 24 wks (95% CI, 62–95)	NR	[20]
	Pembrolizumab (Dako 22-C3)	KEYNOTE-013	Phase Ib	94% (≥1%)	65% (90% CI, 48–79%) ORR for all pts	69% at 24 wks; 46% at 52 wks	NR	[68]

Head + Neck cancer								
	Pembrolizumab (Dako 22-C3)							
	Pembrolizumab	KEYNOTE-055	Phase II	14% (<1%)	17% (95% CI 9–28)	NR	NR	[36]
				82.6% (≥1%)	8% (95% CI, 0.2–36)	NR	NR	
	Pembrolizumab	KEYNOTE-012	Phase Ib	22% (<1%)	NR	NR	NR	[51]
				78% (≥1%)	NR; 18% (95% CI 8–32) for all pts	NR	NR; 13 mo (95% CI 5-NE) for all pts	
	Nivolumab (Dako 28–8)							
	Nivo vs. chemo	CheckMate 141	Phase III	42.7% (<1%)	12.3% vs. 10.5% for nivo vs. chemo	NR	5.7 vs. 5.8 mo; HR = 0.89 (0.54–1.45) for nivo vs. chemo	[199]
				57.3% (≥1%)	17% vs. 1.6%	NR	8.7 vs. 4.6 mo; HR = 0.55 (0.36–0.83) for nivo vs. chemo	
Merkel cell carcinoma								
	Avelumab (Dako 73–10)	JAVELIN Merkel 2000	Phase II	18% (<1%)	18.8% (4.0–45.6)	NR	NR	[37]
	Avelumab			66% (≥1%)	34.5% (95% ci 22.5–48.1)	NR	NR	

Abbreviations: *CI* confidence interval, *HR* hazard ratio, *IC* tumor-infiltrating immune cells, *IHC* immunohistochemistry, *NA* not applicable, *NE* not estimable, *NR* not reported, *NS* not significant, *NSCLC* non-small cell lung cancer, *ORR* objective response rate, *OS* overall survival, *PD*-1 programmed cell death-1, *PD*-1 L programmed cell death-1 ligand, *PFS* progression-free survival, *TC* tumor cells scored as IHC 0 (0% staining), 1 (<1%), 2 (1–9%), 3 (10–32%), 4 (33–65%), and 5 (≥ 66%). Thus, in melanoma, all patients are eligible for pembrolizumab regardless of PD-L1 status.

3.3.1.4 PD-L1 Expression in NSCLC

There is an overwhelming body of evidence demonstrating the superiority of PD-1 drugs compared to chemotherapy in producing superior PFS and OS in the second-line treatment setting of NSCLC. This is illustrated by four important trials, CheckMate 017 and 057 testing nivolumab and KEYNOTE-001 and KEYNOTE-010 using pembrolizumab [25, 26, 32, 34]. Confirming this notion, the updated 2-year survival for these studies shows a maintenance of survival superiority for both squamous and non-squamous histologies with an average of about 30% OS at 2 years, which is unprecedented in this cancer type, although overall response rates still range in the 20% [60]. The task of identifying these long-term responders therefore becomes crucial, and the PD-L1 biomarker has been looked at in this setting, showing again varying results depending on the drug and assay used.

3.3.1.5 PD-L1 Expression in the ≥ Second-Line Setting

More data are known of the PD-L1 biomarker in the second and later lines of therapy for lung cancer and have shown some compelling results.

Nivolumab

In the case of nivolumab, in non-squamous cell carcinoma, the phase III trial CheckMate 057 reported significant differences in overall response rates by PD-L1 expression cutoffs of ≥1%, ≥5% and ≥10% [25]. In addition, significant benefit was reported for OS and PFS at each PD-L1 expression cohort level on this trial, suggesting a positive correlation between this biomarker and response to therapy.

In contrast, the phase III trial in squamous cell carcinoma of the lung, CheckMate 017, did not show a correlation between response to nivolumab and PD-L1 expression at any of the thresholds (≥1%, ≥5%, and ≥10%), and patients all benefitted to some degree more from nivolumab than docetaxel, regardless of PD-L1 expression [26]. This was further exemplified in the phase II trial in squamous cell histology, CheckMate 063, which did show consistently better rates of partial response (PR) and stable disease (SD) across all three threshold levels (≥1%, ≥5%, and ≥10%), but ORR were not statistically different for any level [48].

Pembrolizumab

The KEYNOTE-001 phase I trial (described in detail above) set the stage for FDA approval of pembrolizumab in NSCLC in the second-line setting based on a positivity cutoff of ≥50% for the companion diagnostic assay 22C3 assessed by IHC [32]. Further results from the phase II/III study KEYNOTE-010, which selected patients with at least 1% PD-L1 tumor positivity for treatment with either pembrolizumab (at different doses) or docetaxel, showed a significant benefit in OS and PFS rates for immunotherapy in those patients with at least 50% of tumor cells expressing PD-L1 [34].

This data confirms the utility of the 22C3 assay as a biomarker for patient selection for treatment with pembrolizumab. Furthermore, additional results from the 591 (57.2%) of patients with 1–49% PD-L1 expression in KEYNOTE-010 were recently reported, showing a PFS and ORR benefit for pembrolizumab compared to docetaxel and suggesting a role for broadening the selection of patients for therapy to a lower cutoff for positivity [28]. In this recent report, HR for OS was reported at 0.79 (95% CI 0.61–1.04) or 9.4 months and 0.71 (95% CI 0.53–0.94) or 10.8 months for pembrolizumab, 2 mg/kg and 10 mg/kg, respectively, compared to docetaxel, without significant differences between the two doses. This subsequently led to FDA approval of pembrolizumab for those patients with advanced NSCLC whose tumors express ≥1% PD-L1 after one line of systemic chemotherapy [28, 34].

Atezolizumab

There are currently a number of phase II studies demonstrating a correlation with the IHC SP142 assay and response to atezolizumab in NSCLC patients after first-line therapy. The phase II FIR trial, which selected patients with TC 2 or 3 and/or IC 2 or 3 for PD-L1 positivity and treatment with atezolizumab, enrolled 138 patients [54]. The study demonstrated the highest ORR in patients with high PD-L1 expression (those with TC 3 or IC 3), ranging from 27 to 29%. This would correspond with PD-L1 expression of ≥50% for TCs and ≥10% for ICs. In addition to the FIR trial results, the POPLAR trial, a randomized phase II study of atezolizumab vs. docetaxel, also demonstrated increased efficacy with higher levels of PD-L1 expression on TCs and/or ICs [30].

Durvalumab

Although this drug is not yet FDA approved for lung cancer and no phase III data is yet available, the phase II, ATLANTIC trial recently reported results in two out of its three cohorts [31]. This study initially enrolled all-comers but then restricted enrollment to patients with PD-L1 high tumors determined by membrane staining.

Cohort 2, with 265 patients, was divided into PD-L1 low expressers (<25% PD-L1 expression on tumor cells) and PD-L1 high expressers (≥25% tumoral PD-L1 expression), and patients in cohort 3, containing 68 patients, were PD-L1 high expressers with ≥90% on tumor cells. The ORR with durvalumab increased in line with PD-LI expression. In PD-L1 low or negative patients with PD-L1 expression on <25% of tumor cells, the ORR was 7.5% (95% CI, 3.1–14.5), and ORR was 16.4% (95% CI, 10.8–23.5) in patients with PD-L1 expression ≥25%. But the highest ORR of 30.9% (95% CI, 20.2–43.3) was observed in patients with tumoral PD-L1 expression on ≥90% of tumor cells. In addition, the 1-year OS rates were 48% in patients for PD-L1 ≥ 25% and 51% in patients with PD-L1 ≥ 90%. This would suggest a role for the SP263 assay in the selection of patients but still needs further prospective confirmation. A phase Ib combination study with 102 patients of durvalumab and the anti-CTLA-4 tremelimumab was recently published, demonstrating no superiority in ORR or PFS for PD-L1-positive patients, based on a previously validated cutoff of at least 25% PD-L1 tumoral expression [21]. Although these numbers were small for definitive conclusions to be made, further studies are needed to confirm these findings and the data remains inconclusive.

3.3.1.6 PD-L1 Expression in the First-Line NSCLC Setting

Immune checkpoint inhibitor therapy is now moving into the first-line setting of the lung cancer treatment arsenal, and discrimination of cutoffs for IHC positivity of these different assays is increasingly more important in selecting patients for these therapies.

KEYNOTE-024, a phase III study of 305 previously untreated NSCLC patients selected for strong PD-L1 expression (≥50%), showed superior PFS and OS compared to investigator's choice platinum-based chemotherapy [42]. Based on a PFS benefit of 10.3 vs. 6 months for pembrolizumab (HR for disease progression or death = 0.50; 95% CI 0.37–0.68; p <0.001) and ORR of 44.8% vs. 27.8% for pembrolizumab and chemotherapy, respectively, pembrolizumab was approved in the first-line treatment of NSCLC in those patients with PD-L1 expression ≥50%.

In contrast with the pembrolizumab data, the phase III study of nivolumab vs. investigator's choice chemotherapy in the first-line setting, CheckMate 026, did not meet its primary PFS endpoint [53]. In this trial of 541 patients with PD-L1 expression ≥5%, single agent nivolumab did not improve PFS with a median PFS of 4.2 and 5.9 months for nivolumab and chemotherapy, respectively. A smaller cohort of patients from the CheckMate 012 study treated with combination nivolumab/ipilimumab in the first-line setting had previously shown encouraging responses and PFS compared to nivolumab monotherapy [65]. This early correlation with response was observed for increasing PD-L1 expression levels (≥1%, ≥5%, ≥25%, ≥50%), albeit responses were observed in spite of PD-L1 expression. These disappointing results in the phase III setting after encouraging phase I results highlight the need for determination of well-defined cutoffs for the continued clinical development of this drug in other treatment lines and regimens.

For the anti-PD-L1 drug atezolizumab, a recently reported phase II trial for PD-L1 selected patients (TC 2/3 or IC 2/3) in the first-line setting, BIRCH, demonstrated improved ORRs for higher cutoff levels of TC 3 or IC3, 24–27%, compared to TC 2/3 or IC 2/3, 17–19% response [24]. This improved trend, however, was not as pronounced for PFS or OS, and from these results, the study concluded that PD-L1 expression might be an effective marker.

3.3.1.7 PD-L1 Expression in Renal Cell Carcinoma

A randomized phase III study comparing nivolumab to everolimus in advanced renal cell carcinoma after treatment with antiangiogenic therapy demonstrated about a 5-month OS benefit for immunotherapy and led to the approval of nivolumab in this histology [38]. For this trial, CheckMate 025, 181 of 756 (24%) of patients had PD-L1 expression of at least 1%, and 46 of 756 (6%) had PD-L1 ≥5%. Among those with PD-L1 ≥1%, OS was 21.8 months in the nivolumab-treated patients and 18.8 months in the everolimus group, with a hazard ratio (HR) of 0.79, (95% CI, 0.53–1.17). For those with <1% PD-L1 expression, OS was 27.4 vs. 21.2 months, respectively, with a HR of 0.77 (95% CI 0.60–0.97). Therefore, this cutoff of ≥1% was not predictive of response to therapy with nivolumab. Furthermore, when utilizing a threshold of ≥5%, similar results were noted, although this cohort was too small for further interpretation.

3.3.1.8 PD-L1 Expression in Bladder Cancer

Atezolizumab, the anti-PD-L1 agent that uses the Ventana SP142 IHC assay combining both tumor and immune cells in its scoring system, received the first FDA approval for advanced bladder cancer. This was based on data from a single arm phase II trial of 315 heavily pretreated bladder cancer patients [50]. The PD-L1 status on this study was defined by the percentage of PD-L1-positive immune cells in the tumor microenvironment, where IC0 (<1% immune cell staining), IC1 (≥1% but <5%), and IC2/3 (≥5%). The reported results demonstrated a significantly improved ORR and overall survival (OS) rate for higher levels of PD-L1 IHC expression on immune cells, but not on tumor cells, rendering the IC cutoffs clinically relevant and highlighting the importance of adaptive immunity as a driver of benefit to immune checkpoint inhibitors.

The original results demonstrated an ORR of 27% for the IC 2/3 group (95% CI 19–37, p <0.0001), 18% in the IC 1/2/3 group 95% (CI 13–24, $p = 0.0004$) and 15% in all patients (95% CI 11–20, $p = 0.0058$). A significant difference in response was also maintained for these prespecified cohorts with longer follow-up of 310 patients [50]. Interestingly, although PD-L1 staining by tumor cells was not associated with response to atezolizumab, mutational load was found to strongly correlate with response to therapy. This finding was independent of the association between TCGA subtype or PD-L1 immune cell score and response, supporting the importance of tumor mutational burden as an additional independent and complementary biomarker of response, discussed in detail in further sections.

In addition, nivolumab just received approval based on a phase I/II trial of 86 advanced urothelial cancer patients, CheckMate 032[52]. The study did not select patients on the basis of PD-L1 status but reported an incidence of 32% PD-L1 positivity for cutoff ≥1% and 18% for ≥5% threshold, so small total numbers of patients. Median OS was 16.2 months in those ≥1% and 9.9 months in those <1%. Median PFS was 5.5 months (95% CI 1.4–11.2) in the ≥1% group and 2.8 months (1.4–6.5) in <1% group. Similar results were noted in patients with at least 5% PD-L1 expression. Interestingly, ORR was not higher in the PD-L1-positive population 26.2 for PD-L1 negative vs. 24% for PD-L1 positive (cutoff ≥1%), which might be related to the smaller total number of patients in the trial.

Pembrolizumab has also been tested in bladder cancer in a large randomized phase III trial of 542 patients, KEYNOTE-045, against chemotherapy in the second-line setting, which demonstrated an expected improved survival for the pembrolizumab arm across all groups [23]. Median OS was reported at 10.3 months (95% CI 8.0–11.8) in the pembrolizumab group, compared with 7.4 months (6.1–8.3) in the chemotherapy group (HR for death = 0.73; 95% CI 0.59–0.91; $p = 0.002$). In a further break up of patients into groups with a PD-L1 combined positive score of ≥10% or <10%, median OS was 8.0 months (95% CI 5.0–12.3) in the pembrolizumab group and 5.2 months (4.0–7.4) in the chemotherapy group (HR = 0.57; 95% CI 0.37–0.88; $p = 0.005$). No significant PFS differences were noted in the different groups stratified by PD-L1 status, however. In terms of response rates, superior responses were noted in the immune checkpoint group (21.1%) vs. the chemotherapy group (11.4%), $p = 0.001$, with similar results stratified by the 10% combined PD-L1 score. Taken this data together, one can surmise the 10% threshold is a prognostic one but still not a definitive cutoff point for this drug.

3.3.1.9 PD-L1 Expression in Hodgkin Lymphoma

In May 2016, the FDA-approved nivolumab for the treatment of classical Hodgkin lymphoma relapsed after autologous stem cell transplant and brentuximab vedotin. A small but impressive phase I study demonstrated an ORR of 87%, including 17% complete responses (CR), albeit the study is still ongoing, and only 23 study participants were included in the initial reported analysis [20]. These unusually high response rates noted in Hodgkin lymphoma to single agent nivolumab have been explained in part by a constitutive overexpression of the PD-1 ligand (PD-L1) on Reed-Sternberg cells. The rationale being that a high prevalence of 9p24.1 amplifications and increased JAK2 activity, as well as Epstein-Barr infection, all potentially contribute to induce higher transcription and expression of PD-L1 and PD-L2 on Reed-Sternberg cells, respectively [66, 67]. In this phase I study, ten patients were tested for PD-L1 and PD-L2 via FISH assay and confirmed the presence of 9p amplification and active JAK-STAT signaling [20].

Following this approval, pembrolizumab has recently received approval based on the phase Ib study KEYNOTE-013 of 31 heavily pretreated Hodgkin patients, with an ORR of 65% and an again impressive 16% CR rate [68]. The PFS rate was 69% at 24 weeks and 46% at 52 weeks. Of the 31 patients on trial, 16 had tumor tissue evaluable at baseline, with 15 of those (94%) demonstrating PD-L1 positivity based on a ≥1% cutoff and 90% showing high levels of PD-L2 staining. Again, a small but significant study demonstrating the biology of this tumor type in relation to its immune makeup.

3.3.1.10 PD-L1 Expression in Head and Neck Cancer

Advanced squamous cell carcinoma of the head and neck is the most recent FDA addition to the growing list of histologies for which immune checkpoint agents are approved. The phase II trial of pembrolizumab in recurrent/metastatic head and neck cancer after progression on platinum and cetuximab, KEYNOTE-055, has reported preliminary results of the first 92 patients treated for ≥6 months [36]. Thus far, PD-L1 positivity without reported cutoffs was found in 76/92 and, with 13/92 PD-L1 negative, and ORR of 13/76 (17%) in PD-L1 positive, and 1/13 (8%) in PD-L1 negative have been reported. Although this data is premature and so far non-conclusive with only a small number of patients reported, the phase Ib expansion cohort of KEYNOTE-012 did demonstrate evidence of a statistically significant predictive correlation [69]. With a PD-L1 cutoff for positivity of at least 1% of tumor cells or stroma, they observed an ORR of 22% vs. 4% for PD-L1-positive and PD-L1-negative tumors, respectively ($p = 0.021$). This demonstrates another positive correlation for the pembrolizumab assay.

3.3.1.11 PD-L1 IHC Discussion

Should clinicians rely solely on the tumor's PD-L1 status for treatment decisions regarding immunotherapy? One could argue that if only a minority of patients respond to immune checkpoint inhibition (about 20% throughout most solid tumors) [70], then it would be important to identify those patients most likely to respond, and this is currently our most widely used tool to assess that. On the other hand, we have also seen that some PD-L1-negative patients can still respond to these treatments, which are better tolerated than systemic chemotherapy and cutoffs for positivity can vary widely; therefore those patients should not necessarily be excluded from consideration of immunotherapy drugs. At this point in time many questions remain, and understanding some of the technical and inherent challenges with PD-L1 testing can shed some light as to the predictive utility of this biomarker.

3.3.1.12 Issues with Variability in PD-L1 IHC Assays

The lack of standardization among the different PD-L1 IHC assays has rendered comparison of these different biomarkers throughout clinical trials which is quite challenging; therefore, it is not clear how all the different assays compare with one another on a clinical level [58]. An important issue is that there is no clear consensus on how to measure PD-L1 expression, and this has led to great variability among the different assays [71]. Proprietary companion assays are being developed, and as can be seen in Table 3.1, they can differ in the cell type preferentially being stained for PD-L1 (TC vs. IC), the location and distribution of PD-L1 expression (tumor cell membrane vs. stroma vs. immune cells), and the cutoffs for positivity (ranging anywhere from ≥1 to 50%) [18, 20, 22–31, 33, 36–41, 49, 50, 53, 54, 59, 61, 62, 65, 69, 71]. In addition, the assays also differ in the tissue processing requirements from biopsies (fresh vs. archival) and all use distinct IHC detection antibodies, those being 28–8 (DAKO), 22C3 (Merck), SP142 (Roche/Genentech), and 73–10 (DAKO) [18, 20, 22–31, 33, 36–43, 46, 48–50, 53, 54, 59, 61, 62, 65, 69, 71, 72]. Furthermore, it is also known that due to a paucity of binding sites for IHC detection antibodies on the PD-L1, these antibodies will bind to different sites from the immune checkpoint antibodies on the PD-L1 [73].

3.3.1.13 Inherent Challenges of PD-L1 Testing

There are also biologic limitations to the use of PDL-1 IHC. The first one being the inter- and intratumoral heterogeneity of PD-L1 expression within tumors. PD-L1 expression in tumors has been found preferentially at the tumor surface in proximity to the immune interface and is regulated by both oncogenic and inflammatory signals, highlighting the variability and expression among different tumor types [71]. An increasing number of oncogenic signaling pathways regulating PD-L1 have been identified, such as AKT, PTEN, JAK/STAT, EGFR, MAPK, transcriptional factors (i.e., NF-kB), and epigenetic factors, which are now having an impact in the choice of combination therapies being tested to increase responses to immune checkpoint agents [57, 74]. Another route is through the inflammatory induction of PD-L1 via IFN-γ, which can also vary during disease progression and treatment [16]. Adding to this complexity is the knowledge that not only tumor cells express PD-L1 on their surface but also immune cells, as well as stromal cells, which can be inducible as well as transient, increasing the heterogeneity of the tumor microenvironment [57]. Another factor to take into account is the potential discordance of PD-L1 expression between primary and metastatic tumor sites, which has been described previously [75], which along with the above data highlights the inadequacy of a single temporal evaluation of PD-L1 status of a tumor in making therapeutic decisions. Overall, the variability in expression of PD-L1 makes a particular cutoff for positivity of the assay increasingly challenging and likely explains why no studies have reported a positive or negative predictive value approaching 100% to date.

Although the PD-L1 assay can be useful and is of value in stratifying patients for treatment with an immune checkpoint agent, especially in lung cancer, because of a number of both technical and biologic issues with this assay it is still not a reliable independent predictive biomarker of response to either monotherapy or combination immune checkpoint therapy. Further studies are needed to better understand its intricacies and the addition of other biomarkers will be useful to shedding more light on this issue.

3.3.1.14 Efforts at Harmonizing the Different PD-L1 Biomarkers

More recently, efforts from the scientific community are being made to harmonize these different PD-L1 assays in an attempt at standardization of the biomarker. For instance, the International Association for the Study of Lung Cancer has spearheaded the "BluePrint PD-L1 IHC Assay Comparison Project" in order to shed much needed light on how these assays compare with one another in NSCLC [76, 77]. A recent report of the first phase of this project assessed the clinical performance of the PD-L1 assay by staining 39 NSCLC tumors with four PD-L1 IHC assays (22C3, 28–8, SP142, and SP263) after which independent interpretation of the assays was done by 3 different experts and comparison of results was made [77].

These analytical comparisons showed that the percentage of PD-L1-stained tumor cells was similar in the 22C3, 28–8, and SP263, but not the SP142 assay, which had fewer stained tumor cells overall. Although all assays expressed PD-L1 in the immune cells, there was greater variability in immune cell staining of PD-L1 throughout all four assays, perhaps due to lack of training or alignment on scoring of IC. In 19 of 38 cases or 50%, there was agreement with all four assays regardless of which matched assay cutoff was employed, and these 50% were identified as above the selected cutoffs. There were five cases or 13% identified as below the selected cutoffs for all the assays, with various levels of overlapping agreement between assays for the specified cutoff. Interestingly, for 37% of cases, another PD-L1 classification would have been made depending on the assay or scoring system which was used. The study concluded that in spite of the similarities in performance among 3/4 assays, these were not interchangeable assays, and the appropriate companion diagnostic assays must be used for each drug/company until there is better understanding of these four assays.

3.3.2 The Tumor Immune Cell Landscape

3.3.2.1 TILS: Clinical Applications as a Prognostic and Predictive Biomarker

Retrospective population studies of thousands of tumors have shown that a type I immune response (or T helper 1, Th1) is essential for clinically successful antitumor immunity against cancer [78]. This response involves a distinct immune infiltrate consisting of a high density of infiltrating T cells (i.e., CD8 and memory cells) and a low density of regulatory cells (i.e., Treg, Th2, myeloid-derived suppressor cell, MDSC). The presence of these immune cells in or around the tumor milieu, or tumor-infiltrating lymphocytes (TILs), specifically the type I or Th1 T cells, was associated with improved survival in cancer patients across multiple tumor histologies, regardless of stage, burden of disease, populational risk factors, or even treatments rendered [79–91]. In colorectal cancer, Pages et al. demonstrated that a high density of CD45RO+ memory T cells was an independent predictor of increased overall survival with a 5-year survival and disease-free survival of 46.3% and 43.1% compared to 23.7% and 21.5% in the low density infiltrate group [92]. In this same cohort of patients, Galon et al. showed that stratification by immune cell type, density, and location were a superior predictor of survival when compared to traditional histologic tumor-node-metastasis (TNM) staging [93]. Additional studies also showed the correlation between the immune profile, the primary tumor microenvironment, and decreased findings of metastatic disease for patients with increased innate immune cells (macrophages, dendritic cells, and NK cells) and activated CD4+ T cells [94].

Additional studies evaluating the location of TILs within or around a tumor are also of prognostic significance. For instance, data from the BIG 02–98 clinical trial in 2009 breast cancer patients which tested the addition of docetaxel to doxorubicin-based adjuvant chemotherapy for lymph node-positive breast cancer showed that TILs were prognostic of improved survival when found in the stromal compartment, but not within the tumor of patients who were HER-2+ [85]. The study also found a strong association with improved survival in triple-negative breast cancer (TNBC) patients irrespective of location, but no prognostic association of ER+ breast cancer and TILs, regardless of location. This evidence attests to what's believed to be a higher immunologic activity of TNBC compared to other subtypes of breast cancer and has been explored in several trials of immune checkpoint inhibitors [40, 95].

Furthermore, studies on the clinical utility of specific TIL cutoffs in early stage breast cancer have been done to hopefully identify a TIL cutoff that defines a node-negative subgroup with an excellent outcome who could potentially be spared or given shorter adjuvant chemotherapy [90]. In a retrospective study, for instance, Kaplan-Meyer survival curves for the prognostic value of stromal TILs was reported across three nodal categories of TNBC patients (node negative, N1-3 and >3), and across all data sets, a value of stromal TILs > or 20% signified distinctly improved outcomes in this population [96]. The best prognostic group, those who were node negative with stromal TILs ≥20%, had an estimated 5-year survival of 92%.

The urgent need for clinical TIL criteria was the driving force behind the work of Galon and Pages et al. in addition to several other contributing researchers to the development of "Immunoscore" [97–100]. The goal of the Immunoscore was to harmonize the two lymphocyte populations (CD3/CD8, or CD3/CD45RO, or CD8/CD45RO), both in the core of the tumor and the invasive margin of the tumor, to establish prognosis of clinical outcome in patients. As previously discussed, this scoring system had the potential to provide a prognostic value that may be superior to the AJCC/UICC TNM-classification [98].

Unfortunately, not all data on the topic of TILs is fully consistent, and although TILs can be prognostic of improved survival in breast cancer, they were found to be predictive of pathologic complete response to neoadjuvant chemotherapy only in the HER-2 positive population [81]. In a multivariable analysis adjusted for clinico-pathologic parameters, these lymphocyte predominant tumors (>50% intratumoral TILs) was an independent predictor of pCR. Having a rich lymphocytic infiltrate in the tumor leads to path CR in over 75% of patients receiving carboplatin in addition to standard neoadjuvant chemotherapy in those with HER-2-positive disease only, not TNBC. Similar results were found in the FinHER trial of 1010 early stage TNBC and HER-2+ breast cancer patients, whereby higher levels of TILs at diagnosis were prognostic of improved outcomes in the TNBC group, but only in the HER-2+ group was TILs predictive, with trastuzumab significantly associated with decreased risk of recurrence in HER-2+ patients with high levels of TILs [84]. Analyzing this data together, we can see a strong correlation of baseline levels of TILs as a prognostic marker in several subtypes of breast cancer, specifically TNBC. These findings demonstrate how the clinical use of TILs may be extremely context specific.

Additional concerns with TILs have been identified by Curtis et al. who point out several areas of nonconsensus with TIL evaluation such as what parts of a tumor should be assessed for TILs and if multiple sites would need to be performed to compensate for tumor heterogeneity. They also bring up statistical analysis questions such as whether TIL criteria would be a product of considering TIL data as ordinal data through the use of quantile categories which was employed by Nosho et al. vs. TIL data as a continuous variable which was used by Laghi et al. in demonstrating that higher CD3+ TIL density at the invasive tumor margin correlates with decreased risk of metastasis [101, 102].

Although baseline TIL status has been validated as a prognostic marker of improved survival and can be a valuable predictive biomarker for immune checkpoint inhibitor therapy, it has not yet been prospectively validated as a predictive biomarker. Despite the efforts of groups such as the Society for Immunotherapy of Cancer to promote consensus immune profiling in routine histologic analysis, such methods have not entered pathologic practice. In the future, this will likely change as additional studies demonstrate the utility of the prognostic utility of TILs.

3.3.2.2 Dendritic Cells

Infiltrating DCs, which act as APCs, have been shown to be defective by several mechanisms in cancer. Molecular mediators such as VEGF have been shown to impair DC maturation in numerous experimental models which could potentially affect response to immunotherapy [103]. Signaling mediators such as IL-6 and colony-stimulating factor 1 affect monocyte maturation away from DCs in favor of macrophages which theoretically dampen the adaptive immune response [104]. The effect of these mechanisms on clinical outcomes in cancer is still under investigation.

3.3.2.3 Macrophages

Tumor-associated macrophages (TAMs) are among the most abundant immune cells within the tumor core and surrounding the invasive margins. Macrophages are typically classified as having the phenotypes M1 (pro-inflammatory) vs. M2 (anti-inflammatory and tissue regeneration). In the case of TAMs, the molecular signatures for both phenotypes can be displayed but typically skews toward an M2 phenotype for pro-tumoral effects and an M1 phenotype for antitumor [105]. In general most clinical data supports TAMs as having a pro-tumor effect [106]. Correlation of increased TMA infiltration with poor prognosis or more aggressive disease has been observed in almost all cancer types including NSCLC, gastric, oral, ovarian, breast, prostate, and bladder [107–112]. However, studies also demonstrate TAMs associated with a favorable prognosis in some of the same disease types including NSCLC where M1-like TAMs show a positive effect on survival [113]. For clinical utility, the nonspecificity of M1/M2 markers coupled with phenotypic overlap of TAMs is problematic. Therefore, although the association of M2-like TAMs is well supported by studies, clinical adoption or guidelines will require more definitive identification methods.

3.3.2.4 B Cells

Studies of B cells in tumor immunology have continuously shown conflicting results supporting both pro and antitumor associations. In CRC, Barbera-Guillem et al. demonstrated in a small group of patients that treatment with anti-CD20 (rituximab) reduced tumor burden in half the patients treated [114]. Mouse model studies have also demonstrated antitumor immune effects with B=cell depletion. Afffara et al. treated a transgenic de novo SCC mouse model with rituximab and found synergistic effects when combined with chemotherapy that resulted in tumor reduction, increased T-cell infiltration, and macrophage phenotype switching [115]. However, B-cell depletion has also been associated with pro-tumorigenic effects. Using a mouse melanoma model treated with a mouse anti-CD20 antibody, DiLillo et al. demonstrated that B-cell depletion resulted in impaired T-cell activation and enhanced tumor growth [116]. There are many more studies supporting both effects for B cells and clearly represent an area requiring further investigation.

3.3.2.5 NK Cells

NK cells recognize and kill tumor cells through a number of well-established mechanisms. Increased NK cell infiltration has been associated with improved clinical outcomes in a number of different cancers including CRC, gastric, and NSCLC [117–119]. NK cell studies, however, suffer from nonspecific markers and varying phenotypic criteria used in clinical studies making conclusions difficult to interpret. In NSCLC, NK cells have also been shown to have no association with clinical outcomes [120]. As is the case with B cells, such discrepancies highlight the need for further investigation.

3.3.2.6 Myeloid-Derived Suppressor Cells

MDSCs produce an array of molecules capable of inhibiting CD8+ T cells, DCs, and NKs, and stimulating Tregs creating a pro-tumor microenvironment [121, 122]. Despite their biologic importance, evaluating MDSCs in tumors is technically challenging due to their complex and diverse immunophenotype which has precluded significant clinical evaluation.

3.4 Mismatch Repair Status, Mutation Burden, and Neoantigens

Mismatch repair status, mutational burden, and neoantigenicity are all related elements that exist along a continuum leading to immune activation and response to immunotherapy. The interconnection between these elements is shown in figure (x), which shows the relation of MMR status to the frequency of mutations in a tumor, and then finally to the translation of those mutations into antigens that can elicit an immune response. In the next several sections, each of these elements will be discussed in detail in order to fully explain the underlying biology and potential function as immunotherapy biomarkers.

3.5 Mismatch Repair and Microsatellite Instability

Mismatch repair (MMR) genes function to eliminate base-base mismatches and insertion-deletion loops that arise during DNA replication. Loss of function of these genes, known as MMR deficiency (MMR-D), leads to single base substitutions in non-repetitive DNA and insertion-deletion loops that affect repetitive DNA. The former results in a high frequency of somatic variants leading to hypermutated tumors with 10–100 variants/Mb, also referred to as a mutator phenotype [123]. The latter involves gains and losses of short repeat units within microsatellites referred to as microsatellite instability [124]. Germline mutations in the MMR genes MLH1, MSH2, MSH6, and PMS2 followed by somatic inactivation of the remaining wild-type allele result in Lynch syndrome (LS) or hereditary nonpolyposis colorectal cancer (HNPCC) which accounts for 5% of all colorectal cancers and a significant increased risk of ovarian and endometrial cancer [125–127]. LS is most commonly caused by loss of MLH1 or MSH2 through deletion or point mutation and less commonly from mutation of MSH6 or PMS2. MSH2 function can also be effected through hypermethylation secondary to deletion of the EPCAM gene which is immediately upstream on chromosome 2 and leads to transcriptional suppression. Classical LS however with germline inheritance only explains a subset of patients with both sporadic colon cancer and other cancers that show MMR deficiency and subsequent development of MSI. In colon cancer, biallelic hypermethylation of the promotor region of MLH1 leading to loss of MLH1 transcription and MMR deficiency accounts for 15% of all sporadic colorectal cancer [128]. This pathway is linked to BRAFV600E mutations facilitating high levels of CpG island methylation leading to the CpG island methylator phenotype (CIMP) [129]. Review of the TCGA shows that 16% of colorectal cancers were hypermutated, and the majority of which showed MSI positivity with MLH1 methylation CIMP occurring in the majority of cases [130]. An additional subset of MMR-D/MSI+ patients exist which do not carry MLH1 methylation; in these cases the majority had mutations in POLE/POLD1 genes [131]. POLE/POLD1 mutations can also occur in MSS tumors highlighting the importance of extended genetic testing in suspected patients.

3.6 MMR and MSI Testing Methods

Assessment of MMR and MSI status in the context of colorectal and endometrial cancer has become a common practice given the role in screening for LS and the prognostic value the tests have for chemotherapy and immunotherapy [132, 133]. For MMR assessment, testing can be done using immunohistochemistry during routine pathologic workup with deficiency being classified as lack of expression of any one of the MMR proteins MLH1, MSH2, MSH6, and PMS2 [134]. MSI testing utilizes a multiplex PCR-based assay that amplifies microsatellite markers that consist of mono- and dinucleotide repeats. The NCI/International Collaborative Group-HNPCC has recommended a standard MSI panel that includes BAT26, BAT25, D2S123, D5S346, and D17S250; however, investigators have developed custom panels that may improve on sensitivity or are more applicable to certain demographics [135]. Recently, bioinformatics methods have been developed to identify MSI status from NGS data [136, 137]. Hall et al. in collaboration with Foundation Medicine (FM) developed a novel method to accurately identify MSI status utilizing FM's targeted gene panel [138]. Given the increased use of targeting sequencing in the clinical setting, assessment of MSI status by these methods will surely increase.

Interpretation of MSI is divided into three groups, MSI-high (MSI-H), MSI-low (MSI-L), and MSI-stable (MSS). The importance of MSI-L however is not entirely clear with observed mutations potentially representing background genetic instability in normal and cancerous cells [139]. Therefore, the classification of MSI is routinely limited to MSI+ or MSI− [140]. In the meta-analysis of 7,642 CRC patients that contained 1,277 MSI+ patients, Popat et al. demonstrated that MSI+ was associated with a significant improvement in overall survival [141]. The combined HR estimated associated with MSI was 0.65 (95% CI, 0.59–0.71). This benefit was maintained after restricting analyses to clinical trial patients (HR = 0.69; 95% CI, 0.56–0.85) and patients with locally advanced CRC (HR = 0.67; 95% CI, 0.58–0.78). In patients treated with adjuvant fluorouracil (FU), CRCs with MSI had a better prognosis (HR = 0.72; 95% CI, 0.61–0.84). CRC tumors that are MMR-D/MSI+ show an increased number of tumor-infiltrating lymphocytes and a marked shift in T-cell profile toward activated and cytotoxic phenotype [142]. Interestingly in EC, MSI status did not correlate with a specific T-cell immune profile [143]. Additionally, the prognostic significance of MSI status in EC is not clear with reports indicating a range of findings from increased survival, no difference, and worse prognosis [143–146]. Other cancers known to have MS instability include urogenital, cutaneous, sarcomas, and ovarian cancer although the clinical significance, particularly in relation to tumor immune response, is unclear [147–150].

3.7 Effect of MMR and MSI on Immunotherapy

With the advent of immunotherapy agents such as checkpoint inhibitors, the clinical implication of MMR-D and MSI+ has become increasingly important. In CRC patients being treated with pembrolizumab, Le et al. found an immune-related progression-free survival rate of 40% (four out of ten patients; 95% confidence interval [CI 12–74) at 20 weeks in patients with MMR-D vs. 0% (95% CI, 0–20) at 20 weeks in patients with MMR-P [133]. Additionally, in non-CRC patients that were MMR-D which included ampullary, endometrial, gastric, and biliary tumors, immune-related progression-free survival at 20 weeks was 78% (CI, 40–97). CD8-positive lymphoid infiltrate was increased in both the CRC and non-CRC MMR-D patients compared to the MMR-P CRC patients consistent with immune cell findings from previous mentioned studies.

3.7.1 Mutational Burden and Neoantigens

The concept that tumors of non-viral origin contain "neoantigens" recognizable by the immune system dates back to the 1940s and 1950s. These initial studies showed that inbred mice with carcinogen-induced tumors postsurgical resection were immune to future challenges by those resected tumor cells but not by other tumor cells created using the same carcinogenic model insinuating that the mice had developed immunity to a specific tumor antigen [151, 152]. The second half the century then focused on elucidating the specific mechanism for how neoantigens are generated. Schieber et al. were one of the first to show a direct link that a tumor-specific mutation could function as a tumor neoantigen [153]. During this same period in time, Knuth and the Rosenberg group showed that ex-vivo peripheral blood from patients with melanoma were reactive with melanoma cells in vitro but not normal cells suggesting that cancers possessed tumor-specific antigens [154, 155].

Subsequent work by Boon et al. and Sachin et al. in the development of methodologies for cloning and characterizing tumor antigens led to the understanding that tumor antigens were created through multiple mechanisms including tumor-specific mutant genes, alternative splicing, normal proteins with aberrant quantitative or qualitative expression in tumor cells, and proteins only expressed in germ cells and tumor cells [156–158]. Therefore, neoantigens or tumor-specific antigens (TSAs) comprise a subset of total tumor antigens which includes tumor-associated antigens (TAAs) and cancer germline/cancer-testis antigens (CTAs).

3.7.2 Neoantigens

The general understanding that tumors which contain a proportionally high number of mutations or genomic instability demonstrate tissue-specific immune effects has been empirically understood in the medical community for some time as discussed in the MMR/MSI section. However, it wasn't until the watershed work by the TCGA demonstrating the mutational landscape across all cancers that the concept of mutational burden and the cancer genome truly began to enter common medical knowledge. Initial in silico studies by Allison and Vogelstein et al. demonstrated the ability to predict tumor-specific mutant antigens [159]. Later work by Schumacher et al. using exome sequencing and high-throughput MHC tetrameter screening of T cells from patients with melanoma showed that checkpoint blockade immunotherapy with anti-CTLA facilitated the expansion of preexisting T cells specific for tumor neoantigens [160]. Recently, Rizvi and Chan demonstrated in lung cancer patients treated with anti-PD1 therapy that a high non-synonymous mutational load based on WES correlated with increased durable clinical benefit (DCB) and progression-free survival (PFS) [161]. This relationship has also been demonstrated in patients with melanoma being treated with anti-CTLA-4 therapy [162]. Interestingly though, in both studies, there are patients with high mutational burdens who do not respond to therapy along with patients who have low mutational burden that do respond to therapy. The explanation for these findings, which has tangentially been discussed so far, is that not all mutations create equivocally antigenic products.

The creation of a neoantigen occurs through a three-step process. The first step is the actual point mutation, deletion, insertion, or rearrangement resulting in an altered protein. Next, that protein must be processed into a peptide capable of binding to an MHC molecule, and finally that peptide must be presented to a T-cell receptor (TCR) that binds to an epitope on the peptide. Because of the multiple steps in this process, a cancer mutation can produce a neoantigen through several mechanisms. The most well understood is that a cancer mutation can create a de novo peptide capable of binding to an MHC molecule and TCR, but other mechanisms include a mutation that results in a new TCR contact site for a peptide already recognized by an MHC molecule and the introduction of a proteasomal cleavage site enabling more efficient processing of a potential neoantigen peptide [163]. The intracellular processing of peptides also occurs by different mechanisms depending on MHC class. Peptides processed through MHC class I interact with CD8+ T cells vs. processing for MHC class II is coupled with CD4+ T cells resulting in different neoantigen products from the same peptides [163, 164]. Additionally, since there are three to six HLA molecules for class I and class II in each person, any given mutation can result in multiple epitopes capable of bind to an HLA molecule. It's also important to note that a genes function or impact on oncogenic transformation appears to be unrelated to whether that gene will form a neoantigen [165]. However, driver mutations capable of neoantigenicity have been identified as CD8+ TILs in a colon cancer patient that were reactive against the mutation KRAS G12D [166].

3.7.3 *Neoantigenicity Prediction Methods*

Computational models for neoantigen predication have been designed to assess antigen processing, peptide transport, and peptide binding to MHC-I. Of these approaches, prediction of peptide binding to MHC-I has received the most attention. This method is accomplished by performing WES on a patient's tumor followed by mapping which potential −8 to −11 residue peptides will bind to the patient's HLA sequence [167, 168]. This type of analysis has been utilized in the clinical context to predict response to checkpoint inhibitors [160, 161]. In general, however, these approaches are still very much a technology in development [163]. Improvement in these in silico methods will require overcoming confounding factors such as sequencing errors along with the integration of other types of data including eluted peptides from MHCs identified by mass spectrometry. The Tumor Neoantigen Selection Alliance (TESLA) is currently addressing these challenges through large-scale data sharing. Lastly, it is important to note that these methods are currently designed to use WES data which is what Rizvi et al. utilized to demonstrate mutational burden correlated with predicted tumor neoantigenicity [161]. In clinical practice, tumors are almost always sequenced using targeted panels, which may complicate the application of antigenicity methods. Although as sequencing costs continue to fall, WES may become more common in the clinical setting.

3.7.4 *Tumor Mutational Burden*

The issue of translating WES clinical research data to panel sequencing was until recently also a major question for the application of TMB for routine clinical use. With WES, TMB can be calculated as an absolute number, but for panel sequencing, it must be converted into the frequency metric mutations per megabase (mut/Mb). Frampton et al. analyzed over 60,000 clinical cancer patients across all tumor types using Foundation Medicines comprehensive genomic profiling assay (FM-CGP) and created a mutational burden algorithm that removes germline polymorphisms and functional variants in order to normalize the results. They then tested this pipeline against 7,000 WES patient samples in TCGA and demonstrated significant correlation [169]. In the IMvigor trial, Hoffman-Censits et al. demonstrated similar correlation of mutational load in bladder cancer when comparing FM-CGP to WES [170]. They also showed, when stratifying mutational load by quartiles, patients with the highest TMB had superior response to anti-PD1 therapy with atezolizumab regardless of concurrent treatment with platinum-based chemo. Campesato et al. reanalyzed WES data from melanoma patients' [162] and NSCLC patients' [161] WES data using the genes listed in FM-CGP along with their in-house targeted panel to assess how TMB extrapolation applies to therapeutic response [171]. For the NSCLC patients who had received anti-PD1 therapy, both panel sequencing predictions of TMB correlated with what was shown using WES. In the melanoma patients who received anti-CTLA4, panel sequencing TMB did not show association with response to therapy. In pancreatic cancer, George et al. using FM-CGP demonstrated that TMB as opposed to MSI assessment alone significantly increased the number of patients with metastatic CRC who could benefit from checkpoint inhibitors [172].

Clearly, the use of TMB for therapeutic prediction is an area that requires further investigation. Establishing numerical classifications for TMB will require significant efforts to identify specific TMB criteria for a given tumor and associated immunotherapy. This will become increasingly more difficult as immunotherapies are given in combination such as in melanoma with anti-CTLA4 plus ant-PD1. Another issue to consider related to the interpretation of TMB is the age of the sample being sequenced in the context of when a treatment decision is made. Because of the invasiveness and risk of biopsy procedures, CGP assays are not infrequently performed on samples older than 1 year and posttreatment with DNA damaging/promutagenic therapies. This difference in time means that for some cases, TMB will be underestimated. However, given that the occurrence of a mutation is a stochastic process rather than a linear relationship amendable to extrapolation, attempting to adjust or estimate the effect of time on mutation burden would be difficult and likely inherently flawed [173]. All of these variables together reinforce the importance that clinicians utilize TMB and eventually neoantigenicity metrics within a patient's clinicopathologic context of disease and therapeutic options.

3.7.5 Tumor Microenvironment and Immune Pathway Profiling

The complex molecular relationship between tumor cells and their surrounding environment provides a wealth of potential biomarkers. Genomic, transcriptomic, and proteomic analysis methods offer potential solutions to this complexity by allowing a global assessment from a single assay that can be used to predict metrics such as immune cell infiltration, tumor subtyping, pathway analysis for biologic signatures such as hypoxia or inflammation, and therapeutic prediction algorithms. In the clinical context, all of these applications are in the early phase of development but are worth discussing given their potential impact.

3.7.6 T-Cell Receptor Sequencing

In the context of immunotherapy and oncology, TCR sequencing can to some degree be seen as a convergence of TIL and neoantigen assessment because it provides further resolution into the immune profile while also providing sequence specific information. TCRs consist of a heterodimer of two chains (αβ or γδ) which both undergo somatic recombination of the variable (V), diversity (D), and joining (J) gene segments in addition to addition/subtraction of bases at recombination junctions [174]. This process is analogous to the generation of antibody diversity by somatic recombination of the B-cell receptor locus [175]. The most variable region in the TCR is CDR3 which plays a critical role in antigen recognition. The most abundant T cells in the immune system and the most relevant to cancer immunology are the αβ subtype; therefore the common strategy for TCR profiling involves amplification of the β chain CDR3 locus using predesigned PCR primers followed by deep sequencing [176, 177]. This target TCR sequencing method has been utilized in several clinical applications through use of Adaptive Biotechnologies ImmunoSEQ assay (IS). Tumeh et al. demonstrated in melanoma patients treated with anti-PD-1 therapy that responders showed significant proliferation of preexisting clones posttreatment [178]. Another important finding was that several responders demonstrated high TIL clonality but had an overall low TIL infiltrate count. This finding highlights some of the ambiguity surrounding the use of TIL counts especially if used in isolation. Prins et al. used the assay in GBM patients being treated with a dendritic cell vaccine to show that TCR increased overlap between the tumor and peripheral blood correlated with improved survival [179]. The utility of peripheral blood for TCR sequencing however is not clear. As Page et al. demonstrated in their evaluation of tumor TILs and peripheral blood T cells in breast cancer patients post cryotherapy and anti-CTLA4, the TCR repertoire landscape was independent for intratumoral and peripheral T cells regardless of the degree of intratumoral expansion [180]. Therefore, the use of TCR sequencing from the periphal blood as potential response markers is still unclear at this time. Another important conclusion from their study was the demonstration that a T-cell density metric derived from TCR sequencing of breast core biopsies correlated with TIL counts performed by manual histologic assessment. This finding may be clinically significant because TCR sequencing could provide the uniformity that can be difficult to achieve by manual histologic evaluation. It also allows for TIL evaluation on biopsy samples which given their small size makes histologic evaluation limited. A potential logistical issue for TCR sequencing is that these types of specialized assays could be difficult to utilize in a clinical setting given that the most extensive type of molecular testing typically performed is targeted DNA panel sequencing. This situation is however ripe for change.

As NGS technologies improve, the feasibility and clinical potential of RNA sequencing are rapidly emerging [181, 182]. For TCR sequencing, the clinical adoption of RNA sequencing could be a significant development. The technical limitation is that compared to TCR-seq assays, RNA-seq data results in a disproportionally large number of non-TCR transcripts making clonal identification potentially problematic. Brown et al. compared conventional TCR-seq to RNA-seq data using a novel informatics pipeline to identify unique CDR3β sequences [177]. They found that all high-confidence CDR3β sequences by RNA-seq fell within the top 2.1% of CDR3βs detected by TCR-seq when ranked by abundance. This finding is significant for demonstrating that RNA-seq has the potential to identify the most abundant CDR3β transcripts. Whether or not any of these TCR analysis methods will make it into routine clinical care is unclear. In the current state, they will primarily be used in clinical trial research setting to assess effects of immunotherapies on TILs and peripheral T cells but as sequencing costs continue to fall, the landscape could change.

3.8 Immune Pathway Alterations

Immune suppression can occur via tumor cell intrinsic mechanisms and through interactions with the tumor microenvironment. Recently, Gao et al. demonstrated that tumors lacking copies of interferon pathway-related genes were more likely to not respond to treatment with aCTLA-4 [183]. Using this gene profile, they were able to externally validate the findings in an independent melanoma data set demonstrating the clinical potential of this approach. Relatedly, Shin et al. found that homozygous alteration in JAK2 resulted in the lack of response to aPD-1 therapy. The group demonstrated through in vitro models that the JAK2 alterations led to decreased response to interferons. Currently, JAK2 is covered on most targeted sequencing gene panels [184]. Tumor cell copy number alterations can also be used in a more general capacity to assess antitumor immune response. Davoli et al. evaluated tumor aneuploidy or somatic copy number alterations (SCNA) in TCGA patients and found that tumors with high SCNA levels correlated with a decreased immune signature and increased cell cycle proliferation signature. High SCNA levels also correlated with poorer patient survival. Low SCNA levels demonstrated an inverse effect. These results demonstrate the potential importance of understanding aneuploidy in solid tumors. However, given that targeted panel sequencing is not amenable for SCNA assessment, it is unclear what will be the clinical applicability of these findings.

3.8.1 Immune Cell Infiltrate Prediction Models

Computational methods to deconvolute cell fractions from gene expression profiles (GEPs) have recently been demonstrated to predict cell type-specific contributions from complex tissues [185, 186]. Building off of this concept, Newman et al.'s method was called Cell-type Identification By Estimating Relative Subsets of RNA Transcripts (CIBERSORT), which allows for the resolution of relative fractions of diverse cell subsets in GEPs from complex tissue [187]. By applying CIBERSORT to a GEP metadata set, they were able to demonstrate the ability to identify immune cell subsets associated with prognosis in breast and lung cancer [188]. These approaches may prove to be clinically useful if evidence continues to demonstrate that immune infiltrate hold predictive value as discussed in the immune cell landscape section. Performing this type of profiling by traditional immunohistochemistry methods would create several potential challenges. It would require the use of many tissue sections that could potentially exhaust the material for smaller tissue biopsies. Additionally, quantitation of multiple types of immune cells would be highly operator dependent and unreliable. GEP-based methods would also be prone to sample variability, but the automated process has significant benefits.

3.8.2 Tumor Subtyping and Therapeutic Prediction

The use of expression profiling for tumor subtyping has demonstrated clinical utility. In diffuse large B-cell lymphoma and breast cancer, such expression-related profiles have developed into classification schema that can be used for prognostic and therapeutic prediction [189]. In the context of immune-oncology, such classification methods are in the first phases of development. Using metastatic urothelial cancer subtypes derived from GEP data, Rosenberg et al. identified overlapping microenvironment immune signatures [170, 190]. Coupling the urothelial subtypes with the immune signatures, the group demonstrated that basal type mUC showed an immune suppressed profile with limited response to anti-PD1 therapy. Luminal subtypes showed differential results with type I papillary-like having a profile lacking immune cells and having a limited response to therapy, while type II showed an inflamed profile with good response to therapy.

GEP analysis of immune-related genes has been shown to be useful at identifying markers predictive of response to immunotherapy [35]. Extending this concept, Hugo et al. identified a transcriptional signature they refer to as the innate anti-PD-1 resistance signature (IPRES) which they validated across distinct cancer histologies [191]. The IPRES signature was not predictive of response to anti-CTLA4 treatment suggesting that the underlying biology for therapeutic response is different between immunotherapies.

Proteomic analysis with mass spectrometry (MS) is another method that can provide a comprehensive view of various molecular features. Using a novel MS method called "deep MALDI" on serum samples from NSCLC patients pre- and posttreatment with anti-PD1 therapy, Weber et al. demonstrated that they could stratify patients by response [192].

3.8.3 Host and Germline Biomarkers

The significance of host factors on immunotherapy response is a relatively new area of research in immune-oncology. Environmental exposure to infectious disease can modulate the immune system with downstream effects [193]. Chronic cytomegalovirus infection (CMV) can lead to consumption of memory T cells diminishing the immune system's ability to respond to new antigens [194]. Intestinal flora is another factor that in systemic immune changes can affect antitumor immune responses. Sivan et al. showed in a mouse model that the amount of the bacteria *Bifidobacterium* was directly correlated with the efficacy of anti-PD1 therapy [195]. There are a number of potential strategies for altering the microbiome: antibiotics, probiotics, prebiotics (nondigestible compounds that modulate microbiome), and postbiotics (nonviable products made by microbiome that alter host immune system) [196]. How such strategies can be implemented to optimize response to immune therapies and chemotherapy or radiation will be an interesting area of research in the coming year [150].

3.9 Conclusion

As immunotherapy moves farther into the twenty-first century, continued development of predictive biomarkers will be imperative to ensure that the right patients are selected or excluded to receive these therapies. At this moment, PD-L1 expression seems to be the only FDA-approved biomarker for selection in the setting of first-line therapy for NSCLC.

As evidence of hyperprogression after anti-PD1 therapy continues to emerge, identifying nonresponders will likely become a more focused effort particularly on the basic science front [197]. Key in this effort will be the integration of multiple testing methods relevant to understanding a patient's immune landscape. As has been detailed in the sections of this chapter, there are many different types of immunologic data that can provide insight into how a patient may respond to immunotherapy.

References

1. Ma W et al (2016) Current status and perspectives in translational biomarker research for PD-1/PD-L1 immune checkpoint blockade therapy. J Hematol Oncol 9(1):47
2. Henry NL, Hayes DF (2012) Cancer biomarkers. Mol Oncol 6(2):140–146
3. National cancer institute. http://www.cancer.gov/dictionary?CdrID=45618. 12/28/2016
4. Paik S et al (2004) A multigene assay to predict recurrence of tamoxifen-treated, node-negative breast cancer. N Engl J Med 351(27):2817–2826
5. van't Veer LJ, Paik S, Hayes DF (2005) Gene expression profiling of breast cancer: a new tumor marker. J Clin Oncol 23(8):1631–1635
6. Cohen SJ et al (2008) Relationship of circulating tumor cells to tumor response, progression-free survival, and overall survival in patients with metastatic colorectal cancer. J Clin Oncol 26(19):3213–3221
7. Cristofanilli M et al (2004) Circulating tumor cells, disease progression, and survival in metastatic breast cancer. N Engl J Med 351(8):781–791
8. Goldkorn A et al (2014) Circulating tumor cell counts are prognostic of overall survival in SWOG S0421: a phase III trial of docetaxel with or without atrasentan for metastatic castration-resistant prostate cancer. J Clin Oncol 32(11):1136–1142
9. Allegra CJ et al (2009) American Society of Clinical Oncology provisional clinical opinion: testing for KRAS gene mutations in patients with metastatic colorectal carcinoma to predict response to anti-epidermal growth factor receptor monoclonal antibody therapy. J Clin Oncol 27(12):2091–2096
10. Bang YJ et al (2010) Trastuzumab in combination with chemotherapy versus chemotherapy alone for treatment of HER2-positive advanced gastric or gastro-oesophageal junction cancer (ToGA): a phase 3, open-label, randomised controlled trial. Lancet 376(9742):687–697
11. Piccart-Gebhart MJ et al (2005) Trastuzumab after adjuvant chemotherapy in HER2-positive breast cancer. N Engl J Med 353(16):1659–1672
12. Romond EH et al (2005) Trastuzumab plus adjuvant chemotherapy for operable HER2-positive breast cancer. N Engl J Med 353(16):1673–1684
13. Chen DS, Mellman I (2013) Oncology meets immunology: the cancer-immunity cycle. Immunity 39(1):1–10
14. Ceeraz S, Nowak EC, Noelle RJ (2013) B7 family checkpoint regulators in immune regulation and disease. Trends Immunol 34(11):556–563
15. Sugamura K, Ishii N, Weinberg AD (2004) Therapeutic targeting of the effector T-cell co-stimulatory molecule OX40. Nat Rev Immunol 4(6):420–431
16. Sharpe AH et al (2007) The function of programmed cell death 1 and its ligands in regulating autoimmunity and infection. Nat Immunol 8(3):239–245
17. Latchman Y et al (2001) PD-L2 is a second ligand for PD-1 and inhibits T cell activation. Nat Immunol 2(3):261–268
18. Herbst RS, Gordon MS, Fine GD, Sosman JA, Soria J-C, Hamid O, Powderly JD, Burris HA, Mokatrin A, Kowanetz M et al (2013) A study of MPDL3280A, an engineered PD-L1 antibody in patients with locally advanced or metastatic tumors. Journal of Clinical Oncology 31:3000
19. Pardoll DM (2012) The blockade of immune checkpoints in cancer immunotherapy. Nat Rev Cancer 12(4):252–264
20. Ansell SM et al (2015) PD-1 blockade with nivolumab in relapsed or refractory Hodgkin's lymphoma. N Engl J Med 372(4):311–319
21. Antonia S et al (2016) Safety and antitumour activity of durvalumab plus tremelimumab in non-small cell lung cancer: a multicentre, phase 1b study. Lancet Oncol 17(3):299–308

22. Barlesi F, Park K, Ciardello J et al (2016) Primary analysis from OAK, a randomized phase III study comparing atezolizumab with docetaxel in 2L/3L NSCLC. in ESMO. Copenhagen
23. Bellmunt J et al (2017) Pembrolizumab as second-line therapy for advanced Urothelial carcinoma. N Engl J Med 376(11):1015–1026
24. Besse B, Johnson M, Jänne P et al (2015) Phase II, single-arm trial (BIRCH) of atezolizumab as first-line or subsequent therapy for locally advanced or metastatic PD-L1- selected non-small cell lung cancer (NSCLC). in European cancer congress 2015. Vienna, Austria: abstract 16LBA
25. Borghaei H et al (2015) Nivolumab versus Docetaxel in advanced nonsquamous non-small-cell lung cancer. N Engl J Med 373(17):1627–1639
26. Brahmer J et al (2015) Nivolumab versus Docetaxel in advanced squamous-cell non-small-cell lung cancer. N Engl J Med 373(2):123–135
27. Daud A, Blank CU, Robert C et al (2016) KEYNOTE-006 study of pembrolizumab (pembro) versus ipilimumab (ipi) for advanced melanoma: efficacy by PD-L1 expression and line of therapy. in ASCO. Chicago: J Clin Oncol 34(suppl; abstr 9513)
28. Garon EB, Herbst RS, Kim D-W et al (2016) Pembrolizumab vs docetaxel for previously treated advanced NSCLC with a PD-L1 tumor proportion score (TPS) 1%-49%: results from KEYNOTE-010. in ASCO. Chicago
29. Plimack ER, Bellmunt J, Gupta S et al (2015) Pembrolizumab (MK-3475) for advanced urothelial cancer: updated results and biomarker analysis from KEYNOTE-012. in ASCO. Chicago, IL: J Clin Oncol 33(suppl; abstr 4502)
30. Fehrenbacher L et al (2016) Atezolizumab versus docetaxel for patients with previously treated non-small-cell lung cancer (POPLAR): a multicentre, open-label, phase 2 randomised controlled trial. Lancet 387(10030):1837–1846
31. Garassino MC, Vansteenkiste J, Kim JH et al (2016) Durvalumab in ≥3rd-line locally advanced or metastatic, EGFR/ALK wild-type NSCLC: results from the phase 2 ATLANTIC Study. in IASLC. J Thorac Oncol. Jan 2017
32. Garon EB et al (2015) Pembrolizumab for the treatment of non-small-cell lung cancer. N Engl J Med 372(21):2018–2028
33. Hassan R, Thomas A, Patel MR et al (2016) Avelumab (MSB0010718C; anti-PD-L1) in patients with advanced unresectable mesothelioma from the JAVELIN solid tumor phase Ib trial: safety, clinical activity, and PD-L1 expression. in ASCO. Chicago: J Clin Oncol 34(suppl; abstr 8503)
34. Herbst RS et al (2016) Pembrolizumab versus docetaxel for previously treated, PD-L1-positive, advanced non-small-cell lung cancer (KEYNOTE-010): a randomised controlled trial. Lancet 387(10027):1540–1550
35. Herbst RS et al (2014) Predictive correlates of response to the anti-PD-L1 antibody MPDL3280A in cancer patients. Nature 515(7528):563–567
36. Bauml J, Seiwert TY, Pfister DG et al (2016) Preliminary results from KEYNOTE-055: pembrolizumab after platinum and cetuximab failure in head and neck squamous cell carcinoma (HNSCC). in ASCO. Chicago: J Clin Oncol 34(suppl; abstr 6011)
37. Kaufman HL et al (2016) Avelumab in patients with chemotherapy-refractory metastatic merkel cell carcinoma: a multicentre, single-group, open-label, phase 2 trial. Lancet Oncol 17(10):1374–1385
38. Motzer RJ et al (2015) Nivolumab versus everolimus in advanced renal-cell carcinoma. N Engl J Med 373(19):1803–1813
39. Muro K et al (2016) Pembrolizumab for patients with PD-L1-positive advanced gastric cancer (KEYNOTE-012): a multicentre, open-label, phase 1b trial. Lancet Oncol 17(6):717–726
40. Nanda R et al (2016) Pembrolizumab in patients with advanced triple-negative breast cancer: phase Ib KEYNOTE-012 study. J Clin Oncol 34(21):2460–2467
41. Patel MR, Ellerton J, Infante JR et al (2017) Avelumab in patients with metastatic urothelial carcinoma: Pooled results from two cohorts of the phase 1b JAVELIN Solid tumor trial. in ASCO - Genitorurinary Symposium. Orlando, FL: J Clin Oncol 35(suppl 6S; abstract 330)

42. Reck M et al (2016) Pembrolizumab versus chemotherapy for PD-L1-positive non-small-cell lung cancer. N Engl J Med 375(19):1823–1833
43. Reck M, DeGreen H, Rose AL et al (2016) Avelumab (MSB0010718C; anti-PD-L1) vs platinum-based doublet as first-line treatment for metastatic or recurrent PD-L1-positive non-small-cell lung cancer: the phase 3 JAVELIN Lung 100 trial. in ASCO. Chicago: J Clin Oncol 34(suppl; abstr TPS9105)
44. Ribas A et al (2016) Association of Pembrolizumab with Tumor Response and Survival among Patients with Advanced Melanoma. JAMA 315(15):1600–1609
45. Rittmeyer A et al (2016) Atezolizumab versus docetaxel in patients with previously treated non-small-cell lung cancer (OAK): a phase 3, open-label, multicentre randomised controlled trial. Lancet 389:255–265
46. Rizvi N, Shepherd F, Antonia S et al (2014) First-line monotherapy with nivolumab (anti-PD-1; BMS-936558, ONO-4538) in advanced non-small cell lung cancer (NSCLC): safety, efficacy and correlation of outcomes with PD-L1 status. in Chicago multidisciplinary symposium in thoracic oncology. Chicago: J Radiat Oncol Biol Phys 90(suppl):S31
47. Rizvi NA et al (2016) Nivolumab in combination with platinum-based doublet chemotherapy for first-line treatment of advanced non-small-cell lung cancer. J Clin Oncol 34(25):2969–2979
48. Rizvi NA et al (2015) Activity and safety of nivolumab, an anti-PD-1 immune checkpoint inhibitor, for patients with advanced, refractory squamous non-small-cell lung cancer (CheckMate 063): a phase 2, single-arm trial. Lancet Oncol 16(3):257–265
49. Rizvi NA, B.J, Ou SI et al (2015) Safety and clinical activity of MEDI4736, an anti-programmed cell death-ligand 1 (PD-L1) antibody, in patients with non-small cell lung cancer (NSCLC). in ASCO. Chicago: J Clin Oncol 33(suppl; abstr 8032)
50. Rosenberg JE et al (2016) Atezolizumab in patients with locally advanced and metastatic urothelial carcinoma who have progressed following treatment with platinum-based chemotherapy: a single-arm, multicentre, phase 2 trial. Lancet 387(10031):1909–1920
51. Seiwert TY et al (2016) Safety and clinical activity of pembrolizumab for treatment of recurrent or metastatic squamous cell carcinoma of the head and neck (KEYNOTE-012): an open-label, multicentre, phase 1b trial. Lancet Oncol 17(7):956–965
52. Sharma P et al (2016) Nivolumab monotherapy in recurrent metastatic urothelial carcinoma (CheckMate 032): a multicentre, open-label, two-stage, multi-arm, phase 1/2 trial. Lancet Oncol 17(11):1590–1598
53. Socinski M, Creelan B, Horn L et al (2016) NSCLC, metastaticCheckMate 026: A phase 3 trial of nivolumab vs investigator's choice (IC) of platinum-based doublet chemotherapy (PT-DC) as first-line therapy for stage iv/recurrent programmed death ligand 1 (PD-L1)–positive NSCLC. in ESMO. Copenhagen: Ann Oncol 27 (suppl_6): LBA7_PR
54. Spigel D, C J, Gettinger S et al (2015) Clinical activity and safety from a phase II study (FIR) of MPDL3280A (anti-PDL1) in PD-L1-selected patients with nonsmall cell lung cancer (NSCLC). in ASCO. J Clin Oncol 33(suppl), abstract 8028
55. Topalian SL et al (2012) Safety, activity, and immune correlates of anti-PD-1 antibody in cancer. N Engl J Med 366(26):2443–2454
56. Weber JS et al (2015) Nivolumab versus chemotherapy in patients with advanced melanoma who progressed after anti-CTLA-4 treatment (CheckMate 037): a randomised, controlled, open-label, phase 3 trial. Lancet Oncol 16(4):375–384
57. Gibney GT, Weiner LM, Atkins MB (2016) Predictive biomarkers for checkpoint inhibitor-based immunotherapy. Lancet Oncol 17(12):e542–e551
58. Chae YK et al (2016) Biomarkers for PD-1/PD-L1 blockade therapy in non-small-cell lung cancer: is PD-L1 expression a good marker for patient selection? Clin Lung Cancer 17(5):350–361
59. Liu SV, Powderly JD, Camidge DR, et al (2015) Safety and efficacy of MPDL3280A (anti-PDL1) in combination with platinum-based doublet chemotherapy in patients with advanced non-small cell lung cancer (NSCLC). in ASCO. Chicago: J Clin Oncol 33 abstract 8030

60. Callahan MK, Bendell JC, Chan E, Morse M, Pillai RN, Bono P, Jaeger D, Evans TRJ, Chau I, Calvo E, Le DT, Ott PA, Taylor MH, Sharma P, Antonia SJ, Sharkey B, Christensen O, Amin A (2014) Phase I/II, open-label study of nivolumab (anti-PD-1; BMS- 936558, ONO-4538) as monotherapy or combined with ipilimumab in advanced or metastatic solid tumors. ASCO Meet Abstr 32(15_suppl):TPS3114
61. Larkin J et al (2015) Combined Nivolumab and Ipilimumab or monotherapy in untreated melanoma. N Engl J Med 373(1):23–34
62. Postow MA et al (2015) Nivolumab and ipilimumab versus ipilimumab in untreated melanoma. N Engl J Med 372(21):2006–2017
63. Robert C et al (2015) Nivolumab in previously untreated melanoma without BRAF mutation. N Engl J Med 372(4):320–330
64. Robert C et al (2014) Anti-programmed-death-receptor-1 treatment with pembrolizumab in ipilimumab-refractory advanced melanoma: a randomised dose-comparison cohort of a phase 1 trial. Lancet 384(9948):1109–1117
65. Hellmann MD, Gettinger SN, Goldman JW et al (2016) CheckMate 012: safety and efficacy of first-line (1L) nivolumab (nivo; N) and ipilimumab (ipi; I) in advanced (adv) NSCLC. in ASCO. Chicago: J Clin Oncol 34(suppl; abstr 3001)
66. Green MR et al (2010) Integrative analysis reveals selective 9p24.1 amplification, increased PD-1 ligand expression, and further induction via JAK2 in nodular sclerosing Hodgkin lymphoma and primary mediastinal large B-cell lymphoma. Blood 116(17):3268–3277
67. Green MR et al (2012) Constitutive AP-1 activity and EBV infection induce PD-L1 in Hodgkin lymphomas and posttransplant lymphoproliferative disorders: implications for targeted therapy. Clin Cancer Res 18(6):1611–1618
68. Armand P et al (2016) Programmed death-1 blockade with Pembrolizumab in patients with classical Hodgkin Lymphoma after Brentuximab Vedotin Failure. J Clin Oncol 34:3733–3739
69. Chow LQ et al (2016) Antitumor activity of pembrolizumab in biomarker-unselected patients with recurrent and/or metastatic head and neck squamous cell carcinoma: results from the phase Ib keynote-012 expansion cohort. J Clin Oncol 34:3838–3845
70. Menon S, Shin S, Dy G (2016) Advances in cancer immunotherapy in solid tumors. Cancers (Basel) 8(12)
71. Patel SP, Kurzrock R (2015) PD-L1 expression as a predictive biomarker in cancer immunotherapy. Mol Cancer Ther 14(4):847–856
72. Rebelatto M, Mistry A, Sabalos C et al (2015) Development of a PD-L1 companion diagnostic assay for treatment with MEDI4736 in NSCLC and SCCHN patients. in ASCO. Chicago: J Clin Oncol 33(suppl: abstr 8033)
73. Sznol M, Chen L (2013) Antagonist antibodies to PD-1 and B7-H1 (PD-L1) in the treatment of advanced human cancer. Clin Cancer Res 19(5):1021–1034
74. Chen J et al (2016) Regulation of PD-L1: a novel role of pro-survival signalling in cancer. Ann Oncol 27(3):409–416
75. Callea M, Genega EM, Gupta M, Cheng S, Fay AP, Song J, et al (2014) PD-L1expression in primary clear cell renal cell carcinomas (ccRCCs) and their metastases. in ASCO. Chicago: J Clin Oncol 32: 5s(suppl; abstr 4585)
76. Hansen AR, Siu LL (2016) PD-L1 testing in cancer: challenges in companion diagnostic development. JAMA Oncol 2(1):15–16
77. Hirsch FR et al (2017) PD-L1 immunohistochemistry assays for lung cancer: results from phase 1 of the Blueprint PD-L1 IHC assay comparison project. J Thorac Oncol 12(2):208–222
78. Mittal D et al (2014) New insights into cancer immunoediting and its three component phases--elimination, equilibrium and escape. Curr Opin Immunol 27:16–25
79. Carey LA et al (2016) Molecular heterogeneity and response to neoadjuvant human epidermal growth factor receptor 2 targeting in CALGB 40601, a randomized phase III trial of paclitaxel plus Trastuzumab with or without Lapatinib. J Clin Oncol 34(6):542–549
80. Denkert C et al (2010) Tumor-associated lymphocytes as an independent predictor of response to neoadjuvant chemotherapy in breast cancer. J Clin Oncol 28(1):105–113

81. Denkert C et al (2015) Tumor-infiltrating lymphocytes and response to neoadjuvant chemotherapy with or without carboplatin in human epidermal growth factor receptor 2-positive and triple-negative primary breast cancers. J Clin Oncol 33(9):983–991
82. Gooden MJ et al (2011) The prognostic influence of tumour-infiltrating lymphocytes in cancer: a systematic review with meta-analysis. Br J Cancer 105(1):93–103
83. Ibrahim EM et al (2014) The prognostic value of tumor-infiltrating lymphocytes in triple-negative breast cancer: a meta-analysis. Breast Cancer Res Treat 148(3):467–476
84. Loi S et al (2014) Tumor infiltrating lymphocytes are prognostic in triple negative breast cancer and predictive for trastuzumab benefit in early breast cancer: results from the FinHER trial. Ann Oncol 25(8):1544–1550
85. Loi S et al (2013) Prognostic and predictive value of tumor-infiltrating lymphocytes in a phase III randomized adjuvant breast cancer trial in node-positive breast cancer comparing the addition of docetaxel to doxorubicin with doxorubicin-based chemotherapy: BIG 02-98. J Clin Oncol 31(7):860–867
86. Sasada T, Suekane S (2011) Variation of tumor-infiltrating lymphocytes in human cancers: controversy on clinical significance. Immunotherapy 3(10):1235–1251
87. Schatton T et al (2014) Tumor-infiltrating lymphocytes and their significance in melanoma prognosis. Methods Mol Biol 1102:287–324
88. Solinas C et al (2017) Tumor infiltrating lymphocytes in gastrointestinal tumors: controversies and future clinical implications. Crit Rev Oncol Hematol 110:106–116
89. Teng F et al (2015) Tumor infiltrating lymphocytes (TILs) before and after neoadjuvant chemoradiotherapy and its clinical utility for rectal cancer. Am J Cancer Res 5(6):2064–2074
90. Yu X et al (2016) Prognostic and predictive value of tumor-infiltrating lymphocytes in breast cancer: a systematic review and meta-analysis. Clin Transl Oncol 18(5):497–506
91. Zeng DQ et al (2016) Prognostic and predictive value of tumor-infiltrating lymphocytes for clinical therapeutic research in patients with non-small cell lung cancer. Oncotarget 7(12):13765–13781
92. Pages F et al (2005) Effector memory T cells, early metastasis, and survival in colorectal cancer. N Engl J Med 353(25):2654–2666
93. Galon J et al (2006) Type, density, and location of immune cells within human colorectal tumors predict clinical outcome. Science 313(5795):1960–1964
94. Camus M et al (2009) Coordination of intratumoral immune reaction and human colorectal cancer recurrence. Cancer Res 69(6):2685–2693
95. Adams S, Robinson DJ, Hamilton EP et al (2016) Phase Ib trial of atezolizumab in combination with nab-paclitaxel in patients with metastatic triple-negative breast cancer (mTNBC). in ASCO. Chicago: J Clin Oncol 34(suppl; abstr 1009)
96. Bottai G et al (2016) An immune stratification reveals a subset of PD-1/LAG-3 double-positive triple-negative breast cancers. Breast Cancer Res 18(1):121
97. Galon J et al (2012) The immune score as a new possible approach for the classification of cancer. J Transl Med 10:1
98. Fridman WH et al (2012) The immune contexture in human tumours: impact on clinical outcome. Nat Rev Cancer 12(4):298–306
99. Mlecnik B et al (2011) Histopathologic-based prognostic factors of colorectal cancers are associated with the state of the local immune reaction. J Clin Oncol 29(6):610–618
100. Ogino S et al (2011) Cancer immunology--analysis of host and tumor factors for personalized medicine. Nat Rev Clin Oncol 8(12):711–719
101. Laghi L et al (2009) CD3+ cells at the invasive margin of deeply invading (pT3-T4) colorectal cancer and risk of post-surgical metastasis: a longitudinal study. Lancet Oncol 10(9):877–884
102. Nosho K et al (2010) Tumour-infiltrating T-cell subsets, molecular changes in colorectal cancer, and prognosis: cohort study and literature review. J Pathol 222(4):350–366
103. Gabrilovich DI et al (1996) Production of vascular endothelial growth factor by human tumors inhibits the functional maturation of dendritic cells. Nat Med 2(10):1096–1103

104. Chomarat P et al (2000) IL-6 switches the differentiation of monocytes from dendritic cells to macrophages. Nat Immunol 1(6):510–514
105. Biswas SK, Mantovani A (2010) Macrophage plasticity and interaction with lymphocyte subsets: cancer as a paradigm. Nat Immunol 11(10):889–896
106. Noy R, Pollard JW (2014) Tumor-associated macrophages: from mechanisms to therapy. Immunity 41(1):49–61
107. Zhang J et al (2016) High infiltration of tumor-associated macrophages influences poor prognosis in human gastric cancer patients, associates with the phenomenon of EMT. Medicine (Baltimore) 95(6):e2636
108. Mori K et al (2011) Infiltration of m2 tumor-associated macrophages in oral squamous cell carcinoma correlates with tumor malignancy. Cancers (Basel) 3(4):3726–3739
109. Shimura S et al (2000) Reduced infiltration of tumor-associated macrophages in human prostate cancer: association with cancer progression. Cancer Res 60(20):5857–5861
110. Takayama H et al (2009) Increased infiltration of tumor associated macrophages is associated with poor prognosis of bladder carcinoma in situ after intravesical bacillus Calmette-Guerin instillation. J Urol 181(4):1894–1900
111. Zhang BC et al (2011) Tumor-associated macrophages infiltration is associated with peritumoral lymphangiogenesis and poor prognosis in lung adenocarcinoma. Med Oncol 28(4):1447–1452
112. Zhang Y et al (2013) High-infiltration of tumor-associated macrophages predicts unfavorable clinical outcome for node-negative breast cancer. PLoS One 8(9):e76147
113. Ma J et al (2010) The M1 form of tumor-associated macrophages in non-small cell lung cancer is positively associated with survival time. BMC Cancer 10:112
114. Barbera-Guillem E et al (2000) B lymphocyte pathology in human colorectal cancer. Experimental and clinical therapeutic effects of partial B cell depletion. Cancer Immunol Immunother 48(10):541–549
115. Affara NI et al (2014) B cells regulate macrophage phenotype and response to chemotherapy in squamous carcinomas. Cancer Cell 25(6):809–821
116. DiLillo DJ, Yanaba K, Tedder TF (2010) B cells are required for optimal CD4+ and CD8+ T cell tumor immunity: therapeutic B cell depletion enhances B16 melanoma growth in mice. J Immunol 184(7):4006–4016
117. Coca S et al (1997) The prognostic significance of intratumoral natural killer cells in patients with colorectal carcinoma. Cancer 79(12):2320–2328
118. Ishigami S et al (2000) Prognostic value of intratumoral natural killer cells in gastric carcinoma. Cancer 88(3):577–583
119. Villegas FR et al (2002) Prognostic significance of tumor infiltrating natural killer cells subset CD57 in patients with squamous cell lung cancer. Lung Cancer 35(1):23–28
120. Platonova S et al (2011) Profound coordinated alterations of intratumoral NK cell phenotype and function in lung carcinoma. Cancer Res 71(16):5412–5422
121. Gabrilovich DI, Ostrand-Rosenberg S, Bronte V (2012) Coordinated regulation of myeloid cells by tumours. Nat Rev Immunol 12(4):253–268
122. Almand B et al (2001) Increased production of immature myeloid cells in cancer patients: a mechanism of immunosuppression in cancer. J Immunol 166(1):678–689
123. Shinbrot E et al (2014) Exonuclease mutations in DNA polymerase epsilon reveal replication strand specific mutation patterns and human origins of replication. Genome Res 24(11):1740–1750
124. Peltomaki P (2001) Deficient DNA mismatch repair: a common etiologic factor for colon cancer. Hum Mol Genet 10(7):735–740
125. Pal T, Permuth-Wey J, Sellers TA (2008) A review of the clinical relevance of mismatch-repair deficiency in ovarian cancer. Cancer 113(4):733–742
126. Jang E, Chung DC (2010) Hereditary colon cancer: lynch syndrome. Gut Liver 4(2):151–160
127. Long Q et al (2014) Role of endometrial cancer abnormal MMR protein in screening lynch-syndrome families. Int J Clin Exp Pathol 7(10):7297–7303

128. Grady WM, Carethers JM (2008) Genomic and epigenetic instability in colorectal cancer pathogenesis. Gastroenterology 135(4):1079–1099
129. MAFG mediates CIMP in BRAF-mutant colorectal cancer. Cancer Discov 4(11):OF11 (2014)
130. Cancer Genome Atlas Network (2012) Comprehensive molecular characterization of human colon and rectal cancer. Nature 487(7407):330–337
131. Jansen AM et al (2016) Combined mismatch repair and POLE/POLD1 defects explain unresolved suspected lynch syndrome cancers. Eur J Hum Genet 24(7):1089–1092
132. Benatti P et al (2005) Microsatellite instability and colorectal cancer prognosis. Clin Cancer Res 11(23):8332–8340
133. Le DT et al (2015) PD-1 blockade in tumors with mismatch-repair deficiency. N Engl J Med 372(26):2509–2520
134. South CD et al (2009) Immunohistochemistry staining for the mismatch repair proteins in the clinical care of patients with colorectal cancer. Genet Med 11(11):812–817
135. Yamamoto H, Imai K (2015) Microsatellite instability: an update. Arch Toxicol 89(6):899–921
136. Salipante SJ et al (2014) Microsatellite instability detection by next generation sequencing. Clin Chem 60(9):1192–1199
137. Huang MN et al (2015) MSIseq: software for assessing microsatellite instability from catalogs of somatic mutations. Sci Rep 5:13321
138. Hall MJ, Gowen K, Sanford EM, Ali MA, Kaczmar J, Miller VA, Stephens P, Yelensky R, Daly MB, Sun J (2016) Evaluation of microsatellite instability (MSI) status in gastrointestinal (GI) tumor samples tested with comprehensive genomic profiling (CGP). Poster presented at the 51st American Society of Clinical Oncology (ASCO) annual meeting. J Clin Oncol 34(suppl 4S; abstr 528)
139. Perucho M, Correspondence re*:* Boland CR et al (1998) A National Cancer Institute workshop on microsatellite instability for cancer detection and familial predisposition: development of international criteria for the determination of microsatellite instability in colorectal cancer. Cancer Res 58:5248–5257. Cancer Res 1999 59(1):249–56
140. Kim TM, Laird PW, Park PJ (2013) The landscape of microsatellite instability in colorectal and endometrial cancer genomes. Cell 155(4):858–868
141. Popat S, Hubner R, Houlston RS (2005) Systematic review of microsatellite instability and colorectal cancer prognosis. J Clin Oncol 23(3):609–618
142. Phillips SM et al (2004) Tumour-infiltrating lymphocytes in colorectal cancer with microsatellite instability are activated and cytotoxic. Br J Surg 91(4):469–475
143. Meyer LA, Broaddus RR, Lu KH (2009) Endometrial cancer and lynch syndrome: clinical and pathologic considerations. Cancer Control 16(1):14–22
144. Black D et al (2006) Clinicopathologic significance of defective DNA mismatch repair in endometrial carcinoma. J Clin Oncol 24(11):1745–1753
145. MacDonald ND et al (2000) Frequency and prognostic impact of microsatellite instability in a large population-based study of endometrial carcinomas. Cancer Res 60(6):1750–1752
146. Fiumicino S et al (2001) Microsatellite instability is an independent indicator of recurrence in sporadic stage I-II endometrial adenocarcinoma. J Clin Oncol 19(4):1008–1014
147. van der Post RS et al (2010) Risk of urothelial bladder cancer in lynch syndrome is increased, in particular among MSH2 mutation carriers. J Med Genet 47(7):464–470
148. Risinger JI et al (1995) Microsatellite instability in gynecological sarcomas and in hMSH2 mutant uterine sarcoma cell lines defective in mismatch repair activity. Cancer Res 55(23):5664–5669
149. Orth K et al (1994) Genetic instability in human ovarian cancer cell lines. Proc Natl Acad Sci U S A 91(20):9495–9499
150. Kolodner RD et al (1994) Structure of the human MSH2 locus and analysis of two Muir-Torre kindreds for msh2 mutations. Genomics 24(3):516–526
151. Foley EJ (1953) Antigenic properties of methylcholanthrene-induced tumors in mice of the strain of origin. Cancer Res 13(12):835–837

152. Prehn RT, Main JM (1957) Immunity to methylcholanthrene-induced sarcomas. J Natl Cancer Inst 18(6):769–778
153. Monach PA et al (1995) A unique tumor antigen produced by a single amino acid substitution. Immunity 2(1):45–59
154. Knuth A et al (1984) T-cell-mediated cytotoxicity against autologous malignant melanoma: analysis with interleukin 2-dependent T-cell cultures. Proc Natl Acad Sci U S A 81(11):3511–3515
155. Robbins PF et al (1996) A mutated beta-catenin gene encodes a melanoma-specific antigen recognized by tumor infiltrating lymphocytes. J Exp Med 183(3):1185–1192
156. Boon T et al (1992) Identification of tumour rejection antigens recognized by T lymphocytes. Cancer Surv 13:23–37
157. Sahin U et al (1995) Human neoplasms elicit multiple specific immune responses in the autologous host. Proc Natl Acad Sci U S A 92(25):11810–11813
158. Gubin MM et al (2015) Tumor neoantigens: building a framework for personalized cancer immunotherapy. J Clin Invest 125(9):3413–3421
159. Segal NH et al (2008) Epitope landscape in breast and colorectal cancer. Cancer Res 68(3):889–892
160. van Rooij N et al (2013) Tumor exome analysis reveals neoantigen-specific T-cell reactivity in an ipilimumab-responsive melanoma. J Clin Oncol 31(32):e439–e442
161. Rizvi NA et al (2015) Cancer immunology. Mutational landscape determines sensitivity to PD-1 blockade in non-small cell lung cancer. Science 348(6230):124–128
162. Snyder A et al (2014) Genetic basis for clinical response to CTLA-4 blockade in melanoma. N Engl J Med 371(23):2189–2199
163. Schumacher TN, Schreiber RD (2015) Neoantigens in cancer immunotherapy. Science 348(6230):69–74
164. Roche PA, Furuta K (2015) The ins and outs of MHC class II-mediated antigen processing and presentation. Nat Rev Immunol 15(4):203–216
165. Linnemann C et al (2015) High-throughput epitope discovery reveals frequent recognition of neo-antigens by CD4+ T cells in human melanoma. Nat Med 21(1):81–85
166. Tran E et al (2016) T-cell transfer therapy targeting mutant KRAS in cancer. N Engl J Med 375(23):2255–2262
167. Matsushita H et al (2012) Cancer exome analysis reveals a T-cell-dependent mechanism of cancer immunoediting. Nature 482(7385):400–404
168. Lundegaard C et al (2008) NetMHC-3.0: accurate web accessible predictions of human, mouse and monkey MHC class I affinities for peptides of length 8-11. Nucleic Acids Res 36(Web Server issue):W509–W512
169. Frampton GM, Fabrizio D, Chalmers ZR, Ross JS, Johnson DB, Lovly CM, Sosman JA, Miler VA, Stephens P (2016) Assessment of tumor mutation burden from >60,000 clinical cancer patients using comprehensive genomic profiling. Poster presented at the 51st American Society of Clinical Oncology (ASCO) annual meeting. J Clin Oncol 34 (suppl), abstract 11558 Abstract
170. Hoffman-Censits JH, Grivas P, Van Der Heijden MS, Dreicer R, Loriot Y, Retz M, Vogelzang NJ, Perez-Gracia JL, Rezazadeh A, Bracarda S, Yu EY, Hoimes CJ, Bellmunt J, Quinn DI, Petrylak DP, Hussain SA, Cui N, Mariathasan S, Abidoye OO, Rosenberg JE (2016) IMvigor210, a phase II trial of atezolizumab (MPDL3280A) in platinum-treated locally advanced or metastatic urothelial carcinoma (mUC). Poster presented at the 51st American Society of Clinical Oncology (ASCO) annual meeting. J Clin Oncol (suupl 2S; abstr 355)
171. Campesato LF et al (2015) Comprehensive cancer-gene panels can be used to estimate mutational load and predict clinical benefit to PD-1 blockade in clinical practice. Oncotarget 6(33):34221–34227
172. George TJ, Michael FG, Sun J, Gowen K, Kennedy M, Greenbowe JR, Schrock AB, Ali SM, Klempner SJ, Hezel AF, Ross JS, Stephens P, Miller VA, Fabrizio D (2016) Tumor mutational burden as a potential biomarker for PD1/PD-L1 in colorectal cancer. Poster presented at the 51st American Society of Clinical Oncology (ASCO) annual meeting. J Clin Oncol 34(suppl). Abstract 3587

173. Lipinski KA et al (2016) Cancer evolution and the limits of predictability in precision cancer medicine. Trends Cancer 2(1):49–63
174. Bassing CH, Swat W, Alt FW (2002) The mechanism and regulation of chromosomal V(D)J recombination. Cell 109(Suppl):S45–S55
175. Warren RL et al (2011) Exhaustive T-cell repertoire sequencing of human peripheral blood samples reveals signatures of antigen selection and a directly measured repertoire size of at least 1 million clonotypes. Genome Res 21(5):790–797
176. Li B et al (2016) Landscape of tumor-infiltrating T cell repertoire of human cancers. Nat Genet 48(7):725–732
177. Brown SD, Raeburn LA, Holt RA (2015) Profiling tissue-resident T cell repertoires by RNA sequencing. Genome Med 7:125
178. Tumeh PC et al (2014) PD-1 blockade induces responses by inhibiting adaptive immune resistance. Nature 515(7528):568–571
179. Hsu MS et al (2016) TCR sequencing can identify and track Glioma-infiltrating T cells after DC vaccination. Cancer Immunol Res 4(5):412–418
180. Page DB et al (2016) Deep sequencing of T-cell receptor DNA as a biomarker of clonally expanded TILs in breast cancer after immunotherapy. Cancer Immunol Res 4(10):835–844
181. Byron SA et al (2016) Translating RNA sequencing into clinical diagnostics: opportunities and challenges. Nat Rev Genet 17(5):257–271
182. Cieslik M et al (2015) The use of exome capture RNA-seq for highly degraded RNA with application to clinical cancer sequencing. Genome Res 25(9):1372–1381
183. Gao J et al (2016) Loss of IFN-gamma pathway genes in tumor cells as a mechanism of resistance to anti-CTLA-4 therapy. Cell 167(2):397–404. e9
184. Shin DS et al (2017) Primary resistance to PD-1 blockade mediated by JAK1/2 mutations. Cancer Discov 7(2):188–201
185. Liebner DA, Huang K, Parvin JD (2014) MMAD: microarray microdissection with analysis of differences is a computational tool for deconvoluting cell type-specific contributions from tissue samples. Bioinformatics 30(5):682–689
186. Zhong Y et al (2013) Digital sorting of complex tissues for cell type-specific gene expression profiles. BMC Bioinformatics 14:89
187. Newman AM et al (2015) Robust enumeration of cell subsets from tissue expression profiles. Nat Methods 12(5):453–457
188. Gentles AJ et al (2015) The prognostic landscape of genes and infiltrating immune cells across human cancers. Nat Med 21(8):938–945
189. Nowakowski GS, Czuczman MS (2015) ABC, GCB, and double-hit diffuse large B-cell lymphoma: does subtype make a difference in therapy selection? Am Soc Clin Oncol Educ Book:e449–e457
190. Choi W et al (2014) Intrinsic basal and luminal subtypes of muscle-invasive bladder cancer. Nat Rev Urol 11(7):400–410
191. Hugo W et al (2016) Genomic and transcriptomic features of response to anti-PD-1 therapy in metastatic melanoma. Cell 165(1):35–44
192. Weber J, Roder H, Asmellash S, Meyer K, Sayers K, Steingrimsson A, Roder J (2016) Abstract 4891: a mass spectrometry-based serum test to predict outcome of treatment with nivolumab: analysis of samples taken during therapy. Cancer Res 76(14 Supplement):4891. doi:10.1158/1538-7445.AM2016-4891
193. Spranger S, Gajewski TF (2016) Tumor-intrinsic oncogene pathways mediating immune avoidance. Oncoimmunology 5(3):e1086862
194. Almanzar G et al (2005) Long-term cytomegalovirus infection leads to significant changes in the composition of the CD8+ T-cell repertoire, which may be the basis for an imbalance in the cytokine production profile in elderly persons. J Virol 79(6):3675–3683
195. Sivan A et al (2015) Commensal bifidobacterium promotes antitumor immunity and facilitates anti-PD-L1 efficacy. Science 350(6264):1084–1089
196. Zitvogel L et al (2015) Cancer and the gut microbiota: an unexpected link. Sci Transl Med 7(271):271ps1

197. Champiat S et al (2016) Hyperprogressive disease is a new pattern of progression in cancer patients treated by anti-PD-1/PD-L1. Clin Cancer Res 23:1920–1928
198. Hodi FS et al (2016) Combined nivolumab and ipilimumab versus ipilimumab alone in patients with advanced melanoma: 2-year overall survival outcomes in a multicentre, randomised, controlled, phase 2 trial. Lancet Oncol 17(11):1558–1568
199. Ferris RL et al (2016) Nivolumab for recurrent squamous-cell carcinoma of the head and neck. N Engl J Med 375(19):1856–1867

Chapter 4
Radiographic Evaluation of Immunotherapy

Jennifer Feneis, Seth Kligerman, and Elizabeth Weihe

Abstract For many radiologists, the assessment of oncology patients' response to treatment represents a significant portion of their practice. It has been shown that radiologic responses to immunotherapy can differ from traditional cytotoxic therapy, as do the complications of treatment. Inflammatory response to immunotherapy may mimic actual progression radiologically, an entity known as pseudoprogression. As advances in immunotherapy continue, radiologists need to evolve their practice in order to be able to discern between pseudoprogression and progression. They also need to become familiar with the imaging appearance of specific immune-related adverse events, in order to accurately diagnose these complications so appropriate interventions may be expedited. This chapter will review the standardized methods of radiologically assessing tumor response to traditional cytotoxic chemotherapy as opposed to immunotherapy. It will review the entity and imaging findings of pseudoprogression, and it will also depict the radiologic findings of immune-related pneumonitis and colitis.

Keywords Imaging • Pseudoprogression • RECIST • irAEs • Pneumonitis • Enterocolitis • irRECIST • WHO

4.1 Radiology Technology

In the advent of this new arm of cancer immunotherapy, radiologists have to develop new skills to interpret the changes seen following therapy. While advances in technology continue to improve the tools they use, the imaging modalities used to evaluate response to immunotherapy have not significantly changed over the past decade. Computed tomography (CT) and positron emission tomography-CT (PET-CT) remain primary modalities for the detection and evaluation of tumor

J. Feneis, MD • S. Kligerman, MD • E. Weihe, MD (✉)
Department of Radiology, University of California-San Diego, San Diego, CA, USA
e-mail: jfeneis@ucsd.edu; skligerman@ucsd.edu; eweihe@ucsd.edu

S.P. Patel, R. Kurzrock (eds.), *Early Phase Cancer Immunotherapy*,
Current Cancer Research, DOI 10.1007/978-3-319-63757-0_4

burden in the chest, abdomen, and pelvis (CAP). The Response Evaluation Criteria in Solid Tumors (RECIST) criteria, discussed later, required a minimum CT slice thickness of 5 mm. This is easily met with newer generation CT scanners, which typically acquire submillimeter thick images, which are subsequently reconstructed into thicker slices for interpretation. The American College of Radiology's published practice parameters state that CT scanners should acquire and reconstruct CT scans of the CAP at a maximum of 2 mm and 5 mm, respectively [1, 2], while additional 1–2 mm reconstructions of the thorax using a sharper reconstruction algorithm for bone or lung evaluation are recommended [2]. Having thinner slice thickness allows for more accurate measurements of tumor lesions and improved detection of small lesions [3]. When clinically feasible, intravenous iodinated contrast material should be given to increase sensitivity of lesion detection and allow for better lesion characterization [3].

There is much active research exploring the potential use of immune-based radiotracers that could be visualized with PET, known as ImmunoPET [4]. Although these tools might become routine technology in the future, they have not yet become part of mainstream clinical practice, where F-18 fluorodeoxyglucose (FDG) PET is still the gold standard.

There is a role for magnetic resonance imaging (MRI) in oncologic imaging, particularly in the detection of metastatic disease in certain locations including the liver, brain, and spine. However, this is usually performed to evaluate a specific organ instead of "whole-body" imaging. For example, if a single hepatic metastasis is detected on CT and a partial hepatectomy or metastectomy is being clinically considered, it is appropriate to obtain a liver MRI with a hepatobiliary contrast agent such as gadoxetate disodium to ensure no additional lesions that were occult on CT are in fact present [5]. This exam has greater sensitivity for detection of liver lesions compared to CT due to its improved soft tissue contrast [6]. Similarly, MRI with gadolinium-based intravenous contrast is the imaging gold standard to evaluate metastatic involvement in the brain and spine. While rapid whole-body diffusion MRI is a promising technique for certain malignancies, especially lymphomas, it is not often performed in routine clinical practice [7].

The frequency of image acquisition is variable and may be governed by a specific clinical trial and/or insurance reimbursement. In general, the interval between imaging studies to assess therapeutic response is typically between 8 and 16 weeks. However, as we better understand the radiographic changes that go along with positive and negative responses, this will become more standardized. An important exception to this time frame is if the patient develops new symptoms that suggest an adverse effect of the therapy, in which a targeted CT may provide valuable diagnostic information.

As immunotherapy has emerged as a new arm of cancer treatment, unique radiologic response patterns to immunotherapy and immune related side effects have been observed. These findings are discussed in the rest of this chapter.

4.2 Conventional Imaging Evaluation of Tumor Burden

4.2.1 RECIST

In order to standardize the anatomical assessment of tumor burden and its response to conventional cytotoxic chemotherapies, a large, international group collaborated to develop the RECIST, published in 2000 [8]. The criteria use objective measurement of solid tumors, predominantly on CT studies, to determine a patient's response to therapy. They built on a prior classification scheme developed by the World Health Organization (WHO). The criteria are applied to patients on clinical trials to ultimately see if the therapeutic agent is effective, or if the patient needs to be pulled off the clinical trial. We may now also translate this approach into clinical therapies. A knowledge of these criteria and the ability to incorporate them into daily practice is an essential part of a radiologists' job, and will be summarized here based on the second and most recent revision to the RECIST criteria, version 1.1, published in 2009 [9]. Note that these criteria do not apply to studies for patients with malignant lymphoma or with primary brain tumors, as there are separate guidelines for response assessment in these patient populations, known as the Lugano Classification [10] and Response Assessment in Neuro-Oncology (RANO) criteria [11], respectively.

In order for the RECIST guidelines to be applicable in determining tumor response, a patient has to have "measurable disease," which necessitates at least one solid tumor to meet a minimum size requirement when the longest diameter in the axial plane is measured [9]. This minimum diameter for solid tumors on CT is 10 mm, when the CT slice thickness is 5 mm or less. Lymph nodes should be measured along their short axis, where a minimum diameter of 15 mm is needed to consider it malignant and measureable, where as a short axis diameter of <10 mm is considered normal. All other lesions are classified as "nonmeasurable," and are factored separately into overall determination of patient response [9].

It is essential to estimate the overall tumor burden on baseline studies, which should be acquired as close to initiation of treatment as possible, but no longer than 4 weeks prior to therapy initiation. When patients have multiple measureable tumors, a maximum of five total target lesions should be used in the analysis, with up to only two target lesions taken from the same organ [12]. The diameters of the selected target lesions are summed and reported as the "baseline sum diameters," which are used for comparison to future studies. Additional measureable lesions beyond the five target lesions and all nonmeasurable lesions are considered nontarget lesions. Their presence should still be reported on the baseline study, although measurements do not have to be given [9].

Based on the analysis of the target lesions, RECIST 1.1 describes four possible types of responses to therapy: complete response to therapy (CR), partial response to therapy (PR), progressive disease (PD), and stable disease (SD). In order to qualify as CR, all target lesions must completely disappear, and all pathological lymph nodes (whether target or nontarget) must normalize to <10 mm in short axis. In PR, the baseline sum diameter of the target lesions must decrease by at least 30% [12]. PD can be diagnosed in two ways. In one scenario, the appearance of one or more new lesions diagnoses PD. In the second, two specific criteria must be met. First, there must be a 20% or greater increase in the sum diameter of the target lesions compared to the smallest sum documented to that point. Second, there needs to be an absolute increase in the sum diameter of at least 5 mm. If the sum diameter has not decreased enough to qualify as PR, nor increased enough to qualify as PD, it is classified as SD [9].

In patients with nontarget lesions, there are simplified response categories based on qualitative, not quantitative, analysis of lesion growth/shrinkage, which also take into consideration serum tumor marker levels, if applicable. There are only three categories of response for nontarget lesions: CR, PD, and non-CR/non-PD. To qualify as CR, all nontarget solid organ lesions must disappear, all lymph nodes must measure <10 mm in short axis and serum tumor marker levels must normalize. To be classified as PD, there must be "unequivocal progression" of overall tumor burden, regardless of the response of the target lesions, which would validate cessation of the current therapy. If one or more nontarget lesion persists, and/or serum tumor marker levels remain elevated above normal limits, this should be categorized as non-CR/non-PD [9].

For any given follow-up study, the overall response should take into consideration the responses of target lesions, nontarget lesions (if present) and any new lesions (if present).

4.3 Patterns of Response to Immunotherapy

Unlike traditional cytotoxic chemotherapy agents, immunotherapy agents act to increase or activate the patient's innate antitumor response system. As checkpoint blockade immunotherapy became part of the oncologists' armamentarium, an atypical pattern of tumor response termed as pseudoprogression was observed (Figs. 4.1 and 4.2).

Pseudoprogression is used to describe patients with increased tumor size or radiologic progression after starting immunotherapy in the absence of the clinical decline normally observed from tumor growth [13]. In several clinical trials, investigators have observed patients with an initial increase in total tumor volume after immunotherapy initiation, which was subsequently followed by a long-term decrease in total tumor volume. This subsequent decrease sometimes qualified as either PR or CR by RECIST criteria [14, 15], even though the initial increase in tumor burden would have been classified as PD and the therapeutic agent might have otherwise been withdrawn.

The initial increase in size seen with pseudoprogression may either reflect a surrounding inflammatory response, versus growth until the immune system is adequately activated by the therapy [14, 16]. For example, in a study by Di Giacomo et al., which evaluates the efficacy of the anticytotoxic T lymphocyte-associated

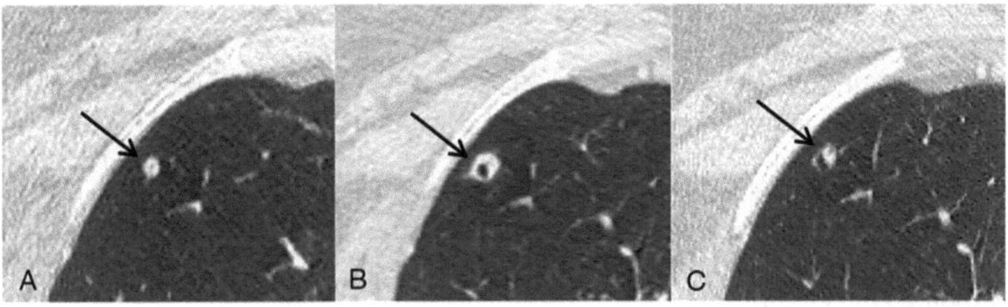

Fig. 4.1 Pseudoprogression. Axial CT images of a patient initially nonresponsive to conventional cytotoxic chemotherapy and subsequently started on immunotherapy. (**a**) 5 days prior to starting immunotherapy, a subcentimeter pulmonary nodule was identified in the right upper lobe (*arrow*). (**b**) 3 months after immunotherapy initiation, the nodule appeared to have enlarged and started to cavitate. (**c**) 5 months after immunotherapy initiation, the nodule shrunk to approximately its pre-initiation size

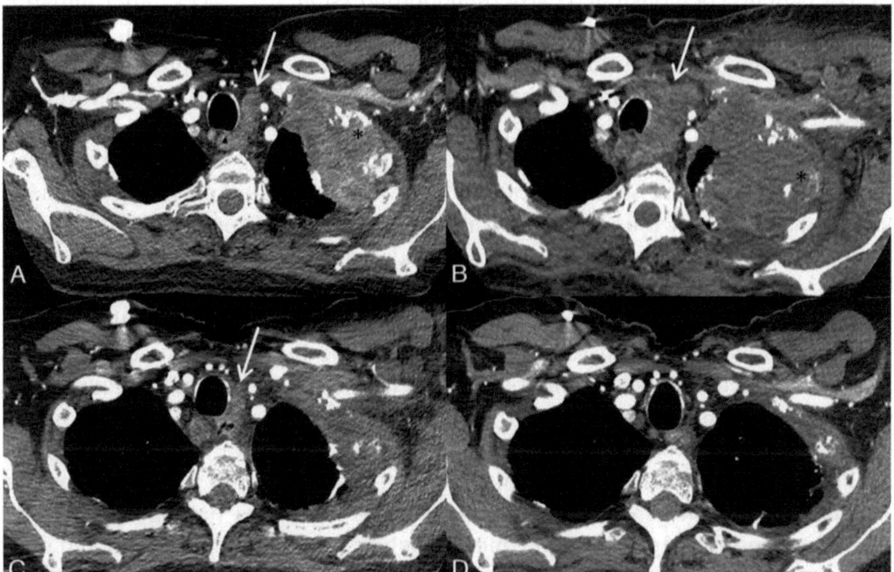

Fig. 4.2 Pseudoprogression. Axial CT images from sequential studies of a patient with a spindle cell tumor on immunotherapy. (**a**) Prior to starting immunotherapy, the patient had a destructive left apical mass with destruction of the superior ribs (*) and associated left paratracheal lymphadenopathy (*arrow*). (**b**) Shortly after initiating immunotherapy, there was apparent marked progression of the primary tumor size. The left paratracheal lymphadenopathy also enlarged (*arrow*), causing worsened left to right mediastinal shift. (**c**) 6 weeks later there was marked response to therapy, with decreased size of the primary tumor and left paratracheal lymphadenopathy. (**d**) 5 months later, the primary tumor and mediastinal lymphadenopathy had nearly completely regressed. Additionally, the invaded ribs have become sclerotic, consistent with a healing response

antigen-4 (CTLA-4) ipilimumab to treat unresectable metastatic melanoma, a biopsy of a lesion that was increasing in size after treatment demonstrated extensive lymphoid infiltrate without malignant cells, consistent with pseudoprogression [16].

Pseudoprogression can also be associated with mixed responses, where several lesions may respond to immunotherapy while other lesions may increase in size or new lesions may appear [14]. In this subset of patients, it is presumed that the appearance of apparently new lesions actually represents T-cell infiltration in small areas of malignancy that were too small to detect on CT before the activated immune response [14, 17, 29].

The appropriate length of time needed to determine if an apparent increase in tumor burden on imaging represents pseudoprogression or true progression is still under evaluation, but many clinical trials use 12 weeks as the first follow-up scan following initiation of therapy. In a study by Hodi et al. in 2016, which assessed responses to the anti-PD-1 agent pembrolizumab in patients with advanced melanoma, 5% of enrolled patients who had at least 28 weeks of imaging follow-up (15 of 327 patients) demonstrated early pseudoprogression at 12 weeks after initiation of therapy. Another 3% (9 of 327) demonstrated late pseudoprogression, which was defined as pseudoprogression evident after 12 weeks following initiation of immunotherapy. Importantly, three of the patients with early pseudoprogression went on to achieve a CR to immunotherapy [15].

The length of time needed between imaging studies during immunotherapy treatment may also depend on the site of tumor involvement. Some current research has shown that lesions within the liver may take longer to demonstrate a decrease in tumor size compared to lesions within the adrenal glands and lymph nodes [18]. There is also emerging evidence that lesions within the adrenal glands, lymph nodes, and then lungs demonstrate a greater overall size reduction with immunotherapy treatment as compared to lesions within the liver [18]. These differences may be related to the specific microenvironments within the different organs but are still undergoing investigation.

Although recognizing pseudoprogression as a pattern of response to immunotherapy is important, it is not frequently observed in clinical practice. Pseudoprogression is seen in only 10–15% of melanoma patients [15] and is much less common in epithelial cancers such as lung cancer and head and neck squamous cell carcinomas where the rate is 2–3% [19, 20].

Two additional patterns of response to immunotherapy identified by Wolchok et al. fit with conventional cytotoxic chemotherapy response patterns: a response in baseline lesions with no new lesions by week 12 and SD [14].

4.4 Immune-Related Response Criteria

As these new patterns of response to immunotherapy became recognized, the tumor response criteria had to be modified accordingly. In December of 2009, new criteria were proposed and published in *Clinical Cancer Research*, termed

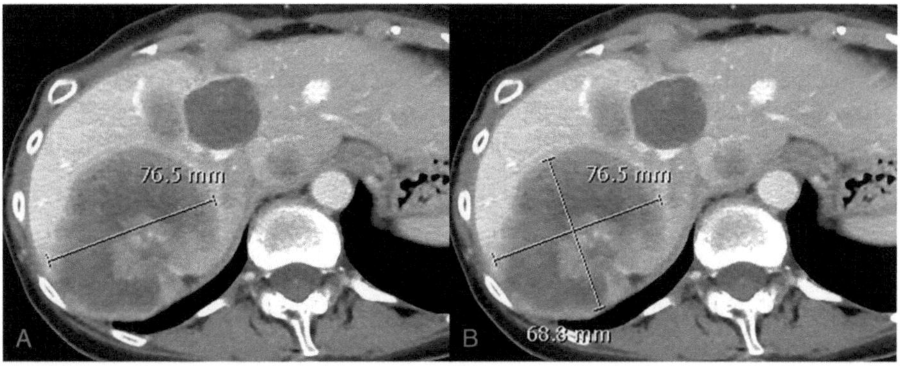

Fig. 4.3 RECIST1.1 versus irRC measurements. Axial CT images from a patient with lung cancer and hypoattenuating liver metastases. (**a**) According to RECIST1.1, only the longest measurement is included, as demonstrated on the segment VII liver metastasis. (**b**) According to irRC, the longest measurement and the longest perpendicular measurement need to be included

immune-related response criteria (irRC) [14]. The irRC were based on data from clinical trials using the anti-CTLA-4 antibody ipilimumab to treat patients with advanced melanoma, and drew from former WHO guidelines, rather than the RECIST1.1 criteria. As such, on baseline studies, up to 10 visceral lesions (with up to 5 lesions per organ) and five cutaneous lesions may be chosen as index lesions. The index lesions are measured as the product of the two largest perpendicular diameters in the axial plane, instead of the single longest diameter used in RECIST1.1. The sum of these products (SPD) is then used for comparison to subsequent studies [14]. The difference between RECIST1.1 measurements and irRC measurements is depicted in Fig. 4.3.

If new lesions arise during immunotherapy treatment, the SPD of the new measurable lesions are summed with the baseline index lesions. A new lesion must measure at least 5 × 5 mm to be considered measureable. Up to 10 new visceral lesions (up to five per organ) and five cutaneous lesions may be added on follow-up studies [14].

The irRC includes the same four types of overall responses, including CR (irCR), PR (irPR), PD (irPD), and SD (irSD), however most definitions are modified. For an irCR, there must be complete disappearance of all lesions (lymph nodes must decrease to <10 mm in short axis) with no new lesions, which is similar to the RECIST1.1 definition. In irPR, however, the decrease in tumor burden must be 50% or greater when compared to baseline, instead of the 30% or greater for RECIST1.1. In irPD, the increase in tumor burden must be at least 25% or greater, instead of 20% or greater for RECIST1.1, and is compared to the nadir recorded (minimum recorded SPD). Note that findings for irCR, irPR, and irPD must first be confirmed by a repeat study at least 4 weeks after first documented. In the absence of irPD, and when the criteria for irCR and irPR are not met, the patient is noted to have irSD [14].

It is important to recognize that under the RECIST1.1 criteria, new lesions always equate to PD. However, under irRC, even with new lesions, the overall response pattern could reflect irPR, irSD, or irPD. Similarly, utilizing the irRC also allows for the diagnosis of pseudoprogression in patients who demonstrate an initial response thought to represent PD, but then show a subsequent decrease in tumor burden. By allowing the correct diagnosis of pseudoprogression to be made, the effective therapy may be continued.

4.5 Immune-Related RECIST

While the irRC was a promising first step in characterizing immune-related tumor response, it has several disadvantages. First, using bidirectional measurements is more cumbersome for the radiologist and has been proven to be more variable than using unidimensional measurements [21]. A study published by Nishino et al. in 2013 also demonstrated high concordance between the utilization of bidimensional measurements compared to unidimensional measurements in 57 patients with advanced melanoma treated with ipilimumab ($K_w = 0.881$), with more reproducibility using unidimensional measurements (95% limits of agreement of (−16.1%, 5.8%) versus (−31.3%, 19.7%)) [22].

Another pitfall with irRC is the high number of target lesions included, which can be double the number of lesions included at baseline as compared to RECIST1.1. A separate study by Nishino et al. evaluated the impact of reducing the number of target lesions from 10 to 5 lesions, evaluated in 90 patients with advanced melanoma also treated with ipilimumab. This study found high concordance between the immune-related response assessment (K_w for best immune-related response = 0.908). They also demonstrated high interobserver agreement of measurements, with a concordance correlation coefficient >0.98 [18].

Taking these and other studies into consideration, another set of response criteria was proposed, which accounted for the new response patterns to immunotherapy treatment initially incorporated into irRC, and also allowed for more direct comparison to the initial RECIST criteria. This was termed immune-related RECIST1.1 (irRECIST1.1) [17, 23, 29].

As in RECIST1.1, irRECIST1.1 again identifies up to five total target lesions at baseline, with up to two lesions per organ. A single, unidimensional measurement in axial plane should again be used to determine the size of target lesions. On follow-up studies, up to five new measureable lesions (two per organ) could be added to the sum of tumor measurements per time point. As in irRC, new lesions are incorporated into the sum of tumor measurements, rather than automatically qualifying as PD as in RECIST1.1 [23].

The overall response categories in irRECIST1.1 use the original numbers described in RECIST1.1, with immune-related PR requiring a ≥30% decrease from baseline, and immune-related PD requiring an increase of ≥20% from the nadir [23].

In addition, there is early evidence suggesting that a change in CT attenuation (measured in Hounsfield units) of a tumor may also aid in assessing treatment response and potentially overall survival [17, 29]. This may be incorporated into the irRECIST criteria in the future, but has not been officially incorporated yet.

4.6 Immune-Related Adverse Effects

irAE encompass any unfavorable and unintended sign, symptom, or disease temporally associated with immune therapy. Some of the more common systems adversely affected by immune therapy include the dermatologic, gastrointestinal, respiratory, and endocrine systems, with musculoskeletal, hematologic, renal, neurologic, and others being reported infrequently [24]. Many of these irAEs can be biochemically discovered as an abnormal laboratory finding or by dermatologic physical exam. However, radiology plays a critical role in diagnosing pneumonitis and colitis.

4.7 Pneumonitis

Pneumonitis is the focal or diffuse inflammation of lung parenchyma [25]. It is one of the most concerning irAE, as it occurs in approximately 5% of patients receiving immunotherapy [25, 26], and severe cases have been shown to lead to patient death in several studies [25, 27].

The CT imaging appearance of pneumonitis can take several forms. A study by Naidoo et al. investigated 915 patients who received either anti-PD-1/PD-L1 monoclonal antibodies as monotherapy or as combination immunotherapy with anti-CTLA-4 monoclonal antibodies specifically for immune-related pneumonitis. Forty-three of the 915 patients (5%) developed immune-related pneumonitis; although most recovered, five of these patients died (one from pneumonitis, three from infections associated with immunosuppression implemented to treat the pneumonitis, and 1 from progressive cancer). The group describes five radiographic patterns of immune-related pneumonitis, including ground glass opacities, cryptogenic organizing pneumonia-like (COP-like), interstitial, hypersensitivity, and pneumonitis not otherwise specified (NOS) [25].

The most common pattern seen in patients with immune-related pneumonitis in the Naidoo study is simply that of new ground-glass opacity (GGO, [25]). GGO is an area of increased attenuation through which the underlying pulmonary architecture may still be visualized (Fig. 4.4). If the opacity obscures the underlying lung architecture, it is then referred to as a consolidation. However, GGO is a nonspecific finding that occurs in a countless number of pathologic states and its presence alone does not make the diagnosis of immune-related pneumonitis. Scattered ground glass opacities usually are asymptomatic. However, ground glass in the setting of the septal thickening and reticulation can signify a more severe form of acute injury known diffuse alveolar damage (DAD) (Fig. 4.5, [28]), which can be seen in the clinical entity of acute respiratory distress syndrome (ARDS). DAD/

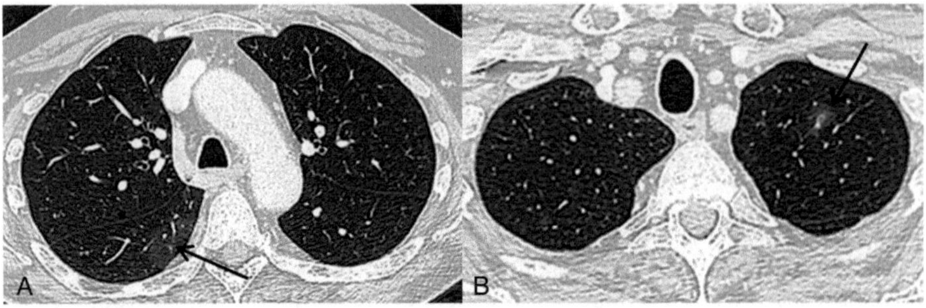

Fig. 4.4 Immune-related pneumonitis with ground glass opacities. Axial CT images (**a, b**) of an asympotmatic patient with metastatic basal cell carcinoma on immunotherapy with development of scattered bilateral ground glass opacities (*arrows*), consistent with subclinical pneumonitis

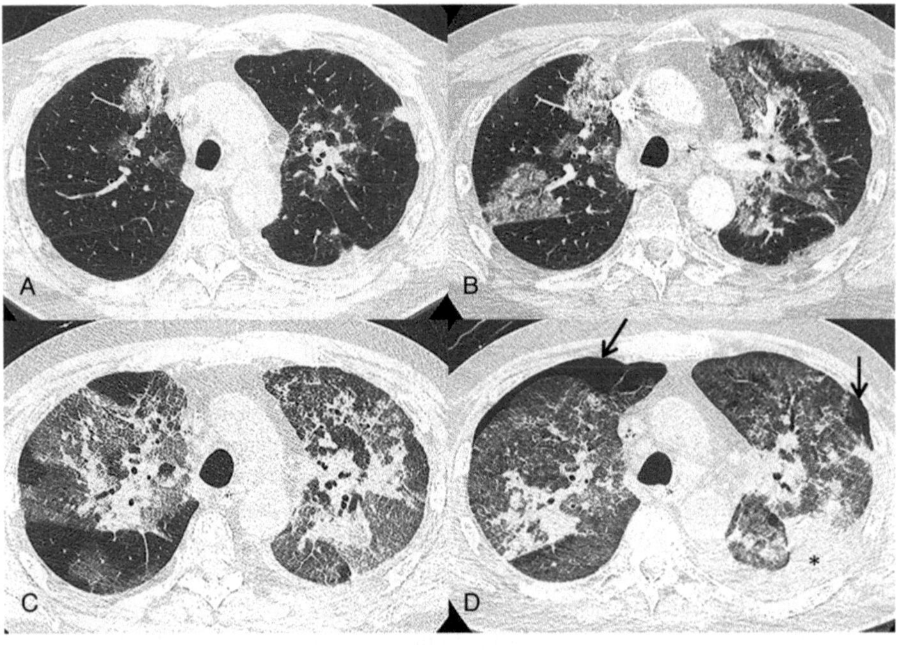

Fig. 4.5 Severe immune-related pneumonitis (diffuse alveolar damage). Axial CT images from sequential CT scans of a patient with metastatic head and neck cancer, on immunotherapy. (**a**) Initial CT images after development of clinical symptoms demonstrated scattered ground glass opacities. (**b**) 4 days later, the patient developed worsening shortness of breath, with CT demonstrating worsening patchy peribronchovascular and peripheral ground glass and consolidative opacities. (**c**) 2 weeks later, the patient required intubation due to fulminant pneumonitis despite cessation of immunotherapy and IV steroid administration. CT demonstrated progressive, near diffuse ground glass and consolidative opacities. (**d**) 10 days later, the patient had also developed bilateral pneumothoraces (*arrows*) and an enlarging left pleural effusion (*)

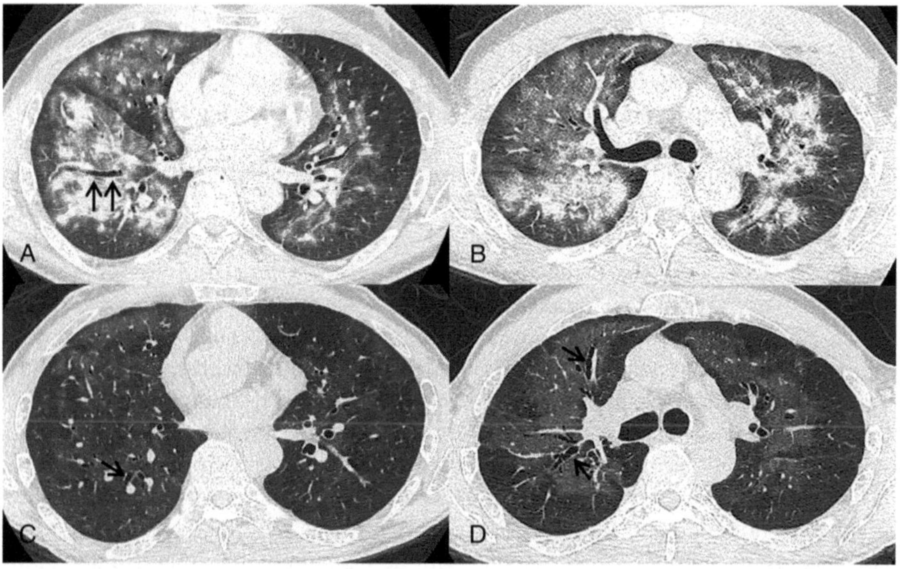

Fig. 4.6 COP-like immune-related pneumonitis. Axial CT images of a patient with mucosal melanoma on immunotherapy with grade 1 pneumonitis demonstrating (**a**, **b**) diffuse bilateral peribronchovascular ground glass nodularity with dense consolidations and bronchiectasis (*arrows*), consistent with COP-like immune-related pneumonitis (**c**, **d**). After holding immunotherapy and completing a course of oral steroids, the opacities have nearly completely resolved, however the bronchiectasis persists, consistent with the development of fibrosis (*arrows*)

ARDS patterned pneumonitis has a more rapid symptomatic onset with extensive parenchymal involvement and can lead to significant fibrosis if the patient survives [17, 28, 29].

Cryptogenic organizing pneumonia can have a varied appearance on CT but most commonly presents as bilateral, peripheral, and peribronchovascular consolidations or GGO. Other features including perilobular opacities, migratory opacities, and more discrete nodularity can be seen [28]. COP-like pneumonitis is another pattern commonly seen in immune-related pneumonitis (Fig. 4.6, [25, 30]). Naidoo et al. noted that patients who developed this particular type of pneumonitis pattern were more likely to need treatment with corticosteroids compared to the other patterns [25].

The "interstitial" subtype refers to a pattern that mimics nonspecific interstitial pneumonia (NSIP), in which there are ground-glass opacities and interlobular septal thickening in a peripheral distribution with possible subpleural reticulation [25, 26, 30]. The hypersensitivity pattern described by Naidoo refers to a pattern than mimics hypersensitivity pneumonitis, with centrilobular nodules and/or tree-in-bud micronodularity [25]. The pneumonitis NOS category includes patients with a combination of nodular and other subtypes on CT, who do not clearly fit into the other subtype categories [25].

Although these described patterns of pneumonitis have been observed in patients on immunotherapy, it is important to note that these patterns are not unique to immunotherapy. Drug-induced interstitial lung disease/pneumonitis can be secondary to both cytotoxic and noncytotoxic drugs with the same wide range of radiologic/histologic patterns including nonspecific ground glass opacities, organizing pneumonia, diffuse alveolar damage, nonspecific interstitial pneumonia, and hypersensitivity pneumonitis [31].

The time of onset of immune-related pneumonitis has been shown to be variable. In the Naidoo study, the mean time to onset was 2.8 months after initiation of immune therapy, with a wide range of 9 days to 19.2 months [25]. The median time of onset in the Tirumani study was 2.3 months, with a range 1.1–8.3 months. Importantly, patients who developed immune-related pneumonitis may or may not develop concomitant respiratory symptoms. In the study by Tirumani, only 50% of patients who developed pneumonitis following therapy were symptomatic at all, with a cough (4 of 8 patients) [26]. One-third of the patients with pneumonitis in the Naidoo study were asymptomatic [25]. It is also important to note that chest radiographs are not adequate to assess for pneumonitis, as they failed to detect a new abnormality in almost 25% of patients with new pneumonitis in the Naidoo study [25]. A chest CT should be obtained in order to better assess for parenchymal changes suggestive of a developing drug-related pneumonitis.

One of the challenges radiologists face is that pneumonitis, particularly when manifested as GGO, can mimic many other diagnoses, including pneumonia, pulmonary edema, diffuse alveolar damage, and tumor progression. In patients, undergoing immunotherapy where there is concern for immune-related pneumonitis, bronchoscopy with lavage +/− biopsy may be undertaken to assist in the diagnosis [24].

Another pulmonic irAE found in a similar number of patients (5%) treated with ipilimumab in the study by Tirumani et al. is that of sarcoid-like lymphadenopathy. This is described as the development of new bilateral symmetric mediastinal and hilar lymphadenopathy occurring in the setting of response to immunotherapy of other sites and in the absence of infection or suspicion for nodal disease (Fig. 4.7). These lymph nodes share a similar histologic appearance of the nonnecrotizing granulomas seen in sarcoid. However, none of the patients develop the clinical manifestations of sarcoidosis, nor do they have elevation of angiotensin converting enzymes or hypercalcemia commonly seen in patients with sarcoid [32]. Note that the findings of new lymph node enlargement in the setting of known cancer should raise concern for worsened/new metastatic disease. However, all patients in this study who had subsequent imaging showed resolution of all lymphadenopathy, supporting but not pathognomonic for a diagnosis of this irAE [26].

4.8 Immune-Related Enterocolitis

As depicted in a systemic review published by Gupta et al. in 2015, studies have shown that approximately one-third of patients who receive anti-CTLA-4 therapy develop some form of gastrointestinal irAE, including esophagitis, gastritis,

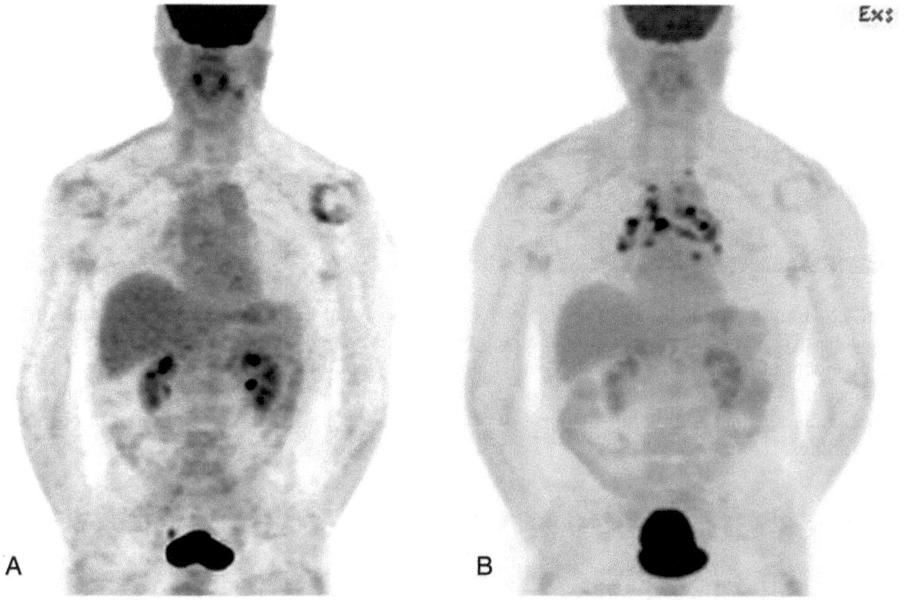

Fig. 4.7 Sarcoid-like pneumonitis. (**a**) Maximum intensity projection (MIP) F18-FDG PET image of a patient with metastatic melanoma prior to starting immunotherapy demonstrating a lack of abnormal mediastinal FDG activity. (**b**) Shortly after the initiation of immunotherapy, the patient developed prominent bilateral, symmetric, FDG-avid mediastinal lymphadenopathy. Although these findings could represent sarcoid-like pneumonitis, progressive metastatic disease should be excluded

diarrhea, and colitis, with diarrhea being the most common and affecting up to 54% of treated patients [33]. Colitis affected between 5% and 33% of treated patients, often proven by biopsy. The time of onset of colitis was variable, in one study ranging from 0 to 59 days, with a median time of onset 11 days after initiation of anti-CTLA4 therapy. In the study by Tirumani et al., the median time to development following initiation of therapy was 1.9 months, with a range of 0.4–4.7 months [26].

It is important to note that diarrhea alone does not mandate the diagnosis of enterocolitis. However, clinical symptoms of abdominal pain, fever, having mucus and/or blood in stools, neutropenia or sepsis all suggest enterocolitis in the presence of diarrhea. In these patients, infectious causes of enterocolitis should be ruled out with laboratory testing of the stool before a diagnosis of immune-related colitis is made. Alternatively, endoscopy/colonoscopy may be performed with mucosal biopsy of sites of visual involvement, which is the gold standard for diagnosis of immune related colitis [33].

Severe cases of immune-related enterocolitis can have life-threatening consequences, including bowel perforation, ischemic bowel, and toxic megacolon. Incidences of these severe consequences are variable in the literature, ranging from <1% of patients [33] to 15% of patients [34]. Dosing of the immunotherapy agent may affect the frequency and severity of the enterocolitis; however, this is still being explored.

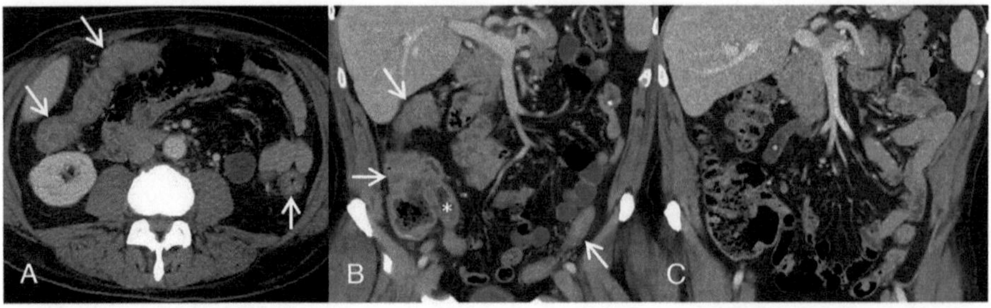

Fig. 4.8 Immune-related pancolitis. (**a**) Axial and (**b**) coronal CT images of a patient with metastatic basal cell carcinoma on immunotherapy who developed immune-related pancolitis with involvement of the terminal ileum (*), with hallmarks of wall thickening (*arrows*), mucosal hyperenhancement and vasorectal edema. (**c**) Coronal CT image 2 months later, after withholding immunotherapy and completing a course of oral steroids, demonstrating resolution of prior imaging findings

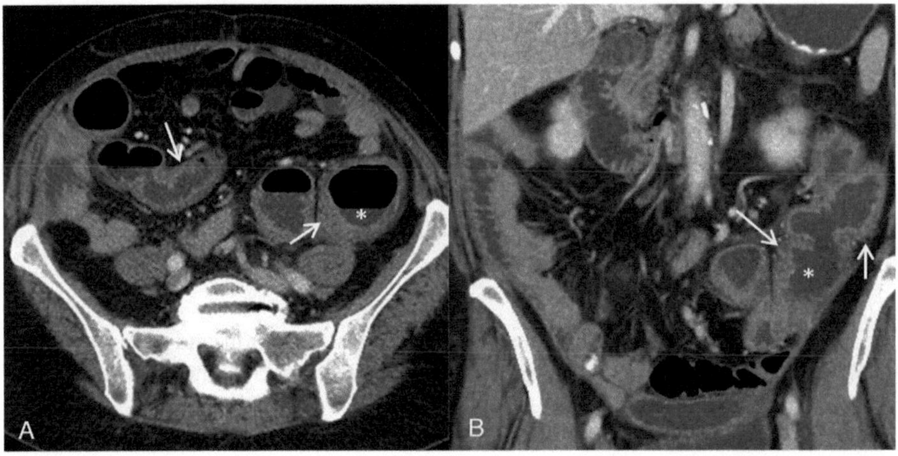

Fig. 4.9 Immune-related pancolitis with acute diarrheal state. Patient with primary peritoneal cancer with postsurgical changes of the abdomen on immunotherapy, with pancolitis also involving the distal ileum. (**a**) Axial and (**b**) coronal CT images demonstrating colonic dilation, colonic wall thickening and mucosal enhancement (*arrows*), consistent with immune-related pancolitis. Also note the fluid within the left hemicolon (*), consistent with an acute diarrheal state

On CT, colitis manifests as bowel wall thickening by more than 4 mm, mucosal hyperenhancement on contrast-enhanced studies, and mesenteric vessel engorgement/hyperemia, with or without free fluid in the abdomen or pelvis (Fig. 4.8). Patients with colitis may or may not have associated diarrhea, which manifests as fluid filling all or part of the colon (Fig. 4.9). There are two types of patterns of involvement described with immune-related colitis: diffuse colonic involvement (pancolitis) or segmental colitis associated with diverticulosis (SCAD), in which the findings of colitis are restricted to a segment of colon with underlying diverticulosis [26, 33]. The pancolitis pattern is seen more commonly than SCAD [26]. Note that the segmental pattern should not correlate to a vascular distribution, which would suggest the presence of an ischemic colitis.

4.9 Conclusion

In summary, immunotherapy is now an established standard of care for many different disease types. Radiologists should be aware of the unique features and imaging characteristics associated with immunotherapy, including the rare incidence of pseudoprogression as well as the unique inflammatory side effects that can progress rapidly. A better understanding of the response characteristics could lead to more accurate reporting of patient responses on immunotherapy.

References

1. Yeh BM, Kambadakone A, Thoeni RF, Towbin AJ, Meyers AB, Smith EA, Thomas KB (2016) ACR-SPR practice parameter for the performance of computed tomography (CT) of the abdomen and computed tomography (CT) of the Pelvis. www.abr.org. Revised 2016, p 1–15
2. Tarver RD, Frush DP, Greenberg SB, Rissing SM, Teague SD, Winer-Muram HT, McAdams HP, Quint LE, Dillman JR, Guillerman RP, Lee EY, Westra SJ (2013) ACR-SCBT-MR-SPR practice parameter for the performance of thoracic computed tomography (CT). www.abr.org. Revised 2013, p 1–10
3. Hooper KD, Singapuri K, Finkel A (2000) Body CT and oncologic imaging. Radiology 215:27–40
4. Mayer AT, Natarajan A, Gordon SR, Maute RL, McCracken MN, Ring AM, Weissman IL, Gambhir SS (2017) Practical ImmunoPET radiotracer design considerations for human immune checkpoint imaging. J Nucl Med 58(4):538–546
5. Seale MK, Catalano OA, Saini S, Hahn PF, Sahani DV (2009) Hepatobiliary-specific MR contrast agents: role in imaging the liver and biliary tree. Radiographics 29:1725–1748
6. Semelka RC, Martin DR, Balci C, Lance T (2001) Focal liver lesions: comparison of dual-phase CT and multisequence multiplanar MR imaging including dynamic gadolinium enhancement. J Magn Reson Imaging 13(3):397–401
7. Lin C, Luciani A, Itti E, Haioun C, Safar V, Meignan M, Rahmouni A (2012) Whole-body diffusion magnetic resonance imaging in the assessment of lymphoma. Cancer Imaging 12(2):403–408
8. Therasse P, Arbuck SG, Eisenhauer EA, Wanders J, Kaplan RS, Rubinstein L, Verweij J, Van Glabbeke M, van Oosterom AT, Christian MC, Gwyther SG (2000) New guidelines to evaluate the response to treatment in solid tumors. European Organization for Research and Treatment of cancer, National Cancer Institute of the United States, National Cancer Institute of Canada. J Natl Cancer Inst 92(3):205–216
9. Eisenhauer EA, Therasse P, Bogaerts J, Schwartz LH, Sargent D, Ford R, Dancey J, Arbuck S, Gwyther S, Mooney M, Rubinstein L, Shankar L, Dodd L, Kaplan R, Lacombe D, Verweij J (2009) New response evaluation criteria in solid tumours: revised RECIST guideline (version 1.1). Eur J Cancer 45:228–247

10. Cheson BD, Fisher RI, Barrington SF, Cavalli F, Schwartz LH, Zucca E, Lister TA et al (2014) Recommendations for initial evaluation, staging, and response assessment of Hodgkin and Non-Hodgkin lymphoma: the lugano classification. J Clin Oncol 32(27):3059–3067
11. Van den Bent MJ, Wefel JS, Schiff D, Taphoorn MJ, Jaeckle K, Junck L, Armstrong T, Choucair A, Waldman AD, Gorlia T, Chamberlain M, Baumert BG, Vogelbaum MA, Macdonald DR, Reardon DA, Wen PY, Chang SM, Jacobs AH (2011) Response assessment in neuro-oncology (a report of the RANO group): assessment of outcome in trials of diffuse low-grade gliomas. Lancet Oncol 12(6):583–593
12. Nishino M, Jagannathan JP, Ramaiya NH, Van den Abbeele AD (2010) Revised RECIST guideline version 1.1: what oncologist want to know and what radiologists need to know. Am J Roentgenol 195:281–289
13. Ferris RL (2017) Evaluating pseudoprogression, atypical responses, and the clinical benefit of cancer immunotherapy. ASCO-SITC clinical immuno-oncology symposium. 16 Feb 2017
14. Wolchok JD, Hoos A, O'Day S, Weber JS, Hamid O, Lebbe C, Maio M, Binder M, Bohnsack O, Nichol G, Humphrey R, Hodi FS (2009) Guidelines for the evaluation of immune therapy activity in solid tumors: immune-related response criteria. Clin Cancer Res 15(23):7412–7420
15. Hodi FS, Hwu WJ, Kefford R, Weber JS, Daud A, Hamid O, Patnaik A, Ribas A, Robert C, Gangadhar TC, Joshua AM, Hersey P, Dronca R, Joseph R, Hille D, Xue D, Li XN, Kang P, Ebbinghaus S, Perrone A, Wolchok JD (2016) Evaluation of immune-related response criteria and RECIST v1.1 in patients with advanced melanoma treated with pembrolizumab. J Clin Oncol 34:1510–1517
16. Di Giacomo AM, Danielli R, Guidoboni M, Calabro L, Carlucci D, Miracco C, Volterrani L, Mazzei MA, Biagioli M, Altomonte M, Maio M (2009) Therapeutic efficacy of ipilimumab, an anti-CTLA-4 monoclonal antibody, in patients with metastatic melanoma unresponseive to prior systemic treatments: clinical and immunological evidence from three patient cases. Cancer Immunol Immunother 58:1297
17. Nishino M, Tirumani SH, Ramaiya NH, Hodi FS (2015) Cancer immunotherapy and immune-related response assessment: the role of radiologists in the new arena of cancer treatment. Eur J Radiol 84(7):1259–1268
18. Nishino M, Gargano M, Suda M, Ramaiya NH, Hodi FS (2014) Optimizing immune-related tumor response assessment: does reducing the number of lesions impact response assessment in melanoma patients treated with ipilimumab? J Immunother Cancer 2:17
19. Ferris RL, Blumenschein G Jr, Fayette J, Guigay J, Colevas AD, Licitra L, Harrington K, Kasper S, Vokes EE, Even C, Worden F, Saba NF, Iglesias Docampo LC, Haddad R, Rordorf T, Kiyota N, Tahara M, Monga M, Lynch M, Geese WJ, Kopit J, Shaw JW, Gillison ML (2016) Nivolumab for recurrent squamous-cell carcinoma of the head and neck. N Engl J Med 375(19):1856–1867
20. Borghaei H, Paz-Ares L, Horn L, Spigel DR, Steins M, Ready NE, Chow LQ, Vokes EE, Felip E, Holgado E, Barlesi F, Kohlhäufl M, Arrieta O, Burgio MA, Fayette J, Lena H, Poddubskaya E, Gerber DE, Gettinger SN, Rudin CM, Rizvi N, Crinò L, Blumenschein GR Jr, Antonia SJ, Dorange C, Harbison CT, Graf Finckenstein F, Brahmer JR (2015) Nivolumab versus Docetaxel in advanced nonsquamous non-small-cell lung cancer. N Engl J Med 373(17):1627–1639
21. McNitt-Gray MF, Kim GH, Zhao B, Schwartz LH, Clunie D, Cohen K, Petrick N, Fenimore C, Lu ZQ, Buckler AJ (2015) Determining the variability of lesion size measurements from CT patient data sets acquired under "no change" conditions. Transl Oncol 8(1):55–64
22. Nishino M, Giobbie-Hurder A, Gargano M, Suda M, Ramaiya NH, Hodi S (2013) Developing a common language for tumor response to immunotherapy: immune-related response criteria using unidimentional measurements. Clin Cancer Res 19(14):3936–3943
23. Nishino M, Ramaiya NH, Chambers ES, Adeni AE, Hatabu H, Janne PA, Hodi FS, Awad MM (2016) Immune-related response assessment during PD-1 inhibitor therapy in advanced non-small-cell lung cancer patients. J Immunother Cancer. 4:84
24. Friedman CF, Proverbs-Singh TA, Postow MA (2016) Treatment of the immune-related adverse effects of immune checkpoint inhibitors a review. JAMA Oncol 2(10):1346–1353

25. Naidoo J, Wang X, Woo KM, Iyriboz T, Halpenny D, Cunningham J, Chaft JE, Segal NH, Callahan MK, Lesokhin AM, Rosenberg J, Voss M, Rudin CM, Rizvi H, Hou X, Rodriguez K, Albano M, Gordon RA, Leduc C, Rekhtman N, Harris B, Menzies AM, Guminski AD, Carlino MS, Kong BY, Wolchok JD, Postow MA, Long GV, Hellmann MD (2017) Pneumonitis in patients treated with anti-programmed death-1/programmed death ligand 1 therapy. J Clin Oncol 35(7):709–717
26. Tirumani SH, Ramaiya NH, Keraliya A, Bailey ND, Ott PA, Hodi FS, Nishino M (2015) Radiographic profiling of immune-related adverse events in advanced melanoma patients treated with Ipilimumab. Cancer Immunol Res 3(10):1185–1192
27. Topalian SL, Hodi FS, Brahmer JR, Gettinger SN, Smith DC, McDermott DF, Powderly JD, Carvajal RD, Sosman JA, Atkins MB, Leming PD, Spigel DR, Antonia SJ, Horn L, Drake CG, Pardoll DM, Chen L, Sharfman WH, Anders RA, Taube JM, McMiller TL, Xu H, Korman AJ, Jure-Kunkel M, Agrawal S, McDonald D, Kollia GD, Gupta A, Wigginton JM, Sznol M (2012) Safety, activity, and immune correlates of anti-PD-1 antibody in cancer. N Engl J Med 366(26):2443–2454
28. Kligerman SJ, Franks TJ, Galvin JR (2013) From the radiologic pathology archives: organization and fibrosis as a response to lung injury in diffuse alveolar damage, organizing pneumonia, and acute fibrinous and organizing pneumonia. Radiographics 33(7):1951–1975
29. Nishino M, Sholl L, Hatabu H, Ramaiya NH, Hodi FS (2015) Anti-PD1-related pneumonitis during cancer immunotherapy. N Engl J Med 373:288–290
30. Hansell DM, Bankier AA, MacMahon H, McLoud TC, Muller NL, Remy J (2008) Fleischner society: glossary of terms for thoracic imaging. Radiology 246(3):697–722
31. Rossi SE, Eramus JJ, McAdams HP, Sporn TA, Goodman PC (2000) Drug toxicity: radiologic and pathologic manifestations. Radiographics 20(5):1245–1259
32. Berthod G, Lazor R, Letovanec I, Romano E, Noirez L, Mazza Stalder J, Speiser DE, Peters S, Michielin O (2012) Pulmonary sarcoid-like granulomatosis induced by ipilimumab. J Clin Oncol 30:e156–e159
33. Gupta A, De Felice KM, Loftus EV Jr, Khanna S (2015) Systematic review: colitis associated with anti-CTLA-4 therapy. Aliment Pharmacol Ther 42:406–417
34. Marthey L, Mateus C, Mussini C, Nachury M, Nancey S, Grange F, Zallot C, Peyrin-Biroulet L, Rahier JF, Bourdier de Beauregard M, Mortier L, Coutzac C, Soularue E, Lanoy E, Kapel N, Planchard D, Chaput N, Robert C, Carbonnel F (2016) Cancer immunotherapy with anti-CTLA-4 monoclonal antibodies induces an inflammatory bowel disease. J Crohns Colitis 10(4):395–401

Chapter 5
Cellular Therapy

Aaron M. Goodman, Tiffany N. Tanaka, and Dan S. Kaufman

Abstract Adoptive cellular therapy includes chimeric antigen receptor (CAR) T cells, natural killer (NK) cells, and tumor-infiltrating lymphocytes. Cellular therapy can be "designed" to target almost any specific tumor antigen to mediate an immune response. This strategy has the ability to overcome or complement some limitations of other immunotherapies such as antibody-mediated checkpoint blockade. Unlike endogenous T cells, CAR T cells recognize tumor-specific antigens independent of HLA-mediated antigen presentation. While CAR T cells have generated excitement to induce long-term remissions or cures in patients with refractory leukemia and lymphoma, the use of CAR-based therapies to effectively treat solid tumors remains in earlier stages. Unlike T cells that must be collected from patients, NK cell-based therapies can function as allogeneic cells. To date, adoptive therapy of allogeneic NK cells have been used most successfully to treat patients with acute myelogenous leukemia. However, many trials and strategies are being developed to engineer NK cells to better target solid tumors. For cell-based therapies to gain widespread clinical utility, optimization of their manufacturing, administration, and characterization of their unique toxicity profiles remain necessary.

Keywords Cellular therapy • CAR T cells • Natural killer cells • Immunotherapy • Tumor infiltrating lymphocytes

A.M. Goodman, MD (✉)
Department of Medicine, Division of Blood and Marrow Transplantation, Division of Hematology/Oncology, University of California, San Diego, CA, USA
e-mail: A1goodman@ucsd.edu

T.N. Tanaka, MD
Department of Medicine, Division of Regenerative Medicine, University of California, San Diego, CA, USA
e-mail: tntanaka@ucsd.edu

D.S. Kaufman, MD, PhD
Department of Medicine, Division of Regenerative Medicine, Division of Blood and Marrow Transplantation, University of California, San Diego, CA, USA
e-mail: dskaufman@ucsd.edu

S.P. Patel, R. Kurzrock (eds.), *Early Phase Cancer Immunotherapy*, Current Cancer Research, DOI 10.1007/978-3-319-63757-0_5

5.1 Introduction

Immune cell reactivity against tumors has been well established and studied for decades. In some cases, spontaneous immune responses can lead to tumor regression, though these are rare in occurrence [1]. Seminal work done by Rosenberg and colleagues at the National Institute of Health (NIH) demonstrates that infusion of autologous tumor infiltrating lymphocytes (TILs), expanded ex vivo, can be successfully utilized to eradicate tumor cells [2, 3]. Allogeneic T cells can result in a graft-versus-tumor effect with the ability to eradicate chemotherapy resistant cells in patients who have undergone allogeneic stem cell transplantation [4, 5]. In addition, the ability of a donor lymphocyte infusion (DLI) to induce long-lasting remissions and cures in patients with hematologic malignancies that have relapsed following allogeneic stem cell transplantation provides further proof of the ability of T cells to eradicate tumor [6].

However, there are inherent limitations to adaptive T-cell transfer. Patients must be able to generate CD8+ cytotoxic T lymphocytes (CTLs) with the ability to recognize tumor antigen presented by major histocompatibility complex (MHC) class I. Furthermore, transferred T cells must have sufficient specificity and numbers to effectively eradicate a tumor [7–10]. Chimeric antigen receptor (CAR) T cells have the ability to overcome these limitations as they can be designed to recognize almost any tumor antigen. Unlike endogenous CTLs, CAR T cells are not restricted to binding antigen bound to MHC class I. The remarkable success of CAR T cells in treating patients with refractory leukemia and lymphoma has generated excitement to use CAR-based therapies to treat a wide variety of cancers [11, 12]. While many studies are ongoing using CAR T cells to treat solid tumors, the challenges seem greater than for treatment of hematological malignancies [10].

Natural killer (NK) cell-based immunotherapy has also been increasingly used in the past few years. Unlike T cells, NK cells do not require self-HLA molecules to recognize tumor targets. Therefore, NK cell-based immunotherapies can work as allogeneic treatments, without risk of graft-versus-host disease. Additionally, NK cells can be engineered to express CARs or other molecules to enhance antitumor activity. Several strategies are being pursued to make NK cell-based immunotherapies suitable for a universal "off-the-shelf" approach capable of treatment of hundreds or thousands of patients from a standardized cell source.

5.2 T-Cell Immunology

Endogenous T-cell receptors (TCRs) consist of an α- and β-chain non-covalently associated with the CD3 complex on the T-cell surface (Fig. 5.1) [13]. Activation of T cells occurs when the TCR recognizes peptides non-covalently bound to MHC on the surface of antigen-presenting cells (APCs) [14] within lymph tissue (lymph nodes). This results in activation of intracellular signaling pathways such as

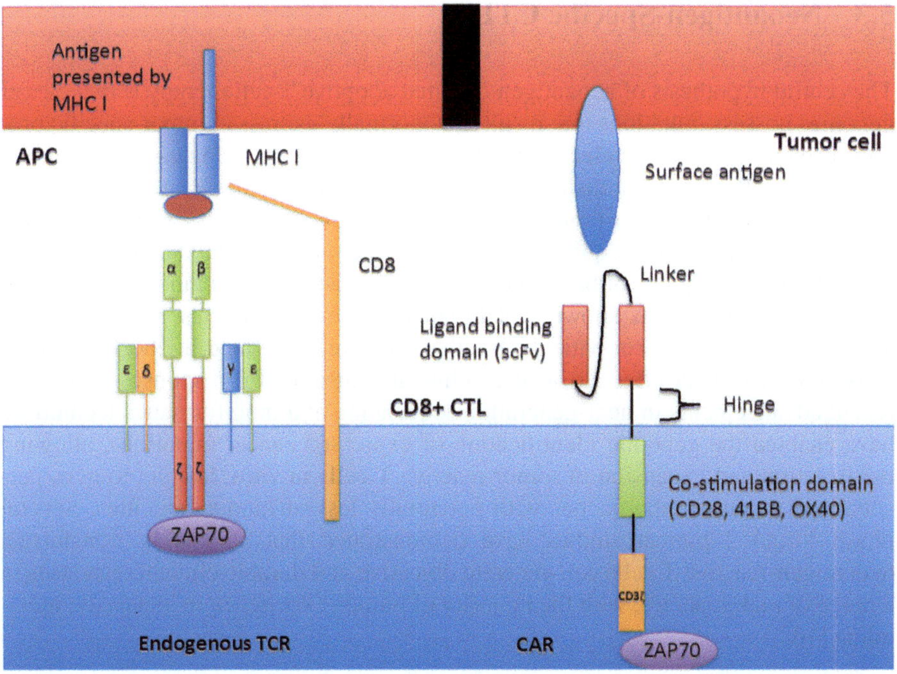

Fig. 5.1 Endogenous TCR versus CAR. Abbreviation: *APC* antigen-presenting cell, *CAR* chimeric antigen receptor, *CTL* cytotoxic T lymphocyte, *scFv* single-chain variable fragment, *TCR* T-cell receptor, *ZAP70* ζ-associated protein 70 (Adapted from Fesnak et al. *Nature Review Cancer*. 2016 [10])

phosphorylation of immunoreceptor tyrosine-based activation motifs (ITAMs) on the CD3ζ chains. Phosphorylation of CD3 ITAMs results in localization of the ζ-chain associated protein kinase (ZAP70) to the TCR-CD3 complex. ZAP70 is then phosphorylated and activated by LCK resulting in activation of numerous downstream signaling molecules culminating in T-cell activation and proliferation.

Activated effector CTLs are able to leave the lymph tissue and survey the environment for target antigen. Upon recognition and binding to a target peptide bound to MHC I, CTLs are able to initiate target cell lysis using perforin and granzymes (Fig. 5.1) [15]. This entire process is highly regulated by both central and peripheral checkpoints. The central checkpoint occurs in the lymph tissue and is mediated by the interaction between cytotoxic T-lymphocyte-associated antigen 4 (CTLA-4) on the surface of T cells and B7-1 and/or B7-2 on APCs. Expression of CTLA-4 on the surface of naive T cells is upregulated upon strong antigen stimulation, and this protein competes with CD28 for binding to B7-1/B7-2 on APCs, thereby inducing peripheral tolerance/anergy [16]. The peripheral checkpoint regulates CTL activation upon TCR binding to MHC-bound peptide presented on the target cell. It involves programmed cell-death protein 1 (PD-1) expressed on T cells and its ligands programmed cell-death 1 ligand 1 (PD-L1) and/or PD-L2, which can be expressed on target cells.

5.3 Neoantigen-Specific CTLs

The central hypothesis of neoantigen-directed adoptive T-cell therapy is that cancer genomes possess mutations that result in abnormally expressed tumor-specific proteins capable of eliciting selective responses from T cells. During cancer initiation, neoplastic cells acquire transformative genetic mutations that give rise to altered proteins. This genomic instability persists as the cancer progresses and additional passenger mutations are acquired. These neoantigens are presented in MHC on cancer cells and are capable of being recognized by an adaptive immune response [17]. Increasing evidence has shown that tumor-reactive lymphocytes pre-exist in the T-cell repertoire of cancer patients, but that they are either held in check or do not cause enough of an effect to lead to clinically meaningful responses. However, recent advancements in next-generation sequencing and bioinformatics techniques have enabled the genomic identification of expressed cancer mutations, allowing the isolation and expansion of tumor-reactive T cells in vitro, leading to new, personalized treatment approaches with potentially less off-tumor toxicities. Several phase 1 and 2 human studies have demonstrated that adoptively transferred, neoantigen-reactive T cells can generate objective and durable clinical responses in a range of malignancies, with the majority of human experience in metastatic melanoma [18].

5.3.1 Tumor Antigen Classification

Genomic instability is one of the cornerstones of oncogenesis. Tumor-specific antigens (TSAs) are abnormally expressed proteins that are not encoded by the host's normal genome, and are the result of mutations acquired by cancer cells. These mutated proteins are perceived as non-self by the immune system and are targets for immune-mediated tumor control or elimination [19]. For virally mediated malignancies, such as cervical cancer and a subpopulation of head and neck cancers, peptide epitopes are derived from viral open reading frames and also give rise to TSAs.

In contrast to TSAs, tumor-associated antigens (TAAs) include proteins encoded by the normal host genome but may be aberrantly expressed or have undergone abnormal posttranslational modifications. For example, Her-2/neu is an overexpressed normal protein in a range of solid malignancies that is associated with enhanced proliferative and survival properties [20]. Since TAAs are normal proteins, their immunogenic potential is dependent on their degree of aberrant expression.

Lastly, cancer germ line or cancer testis antigens (CTAs) are similarly encoded by the normal host genome and are expressed in the testis, fetal ovaries, and trophoblasts but may also be expressed in malignant cells. Although present in normal tissue, CTAs are also potential therapy targets as their tissue expression is relatively restricted [21].

5.3.2 Predicting Neoantigen from Tumor-Specific Mutations

Using massively parallel sequencing, tumor-specific mutations can be identified from millions of protein-encoding genomic fragments (whole exome sequencing) and confirmed to be expressed antigens (RNA sequencing). Since a large proportion of mutations in human malignancies are not shared between patients, these genomic variants are considered to be patient-specific, and thus T-cell reactivity against mutation-derived neoantigens is currently based off of sequencing data on an individual basis. This method of analysis has revealed that tens to thousands of nonsynonymous somatic mutations exist in tumor tissue and are potentially targetable [22]. The set of tumor mutations within expressed genes is a starting point, and tumor mutation calling is achieved by aligning the patient's exome sequencing reads to the reference genome. Tumor variant calls are then obtained by comparing these results to data from a matched normal tissue DNA to identify tumor-specific mutations. Variations in amino acid sequence are then determined from identified changes in nucleic acid sequence, providing the framework to predict the immunogenicity potential of these putative neoantigens. RNA sequencing of tumor tissue not only confirms that the mutated proteins are expressed but may also identify and/or confirm structural variants (e.g., insertions or deletions, or fusion genes that result from chromosomal translocations or inversions) that may be more challenging to characterize with exome sequencing alone.

There are multiple in silico prediction algorithms that have been validated to identify putative neoantigens and predict their immunogenicity based on MHC-binding affinity, which is known to correlate with immunogenicity [23]. Using artificial neural networks and affinity measurements in the Immune Epitope Database and Analysis Resource, these algorithms predict MHC-peptide binding [24]. Once this initial list of candidate neoantigens is generated, further investigation on antigen abundance, antigen processing, and TCR affinity should be completed to prioritize neoepitopes that have the highest ability to elicit an immunogenic, and therefore cytotoxic, response from effector T cells. The neoantigens with the highest immunogenic potential should then be assessed with immunologic assays such as cytokine release assays or enzyme-linked immunosorbent assays (ELISPOT), where peptides are co-cultured with autologous lymphocytes, and mutant epitope recognition and effector function is quantified. Wild-type epitopes should serve as a negative control and be tested concurrently to assure that the T-cell response is specific to the tumor epitope.

5.3.3 Clinical Studies of Neoantigen-Specific T Cells

There is a significant amount of phase 1 or 2, non-controlled human experience with adoptive cell therapy (ACT) using neoantigen-specific T cells, with the most extensive experience in patients with metastatic melanoma [18]. The majority of these trials involved the infusion of T cells generated by isolation of TILs that are subsequently expanded several thousand-fold by ex vivo culture with cytokines. The T-cell infusion is typically followed by administration of IL-2 to enhance T-cell persistence in vivo. There are several practical advantages of ACT: in vitro testing can specifically identify T cells that have antitumor cytotoxicity, T cells can be activated in the laboratory without endogenous inhibitory factors, a small number of tumor-reactive cells are sufficient to expand to quantities sufficient for treatment, and the host can be conditioned prior to ACT. Most of all, neoantigen-specific T cells has proven safe and tolerable by human subjects, with minimal off-tumor toxicity as neoantigen targets are specifically expressed by tumor cells and not by normal tissue.

ACT-based immunotherapy was first described in humans in 1988, when 20 patients with metastatic melanoma were treated with adoptive transfer of tumor-infiltrating lymphocytes (TILs) followed by IL-2 [25]. A follow-up report in 1994 discussed the results of a total of 86 patients with metastatic melanoma treated with TIL followed by IL-2, with 57 patients also receiving a one-time dose of cyclophosphamide 25 mg/m^2 prior to ACT. An objective response rate (ORR) was seen in 29 of 86 patients (34%), and there was no significant difference in ORR between patients who did and did not receive cyclophosphamide conditioning [26]. TIL were administered to patients in this trial regardless of in vitro activity, although a retrospective analysis showed a significant correlation between clinical response and specific in vitro lysis of fresh autologous tumor by TIL ($p = 0.0008$).

A significant improvement in efficacy was seen in 2002 with the introduction of a non-myeloablative preparative regimen prior to ACT, with a proportion of patients also receiving total body irradiation (TBI) [2, 27]. Lymphodepletion prior to ACT helps to eliminate T regulatory cells and lymphocytes that compete with the infused cells for homeostatic cytokines such as IL-7 and IL-15. Patients in these studies were refractory to other available treatments, yet objective responses were seen in 21 of 43 patients (49%) who did not receive TBI, 13 of 25 patients (53%) who received 2 Gy, and 18 of 25 patients (72%) who received 12 Gy. Among these patients, 10 achieved complete response by response evaluation criteria in solid tumors (RECIST), and the 3-year survival of patients who received the lymphodepleting regimen alone or with 2 Gy TBI was 25% and 42%, respectively. In contrast, patients who did not receive a lymphodepleting regimen prior to ACT had a significantly lower 3-year survival rate of 14% ($p = 0.007$), although it should be noted that this was not a randomized comparison.

In a recent review of TIL therapy, which included 194 metastatic melanoma subjects at the National Cancer Institute, the response rate exceeded 50%, with 20–40% complete remissions and 20% durable responses [18]. While acute T-cell infusion related adverse events (AEs) are reported in most of these trials, neoantigen-specific T-cell therapy is overall well tolerated and safe. Several groups noted that acute infusion reactions were not correlated with cell dose or other T cell related factors, such as T-cell phenotype. The most notable non-acute AEs included autoimmune vitiligo and uveitis, an effect thought to be mediated by autoimmune melanocyte destruction, but fortunately, most patients responded well to topical or intraocular corticosteroids.

Outside of the melanoma experience, there have been a few notable studies that have utilized ACT to target tumor-specific peptides. One of the most commonly mutated genes in acute myeloid leukemia (AML) is nucleophosmin (NPM1), for which 50 variants have been characterized. In a study of 27 AML patients, a total of 33% showed immune responses against mutated NPM1 proteins [28]. A recent report on three patients with relapsed Philadelphia chromosome-positive acute lymphoblastic leukemia described the feasibility of generating BCR-ABL-specific CTLs that demonstrated specific antileukemic activity in vitro that translated into molecular or hematologic CR, without significant toxicity [29].

Overall, a few conclusions can be drawn from the human experience with ACT using autologous, neoantigen-reactive, non-engineered T cells: (1) objective, durable clinical responses lasting from a few months to several years are obtainable, (2) high doses of autologous T cells is safe and well tolerated, and (3) T-cell persistence has varied from days to years in vivo, sometimes correlating with the induction and duration of a clinical response.

5.4 CAR T-Cell Design

5.4.1 Structural Differences Between Endogenous T-Cell Receptors and CARs

Unlike CTLs, CAR T cells are highly specific for antigen in an MHC-independent fashion. CARs consist of an extracellular single-chain variable fragment (scFv) of an antibody connected, by a hinge region, to the intracellular signaling components of a TCR [30]. The initial CAR constructs consisted of the variable binding region of a monoclonal antibody and the constant region of the TCR α and β chains [31, 32]. This was later modified to consist of a scFv from both heavy and light chains of an antibody, a hinge region, a transmembrane domain, and a signaling endodomain derived from CD3ζ [33].

Like therapeutic monoclonal antibodies, CARs can be engineered to target a wide range of protein epitopes. The extracellular portion of a CAR (ectodomain) consists of an scFv that determines the CARs specificity and affinity for antigen. Increasing the scFv affinity for antigen results in more potent CAR T-cell activation. Furthermore, CARs with higher affinity immunoreceptors are more easily activated in the presence of lower exposure to target surface antigen [34].

The position of the target antigen epitope within the target protein dictates the efficiency of CAR T-cell activation. Like endogenous TCRs, CARs exhibit decreased signaling proficiency and activation as the distance of the epitope from the target cell membrane increases [35]. For example, CARs targeting an epitope of CD22 proximal to the cell membrane demonstrated superior anti-leukemic activity compared to those targeting a more distal epitope [36]. Modulation of CAR specificity and affinity can be achieved by introducing a flexible serine or glycine linker sequence between the variable heave and light chain of the scFV ectodomain [37].

The hinge domain, based on the constant region of either IgG1 or IgG4, connects the antigen-binding ectodomain to a membrane-spanning domain. Although the hinge region lacks signaling function, its characteristics are crucial in determining a CAR's efficacy [38]. For example, membrane distal epitopes do not require a hinge region within the CAR to successfully activate CAR T cells, while membrane proximal epitopes generally require a long hinge region to be reached [39]. In addition, it has been demonstrated that the IgG4-Fc hinge of CAR T cells can bind to off-target Fcγ receptors, which results in increased clearance of the transferred CAR [40]. CARs with mutations introduced into the hinge region are able to avoid this clearance and demonstrate improved persistence and antitumor response [40].

The transmembrane domain links the extracellular portion of the CAR to the T-cell intracellular signaling machinery. This linker peptide can be derived from either CD3ζ, CD4, or CD28 molecules [31]. Most CAR have been designed using a CD3ζ transmembrane sequence as this enables the CAR to bind endogenous TCR CD3ζ allowing enhanced T-cell signaling activation [41].

5.4.2 CAR T-Cell Generations

T cells require two signals to become "primed" and carry out their effector functions: "signal 1" is activated upon interaction of the TCR with MHC-bound antigen presented on the surface of APCs, giving specificity to the immune response; "signal 2" is a co-stimulatory signal mediated by the binding of B7-1 (CD80) or B7-2 (CD86) on the surface of the APC to CD28 on the surface of the T cell. Without this second stimulus, the T cell will become anergic [42]. First-generation CARs (Fig. 5.2) consist solely of CD3ζ without any co-stimulatory molecules designed into the construct. Trials evaluating first-generation CARs in renal cell carcinoma, ovarian carcinoma, neuroblastoma, as well as other advanced tumors were uniformly disappointing with minimal in vivo expansion and persistence of CAR T cells resulting in minimal antitumor activity [44–48].

To improve CAR T-cell persistence and efficacy, second-generation CARs (Fig. 5.2) were constructed to include co-stimulator molecules in addition to CD3ζ within the endodomain. The initial second-generation CARs developed utilized CD28 or 41BB (CD137) as co-stimulators; however, multiple different co-stimulatory molecules, including OX40 (CD134) and CD27 have been incorporated into second-generation CARs [49–53]. Second-generation CARs have demonstrated superior in vivo expansion and persistence compared to first-generation CARs [54]. Furthermore, the introduction of co-stimulatory molecules to CARs has proven critical for their clinical efficacy. Numerous studies have now been reported describing the efficacy of second-generation CARs across multiple malignancy types including B-cell acute lymphoblastic leukemia (ALL), chronic lymphocytic leukemia (CLL), and B-cell non-Hodgkin lymphoma (NHL) [11, 55].

CARs that incorporate two co-stimulatory molecules into their endodomain are termed third-generation CARs. Third-generation CARs have been developed using

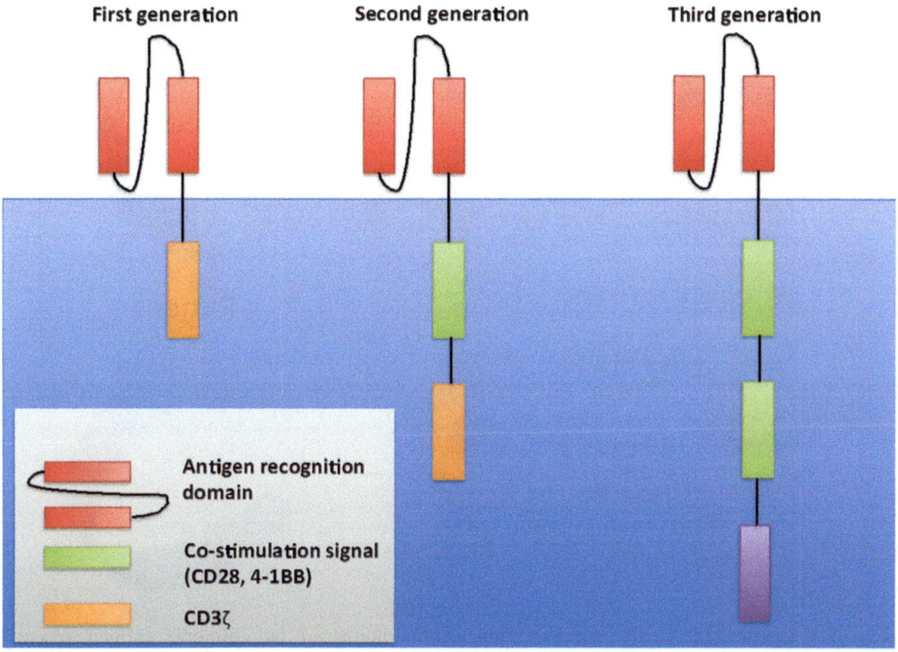

Fig. 5.2 CAR T-cell design (Adapted from Jackson et al. *Nature Review Clinical Oncology*. 2016 [43])

both CD28 and 41BB co-stimulator domains and are beginning to be tested in clinical trials [56, 57]. CARs designed to constitutively express CD40L (CD154) have demonstrated increased proliferation and secretion of pro-inflammatory cytokines with increased cytotoxicity against CD40+ tumors [58]. At this point in time, it is still unclear whether the addition of a second (or more) co-stimulatory domain will improve CAR persistence and efficacy.

5.5 CAR T-Cell Manufacturing and Administration

5.5.1 CAR T-Cell Manufacturing

Manufacturing of clinical grade CAR T cells is an involved multistep process (Fig. 5.3) [59, 60]. Autologous or allogeneic leukocytes are first collected by leukapheresis and enriched for lymphocytes by centrifugal elutriation [61]. T cells, within the pool of collected lymphocytes, are then activated and expanded ex vivo. Multiple methods can be used for T-cell expansion including dendritic cell-based activation, artificial antigen-presenting cell (aAPC)-based activation, bead-based activation, anti-CD3 antibodies, and other technologies. Dendritic cell potency differs among

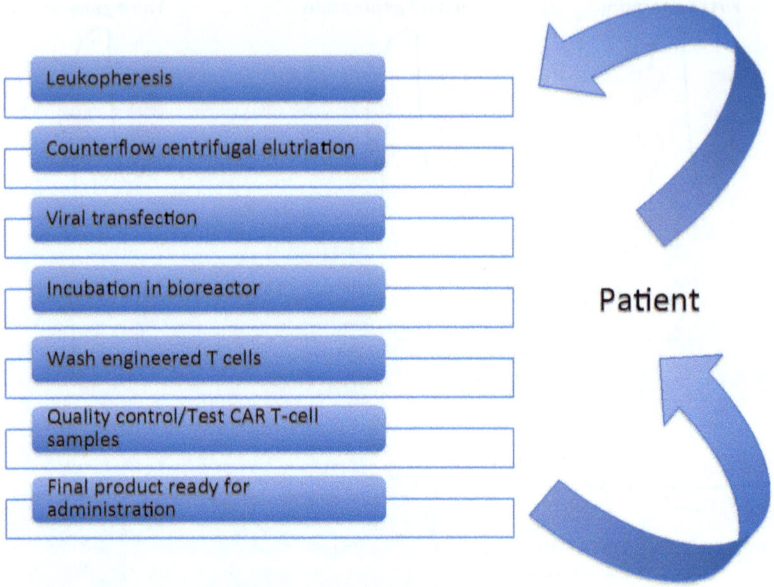

Fig. 5.3 Engineered T-cell manufacturing. Abbreviations: *CAR* chimeric antigen receptor (Adapted from Fesnak et al. *Nature Review Cancer.* 2016 [10])

patients, and this has limited the use of dendritic cell-based T-cell activation in clinical grade CAR manufacturing. aAPCs can overcome this problem; however, they are difficult to use. Their generation requires numerous resources, and it can be challenging to select HLA-matched aAPC lines [62]. Bead-based activation involves placing the patient's collected T cells in culture and incubating with beads coated with CD3 and CD28 (or monoclonal antibodies to CD3 and CD28). CD3- and CD28-coated beads act as aAPCs resulting in activation and expansion of the collected T cells, and this technology is being used in many CAR protocols [63, 64].

Following activation and expansion of the product, the T cells are genetically modified to express CARs. This can be achieved by using ϒ-retroviral or lentiviral transfection, a transposon/transposase system, or messenger RNA (mRNA) transfer via electroporation. Currently, ϒ-retroviral and lentiviral transfection is the most widely used method. However, uncontrolled viral integration into host genomes resulting in insertional mutagenesis and upregulation of proto-oncogenes leading to malignant transformation of the transfected cells is a potential complication of this technology [65, 66]. In addition, ϒ-retrovirus and lentivirus are biological agents that require strict and expensive biosafety testing and monitoring [60].

Given the complexity and risks of viral transfection, other options for genetically modifying T cells are being explored. mRNA transfer involves introducing mRNA into cells by either electroporation or endocytosis. Electroporation involves the use of high voltage electrical shocks allowing cell membranes to become permeable to DNA and RNA [67]. Unlike viral transfection, which yields permanent expression of the transgene, mRNA transfer only results in temporary expression of the coded protein. Furthermore, no genomic integration occurs, which would eliminate the possibility of malignant transformation of the T cells. A limitation of this method is that it would only allow for temporary expression of the transgene (approximately a week) [68].

After the cells have been genetically modified to express CARs, the product is expanded in a bioreactor for a few days. This is followed by cell washing, concentration, and quality control testing [10]. The entire process takes approximately 2–4 weeks from cell collection to patient infusion. However, there are considerable research efforts to shorten this interval and potentially provide "on-site" CAR T-cell production.

5.5.2 *Lymphodepletion*

Most CAR T-cell protocols use some form of lymphodepleting conditioning regimen prior to CAR T-cell infusion (Table 5.1). No standard regimen exists, and it currently remains unclear if there is an optimal regimen to improve CAR T-cell persistence and efficacy [31]. Lymphodepletion involves administrating one or multiple chemotherapeutics prior to administration of the CAR T cells (Fig. 5.4).

Table 5.1 Examples of lymphodepleting conditioning regimens used in B-cell malignancies

Malignancy	Conditioning	Reference
B-ALL	Cyclophosphamide 1000 mg/m^2 daily × 1 day	[11]
B-ALL	Cyclophosphamide 300 mg/m^2 every 12 h × 3 days	[11]
B-ALL	Etoposide 150 mg/m^2 daily × 1 day Cytarabine 300 mg/m^2 × 1 day	[11]
B-ALL	Cyclophosphamide 440 mg/m^2 × 2 days Etoposide 100 mg/m^2 × 2 days	[11]
B-ALL	Fludarabine 30 mg/m^2 × 4 days Cyclophosphamide 300 mg/m^2 × 3 days	[11]
B-ALL	Methotrexate 1000 mg/m^2 day 1 Cytarabine 1000 mg/m^2 every 12 hours days 2,3	[11]
B-ALL	Cyclophosphamide 300 mg/m^2 every 12 hours days 1–3 Vincristine 2 mg day 3 Adriamycin 50 mg/m^2 x day 3	[11]
B-ALL	Clofarabine 30 mg/m^2 daily × 5 days	[11]
B-ALL	Cyclophosphamide 1500–3000 mg/m^2 daily × 1 day	[69]
B-ALL	Cyclophosphamide 2000–4000 mg/m^2 × 1 day	[70]
B-ALL	Cyclophosphamide 2000–3000 mg/m^2 day 1 Etoposide 100 mg/m^2 days 1–3	[70]
B-ALL	Cyclophosphamide 60 mg/kg day 1 Fludarabine 25 mg/m^2 days 2–4	[70]
B-ALL	Fludarabine 25 mg/m^2 days 1–3 Cyclophosphamide 900 mg/m^2 day 3	[71, 72]

(continued)

Table 5.1 (continued)

Malignancy	Conditioning	Reference
B-ALL	Fludarabine 30 mg/m^2 days 1–3 Cyclophosphamide 250 mg/m^2 days 1–3	[73]
CLL	Pentostatin 4 mg/m^2 × 1 day Cyclophosphamide 600 mg/m^2 × 1 day	[12]
CLL	Cyclophosphamide 30–60 mg/kg day 1 Fludarabine 25 mg/m^2 days 1–3	[74]
CLL	Fludarabine 25 mg/m^2 daily × 3 days	[74]
NHL	Cyclophosphamide 1000 mg/m^2 daily × 1 day	[57]
NHL	Cyclophosphamide 60 mg/kg days 1–2 Fludarabine 25 mg/m^2 days 3–8	[75]
NHL	Cyclophosphamide 60–120 mg/kg day 1 Fludarabine 25 mg/m^2 days 2–7	[55]
NHL	Cyclophosphamide 500 mg/m^2 days 1–3 Fludarabine 30 mg/m^2 days 1–3	[76]

Abbreviations: *ALL* acute lymphoblastic leukemia, *CLL* chronic lymphocytic leukemia, *NHL* non-Hodgkin lymphoma

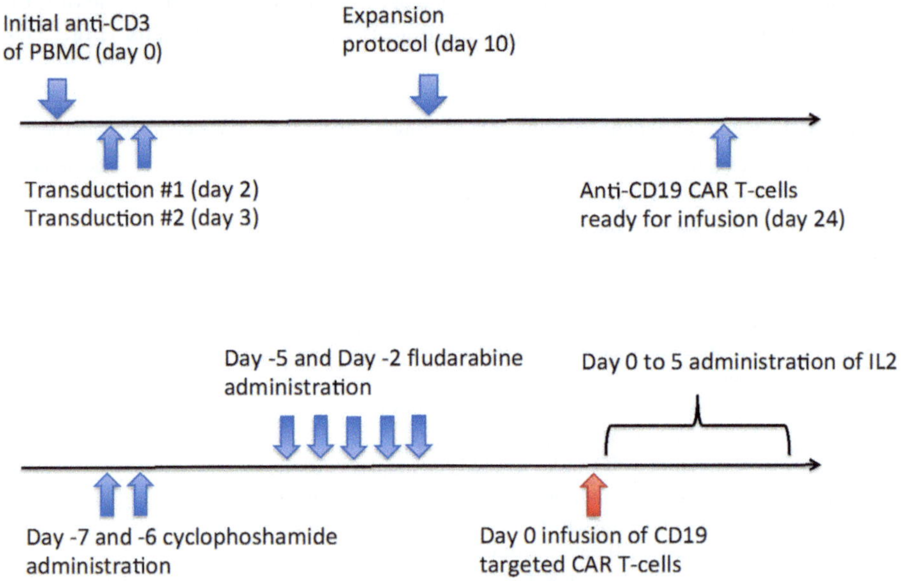

Fig. 5.4 Example of CAR T-cell production and clinical treatment protocol (Adapted from the NCI protocol published by Kochenderfer et al. in *Blood*, March 2012 [75])

Hypothesized benefits of lymphodepletion include transient elimination of CD4 + FOXp3 + T regulatory cells and, possibly, enhanced activity of APCs [77–79]. In fact, preclinical models have demonstrated that lymphodepletion increases cytotoxic T-cell functionality by removing lymphocytes competing for stimulatory cytokines [80]. Studies have also shown an inverse correlation between the likelihood of responding to autologous T-cell transfer and the return T regulatory cells [81]. Finally, lymphodepletion with fludarabine and cyclophosphamide has been shown to downregulate indoleamine 2,3-dioxygenase (IDO), an intracellular enzyme that converts tryptophan into metabolites that inhibit T-cell activity [82].

Clinical evidence does exist that lymphodepletion is necessary for CAR efficacy. Initial studies using the second-generation 19–28z CAR (CD28/CD3ζ) without prior lymphodepletion failed to produce any responses in three patients with CLL [83]. However, among four subsequent patients who received lymphodepletion with cyclophosphamide, one patient achieved a partial response and two others had stable disease [84]. Poor results were also attributed to inadequate lymphodepletion in one study of CD19-targeted CAR T cells in patients with B-cell malignancies following allogeneic stem cell transplantation [85]. At the University of Washington, higher CAR T-cell numbers were seen 28 days after infusion in adults with B-cell acute lymphoblastic leukemia (ALL) who received fludarabine in addition to cyclophosphamide, as opposed to cyclophosphamide alone. A trend toward increased disease-free survival was also observed in the group of patients who received fludarabine in addition to cyclophosphamide [86, 87]. However, in contrast to the above data, responses were seen in 8 of 20 patients with relapsed/refractory B-cell malignancies who received a single infusion of allogeneic anti-CD19 CAR T cells without prior lymphodepletion. In this study, patients had previously received an allogeneic hematopoietic cell transplant, and the CAR T cells were produced from the same allogeneic donor [88]. Interestingly, no cases of graft-versus-host disease were seen despite the administration of allogeneic T cells. Further research remains necessary to better define the optimal agent(s), dose, and timing of lymphodepletion prior to CAR administration.

5.5.3 CAR T-Cell Dose

No standard dose exists among published trials CAR T-cell trials, and it is currently unclear whether higher CAR doses results in increased efficacy [86, 87, 89, 90]. However, a direct correlation between CAR T-cell dose and the rates of cytokine release syndrome (CRS) has been observed across several trials [69, 83, 89]. Doses vary across studies but generally range from 1×10^6 to 11×10^8 cells per kilogram [83]. Interestingly, less vigorous expansion of CARs has been observed in patients with B-ALL who were minimally residual disease (MRD)-positive as opposed to having more overt morphologically positive disease at the time of CAR infusion [69, 91]. These findings suggests that MRD+ patients may be receiving an effectively lower dose of CAR T cells per fixed infused dose due to fewer tumor cells enabling antigenic stimulation of the CAR T cells. This had led some investigators to reserve higher doses of CARs for patients with MRD+ disease while using lower doses for those with morphologically positive disease [83].

5.6 CAR T-Cell Use in Hematologic Malignancies

5.6.1 *B-Acute Lymphoblastic Leukemia (B-ALL)*

To date, CAR T cells have been most successfully used in the clinic for the treatment of patients with B-ALL. ALL represents approximately 2% of lymphoid neoplasms diagnosed annually in the United States. It most frequently occurs in children, but can also be seen in adults with a median age of 39. With aggressive treatment, many patients with ALL can be cured. However, treatment outcomes for relapsed/refractory disease remain dismal. Allogeneic hematopoietic cell transplantation (HCT) can effectively treat and cure some patients with high-risk B-ALL or those that have relapsed disease [92]. Additionally, blinatumomab, a bi-specific T-cell engager (BiTE), has been demonstrated to induce durable remissions in patients with CD19+ B-ALL [93–95], though cures remain relatively rare. However, there remain few good options, other than further chemotherapy, for those who progress after HCT or blinatumomab.

CAR T cells have now been shown by multiple groups to induce durable remissions in patients with B-ALL (Table 5.2), including those who were refractory to blinatumomab and allogeneic HCT. Current targets being explored in clinical trials include CD19 and CD22 [43]. CD19 is expressed on nearly all B cells (excluding plasma cells), including the earliest precursor B cells that are transformed in ALL [102, 103]. CD19 expression is crucial in B-cell development and facilitates the transition from the pro-B to pre-B-cell phase [104]. CD22 is a cell surface glycoprotein that is expressed on over 90% of patients with B-ALL and is not shed into the extracellular matrix [105]. CD22 has been successfully targeted by the anti-CD22 antibody conjugated to calicheamicin, inotuzumab ozogamicin, in patients with relapsed/refractory B-ALL [105].

Two adults were treated in an initial phase I trial evaluating the second-generation 19–28ζ CD19-targeted CAR (CD28/CD3ζ) developed at Memorial Sloan Kettering (MSK). Neither patient received lymphodepleting conditioning prior to CAR infusion; however, one of the patients was in complete remission when treated with the CAR. The patient in remission developed persistent B-cell aplasia, while the other patient progressed. In a larger study using the same 19–28ζ construct, patients with relapsed/refractory B-ALL were first treated with cyclophosphamide followed by infusion of the CAR [91]. All five patients achieved a complete response (CR). Furthermore, all patients with persistent morphological disease or MRD-positive disease upon CAR infusion achieved MRD-negative CRs as assessed by deep sequencing. In a follow-up study using the same 19–28ζ CAR construct, involving 16 patients with relapsed/refractory B-ALL, 88% of patients achieved a CR [69]. There were no incidences of graft-versus-host disease in the four patients treated for relapse after allogeneic stem cell transplantation. Long-term follow-up of 32 adults with B-ALL treated with the 19–28ζ CAR has demonstrated a CR rate of 91% [98]. With a median follow-up of 5.1 months, the 6-month overall survival (OS) rate was 58%. Among patients who achieved a CR, the 6-month OS was 70% for those

Table 5.2 Clinical trials using CAR T cells in hematologic malignancies

CAR design	Target	Patients	Response rate of patients evaluable for response	Toxicities	Reference
B-ALL					
4-1BB CD3ζ (UPENN:CTL019)	CD19	2 children	2/2 (100%)	CRS (severe in 27% of patients) B-cell aplasia	[96]
4-1BB CD3ζ (UPENN:CTL019)	CD19	30 children and adults	27/30 (90%)	CRS B-cell aplasia	[11]
4-1BB CD3ζ (UPENN:CTL119)	CD19	30 children and young adults	26/30 (87%)	CRS (severe in 4 patients) Encephalopathy B-cell aplasia	[97]
CD28 CD3ζ (MSK:19–28z)	CD19	2 adults	1/2 (50%)	CRS B-cell aplasia	[84]
CD28 CD3ζ (MSK:19–28z)	CD19	5 adults	5/5 (100%)	CRS B-cell aplasia	[91]
CD28 CD3ζ (MSK:19–28z)	CD19	16 adults	14/16 (88%)	CRS B-cell aplasia	[69]
CD28 CD3ζ (MSK:19–28z)	CD19	33 adults (includes patients from some of above trials)	29/32 (91%)	CRS (7 patients required vasopressors or mechanical respiration) B-cell aplasia	[98]
4-1BB CD3ζ (UW/JUNO)	CD19	29 adults	27/29 (93%)	CRS (7 patients required ICU care) Severe neurotoxicity in 50% of patients B-cell aplasia	[70]
CD28 CD3ζ (NCI)	CD19	21 children and young adults	14/20 (70%)	CRS B-cell aplasia	[89]

(continued)

Table 5.2 (continued)

CAR design	Target	Patients	Response rate of patients evaluable for response	Toxicities	Reference
CD28 CD3ζ (NCI)	CD19	53 children and young adults	31/51 (61%)	CRS B-cell aplasia	[72]
CD28 CD3ζ (NCI)	CD22	9 children and young adults	4/9 (44%)	CRS	[71]
4-1BB CD3ζ	CD19	47 children and adults	31/35 (89%)	CRS 1 death from intracranial bleed	[73]
CD28 CD3ζ (19–28z)	CD19	8 adults	1/8 (13%)	CRS B-cell aplasia	[84]
4-1BB CD3ζ (UPENN: CTL019)	CD19	1 adult	1/1 (100%)	CRS B-cell aplasia	[12]
4-1BB CD3ζ (UPENN:CTL019)	CD19	4 adults	3/4 (75%)	CRS B-cell aplasia	[99]
4-1BB CD3ζ (UPENN:CTL019)	CD19	14 adults	8/14 (57%)	CRS B-cell aplasia	[100]
4-1BB CD3ζ (UPENN:CTL019)	CD19	49 adults	15/41 (37%)	CRS B-cell aplasia	[90]
4-1BB CD3ζ (UW/JUNO)	CD19	18 adults	13/17 (76%)	CRS Neurotoxicity	[74]

B-cell NHL					
CD3ζ	CD20	9 adults (8 with follicular lymphoma and 1 with mantle cell lymphoma)	2/7 achieved CR prior to CAR T-cell infusion 1 PR after CAR T-cell infusion	None thought to be related to CAR T cell	[101]
4-1BB CD28 CD3ζ	CD20	4 adults	2 patients without measurable disease remained free of progression for 1 and 2 years. 1 patient had a PR	Infusion reactions	[57]
CD28 CD3ζ (NCI)	CD19	1 adult with follicular lymphoma	1 (100%)	B-cell aplasia	[130]
CD28 CD3ζ (NCI)	CD19	8 adults (follicular lymphoma, CLL, and marginal zone lymphoma)	6/7 (86%)	CRS B-cell aplasia	[75]
CD28 CD3ζ (NCI)	CD19	15 adults (9 with DLBCL)	12/15 (80%)	CRS Neurologic toxicity	[55]
CD28 CD3ζ (KTE-C19)	CD19	6 adults (PMBCL and follicular lymphoma)	6/6 (100%)	CRS Neurologic toxicity	[76]
4-1BB CD3ζ (UPENN:CTL019)	CD19	29 adults (DLBCL, follicular lymphoma, and mantle cell lymphoma)	12/18 (67%)	CRS Neurologic toxicity	[305]

(continued)

Table 5.2 (continued)

CAR design	Target	Patients	Response rate of patients evaluable for response	Toxicities	Reference
CD28 CD3ζ (MSK:19–28z)	CD19	7 adults (DLBCL, transformed lymphoma, Burkitt lymphoma)	5/8 (63%)	CRS	[136]
Multiple myeloma					
4-1BB CD3ζ (UPENN:CTL019)	CD19	9 adults	5/9 (56%)	B-cell aplasia	[154]
4-1BB CD3ζ	CD138	5 adults	0/5 (4 with SD)	Infusion reactions	[152]
4-1BB CD3ζ	NY-ESO-1	20 adults	16/20 (80%) (CAR T cells were administered after ASTC)	Autologous graft-versus-host disease	[158]

Abbreviations: *ALL* acute lymphoblastic leukemia, *ASCT* autologous stem cell transplantation, *CAR* chimeric antigen receptor, *CLL* chronic lymphocytic leukemia, *CR* complete response, *CRS* cytokine release syndrome, *DLBCL* diffuse large B-cell lymphoma, *NHL* non-Hodgkin lymphoma, *PMBCL* primary mediastinal B-cell lymphoma, *PR* partial response, *SD* stable disease receiving allogeneic stem cell transplant and 61% for those who did not. Notably, severe CRS requiring vasopressor or mechanical ventilator support occurred in seven patients.

The second-generation CTL019 CD19-targeted CAR (41bb/CD3ζ), developed at the University of Pennsylvania (UPENN), was originally demonstrated to be effective in two children with relapsed/refractory B-ALL [96]. CRS and B-cell aplasia developed in both patients. In one patient, CRS was severe, requiring cytokine blockade with etanercept and tocilizumab, which effectively reversed the syndrome without effecting CAR T-cell expansion. One patient sustained a CR ongoing at 11 months, while the other patient relapsed with CD19-negative blasts 2 months after treatment. A follow-up study reported the results of 30 children and adults with relapsed/refractory B-ALL treated with CTL019 [11]. A CR was achieved in 97% of patients, and at 6 months, the probability of CTL019 persistence was 68%. CRS was seen in all responding patients and was severe in 27% of patients.

The University of Washington (UW) has developed a second-generation CD19-targeted CAR (41bb/CD3ζ) which has been tested in patients with relapsed/refractory B-ALL. These CARs were manufactured from both CD4+ and CD8+ memory T cells distinguishing it from other second-generation CARs. Twenty-seven of 29 patients (93%) achieved a CR after lymphodepleting chemotherapy and infusion of the CAR. Of note, severe neurotoxicity developed in 50% of patients, which was irreversible in one patient resulting in death.

Finally, the National Cancer Institute (NCI) has produced a CD19-targeted second-generation CAR (CD28/ CD3ζ) which resulted in a response rate of 70% of 21 children and young adults with relapsed/refractory B-ALL. CRS was reported and was severe in three patients. Long-term follow-up of this study included 51 patients treated with various lymphodepleting regimens. The overall response rate for the cohort was 61%. Twenty-eight of 31 responders became MRD-negative after treatment with CAR. CRS was seen; however, there were no cases of grade 4 neurotoxicity.

CD19-negative escape has been seen in patients with B-ALL who relapse following CD19-directed CAR T-cell therapy. To overcome this, the NCI recently tested a second-generation CAR (CD28/CD3ζ) directed against the CD22 antigen [71]. Nine heavily pretreated patients who had all received prior allogeneic HCT were enrolled in this study. Seven of these patients had been treated with a CD19-directed CAR T cell of which six had CD19-negative escape. Four patients (44%) attained a MRD-negative CR. This approach appears to be a promising treatment for those who relapse following CD19-directed CAR T-cell therapy, and accrual is ongoing.

5.6.2 Chronic Lymphocytic Leukemia (CLL)

Over the last few years, new promising therapies have been developed including the anti-CD20 monoclonal antibodies ofatumumab [106–108] and obinutuzumab [109], Bruton's tyrosine kinase inhibitor (BTK) ibrutinib [110, 111], and the PI3Kδ inhibitor idelalisib [112, 113]. These therapies have dramatically improved outcomes in all patients with CLL, especially in the elderly and those with 17p deletions. However, despite the recent successes, many patients will likely acquire resistance to therapy [114, 115] resulting in relapse and require lifelong therapy. Patients with CLL who progress after receiving ibrutinib can have few good treatment options. Recently, the FDA approved the BCL-2 inhibitor venetoclax for patients who have 17p mutations and have progressed on ibrutinib [116]. However, further treatment options are limited.

Current CAR targets being explored in CLL include CD19, CD20, ROR1, and Igκ. ROR1 is an orphan-receptor tyrosine kinase-like antigen that is predominately expressed on tissue during embryogenesis [117]. Expression of ROR1 has also been identified in numerous tissue histologies including non-Hodgkin lymphoma (NHL) and uterine, lung, ovarian, pancreatic, and bladder cancer [117]. However, ROR1 expression has been identified on a subset of normal B-cell hematopoietic precursors and pancreatic and lung tissues [118, 119]. A ROR1-targeted CAR has been demonstrated to be highly effective in a preclinical study [119].

B cells express surface immunoglobulin composed of a heavy chain and either a κ or λ light chain. At any given time, approximately 20–80% of B cells will express either a κ or λ light chain [10]. Clonal processes involving B lymphocytes are light chain restricted and express either a κ or λ light chain. CARs targeting either the κ or λ light chain will therefore spare some normal B lymphocytes. Furthermore, Igκ deficiency does not result in an increased susceptibility to infection [120]. Igκ is emerging as an attractive target, and a CAR targeting Igκ has demonstrated activity against CLL in a preclinical study [121].

In one early study, eight patients with CLL were treated with a 19–28z CD19-targeted CAR (CD28/CD3ζ) resulting in one patient having a partial response (PR) that persisted for 6 months and two patients having stable disease for greater than 2 months. Minimal toxicity was observed [121]. Studies at University of Pennsylvania using CTL019 CAR first demonstrated efficacy in a single patient with CLL who sustained a CR greater than 10 months in duration. This was followed by a larger study using 14 patients with relapsed/refractory CLL [100]. The overall response rate was 57% with four CRs and four PRs. All responding patients experienced CRS. In two patients who achieved a CR, the CAR T cells persisted and remained functional for over 4 years. No patients who achieved a CR relapsed. Finally, follow-up of 49 adults with CLL who received CTL019 has recently been reported [90]. Forty-one patients were evaluable for response assessment with 15 patients achieving a response. Five patients remain in CR with a median follow-up of 26 months. Response did not correlate with typical prognostic factors including age, prior therapies, or mutated *TP53*; however, responses did correlate with CTL019 in vivo expansion. Results have also been reported using the University of Washington's second-generation CD19-targeted CAR (4-1BB/CD3ζ) in 18 adults with heavily pretreated CLL who had been previously treated with ibrutinib. The median number of treatments prior to CAR infusion was five, and three patients had progressed after allogeneic stem cell transplantation. Seventy-six percent of patients achieved a response, with 5 CRs. In addition, two of four patients who had received prior venetoclax had a PR. CRS and severe neurotoxicity was reported.

5.6.3 Indolent B-Cell Non-Hodgkin Lymphoma (NHL)

Follicular lymphoma is the most common indolent NHL in countries of the Western hemisphere [122]. Approximately 85% of follicular lymphoma harbor the t(14;18) chromosomal rearrangement, which results in overexpression of the antiapoptotic protein B-cell lymphoma-2 (BCL-2) [123] and thus B-cell immortalization. Most patients with FL have advanced-stage disease at presentation, which is generally incurable with convention therapy [122]. Frontline therapy often consists of combination chemotherapy followed by maintenance treatment with rituximab for those who present with a high tumor burden [124]. Unless treated with allogeneic HCT, relapse is almost inevitable. Novel therapies, including lenalidomide [125] and the PI3Kδ inhibitor idelalisib [126], have been shown to induce durable responses in patients with relapsed and/or refractory disease, although remissions are often not durable. FL is predominately a disease of the elderly, in whom aggressive chemotherapy followed by allogeneic HCT, although potentially curative [127], is usually not feasible; thus, novel treatments are needed.

CARs targeting both CD19 and CD20 have been studied in patients with B-cell NHLs. CD20 is a cell surface glycoprotein expressed on B cells at the beginning of the pro-B-cell phase and is expressed up until the plasma cell stage. CD20 is well known to be expressed on numerous B-cell lymphomas and has been successfully targeted by the antibody rituximab [57, 128].

In a proof of concept trial, seven patients with follicular lymphoma were treated with a first-generation CD20-directed CAR T cell [101]. After infusion of the product, all patients received 14 days of subcutaneous low-dose interleukin-2 (IL2). Two of the seven patients achieved a CR to cytoreductive chemotherapy prior to CAR T-cell infusion. One patient achieved a PR lasting 3 months after CAR infusion, while four patients had stable disease lasting 3, 5, 6, and 12 months. Another study performed by the same group using a third-generation (CD28/41BB/CD3ζ) CD20-directed CAR resulted in a PR in one patient [57].

The National Cancer Institute first reported on successfully treating one adult with follicular lymphoma with a second-generation (CD28/CD3ζ) CD19-targeted CAR T cell [130]. This was followed by a larger study in eight adults with indolent B-cell NHLs using the same second-generation CAR [75]. Responses were seen in six of seven patients evaluable for response. Responses were durable with one response ongoing at 18 months. Toxicity included CRS and B-cell aplasia.

5.6.4 Diffuse Large B-Cell Lymphoma

DLBCL is the most common histological subtype of NHL, accounting for approximately 30% of all NHL cases [131]. Chemotherapy with rituximab, cyclophosphamide, doxorubicin, vincristine, and prednisone (R-CHOP) regimen is the current standard-of-care treatment for patients with this disease [132]. In the rituximab era, 3-year survival is approximately 90% and 60% for patients with low-risk and high-risk disease, respectively, and many patients are in fact cured of the disease [133]. Outcomes in the relapsed and/or refractory setting, however, are generally poor, with approximately 30% of patients experiencing a 3-year event free survival (EFS). Relapsed patients are often treated with a salvage chemotherapy regimen followed by autologous HCT [134]. Almost all patients receive rituximab as part of their initial treatment regimen, and patients in this group have poorer outcomes after relapse, with a 3-year EFS rate of only 20% with salvage therapy followed by autologous HCT.

The National Cancer Institute has reported on the treatment of 15 patients with B-cell NHLs with their second-generation (CD28/CD3ζ) CD19-targeted CAR [55]. Twelve patients (80%) had a response to treatment with eight patients having CRs. Six of 9 patients with DLBCL had a response. CRS was observed and one patient died 16 days after infusion of the CARs from an unknown cause. A follow-up of this study reporting on 27 evaluable patients demonstrated responses in 22 of 27 (81%) patients treated with ongoing CRs of 1–37 months duration [135]. Another follow-up study using this CAR reported results in six patients with either primary mediastinal B-cell lymphoma or transformed follicular lymphoma [76]. The objective response rate was 100% with all patients obtaining ongoing CRs. Toxicity included CRS and neurotoxicity that was reversible.

Studies at Memorial Sloan Kettering evaluated the use of a 19–28z CAR T cell as consolidation after BCNU, etoposide, cytarabine, and melphalan (BEAM) autologous HCT [136]. Eight patients with either DLBCL, transformed lymphoma, or Burkitt lymphoma were enrolled. Five of eight patients remain progression-free at the time of data analysis. Severe CRS was seen in 50% of patients and all patients engrafted their neutrophils.

Finally, studies at University of Pennsylvania evaluated the second-generation CTL019 CAR in 29 patients with B-cell NHLs (DLBCL, follicular lymphoma, and mantle cell lymphoma). Twelve of the 18 patients evaluable for response have responded, and at a median follow-up of 6 months, progression-free survival was 59%.

5.6.5 Multiple Myeloma

Multiple myeloma, a plasma cell neoplasm, represents approximately 1% of all malignancies and 10% of all hematologic malignancies. Over 20,000 cases are diagnosed annually in the United States with a median age of diagnosis of 65 [137].

Treatment for multiple myeloma is complex and tailored toward patient's comorbidities and risk status. Therapy usually involves combining multiple agents including immunomodulators, proteasome inhibitors, and chemotherapy with administration of high-dose chemotherapy followed by autologous HCT for those eligible [137–139]. Almost all patients will relapse as multiple myeloma is incurable unless allogeneic stem cell transplantation is employed [140]. With each subsequent relapse, the disease gets more difficult to treat, resulting in shorter remissions and eventually refractory disease [141, 142].

Current CAR targets being explored in multiple myeloma include CD19, CD38, CD138, NY-ESO-1, and B-cell maturation antigen (BCMA) [43]. CD38 is a type II transmembrane glycoprotein that regulates calcium efflux and signaling in B lymphocytes and is widely expressed on malignant plasma cells [143, 144]. Daratumumab, a monoclonal antibody that targets CD38, has proven successful as a single agent and in combination with lenalidomide and bortezomib in patients with relapsed/refractory multiple myeloma [144–146]. Furthermore, CD38 is expressed on T regulatory cells and treatment with daratumumab results in depletion of T regulatory cells and increased cytotoxic T-cell number and activity [147, 148]. A second-generation CAR T-cell (41BB/CD3ζ) targeting CD38 successfully lysed primary multidrug-resistant malignant plasma cells in preclinical models [149].

BCMA is expressed on both malignant plasma cells and also a subset of mature B cells [150]. In a preclinical study, BCMA was expressed on primary multiple myeloma plasma cells from five of five patients, and a second-generation (CD28/CD3ζ) CAR T cell targeting this antigen has been developed [151]. CD138 (syndecan-1) is expressed highly on malignant plasma cells; however, it has also been identified on differentiated bronchial epithelial cells. A trial using a second-generation (41BB/CD3ζ) CAR-targeting CD138 resulted in stable disease in four of five patients treated [152].

Although CD19 is not expressed on the malignant plasma cells, several reports have suggested that CD19 is expressed on drug-resistant disease-propagating clones [153]. A case report demonstrated the efficacy of the CD19-directed CTL019 CAR in a patient with heavily pretreated multiple myeloma [154]. In this report, the patient was treated high-dose chemotherapy and autologous stem cell transplantation followed by infusion of CTL019. The patient achieved a CR that is ongoing at 12 months. Supplementary data from this publication presented an additional eight patients, of which four achieved PRs.

NY-ESO-1 is an immunogenic cancer testis antigen that has been associated with both spontaneous and vaccine induced cancer eradication [155, 156]. Approximately 60% plasma cells from patients with advanced multiple myeloma express NY-ESO-1 [157]. A study using an NY-ESO-1-targeted CAR in patients with relapsed/refractory multiple myeloma has been performed by the University of Pennsylvania group [158]. Twenty patients underwent autologous HCT with melphalan conditioning followed by CAR infusion. Sixteen of 20 patients had a response. Surprisingly, three patients experienced autologous graft-versus-host disease of the gut, which has been previously observed after the transfer of activated, but non-gene-modified, T cells [159].

5.6.6 *Acute Myeloid Leukemia (AML)*

In the United States, approximately 12,000 individuals are diagnosed with acute myeloid leukemia (AML) annually, and the majority of them will die from their disease [160]. The median age for individuals with AML is 70, and treatment outcomes become progressively dismal with increasing age [161]. Risk stratification is incredibly important in determining treatment decisions in AML and is based on patient related factors, including age [162] and comorbidities, and disease related factors such as cytogenetics [163], molecular features [164–168], and AML subtype [169].

Standard therapy for AML has not changed substantially for over the last 30 years and consists of intensive induction chemotherapy with cytarabine and an anthracycline [170, 171]. Approximately 60–80% of patients treated with intensive therapy obtain a CR; however, almost all will relapse without further chemotherapy [172]. Depending on risk status, consolidation therapy consists of high-dose cytarabine or allogeneic HCT [173, 174]. Many patients with AML are either elderly and/or comorbid and are unable to tolerate intensive induction therapy, have primary refractory disease, or relapse following induction. Outcomes for these populations are poor. Treatment options for these groups consist of re-induction with intensive salvage therapy [175–179], hypomethylating agents [180–183], and/or best supportive care. Those who relapse following allogeneic HCT generally have dismal outcomes unless relapse was 1 or more years after transplantation [184]. Limited treatment options exist for this group of patients including donor lymphocyte infusion (DLI) [185] to maximize the graft-versus-leukemia effect, re-induction, and, for a minority, a second allogeneic HCT.

CAR T-cell development has proven more difficult in AML then in B-cell malignancies as many antigens found on myeloid blasts are also found on healthy tissue. Targets currently being explored include IL-3R (CD123), CD33, and LeY. Limited data on the safety and efficacy of CAR therapy for patients with AML has been published.

CD33 is expressed in close to 90% of all AML cases [186]. Preclinical data has demonstrated the efficacy of CD33-directed CAR T cells against both cell lines and xenografts [187–190]. However, CD33 is present on normal tissue and hematopoietic precursors. For example, CD33 is expressed on Kupffer cells in the liver and hepatotoxicity has been observed with the use of an antibody-drug conjugate directed against CDD33 [191, 192]. A case report has been published using an anti-CD33 second generation (41BB/TCR-ζ) in a patient with relapsed AML [193]. The CAR T cells were administered without any prior conditioning chemotherapy. Grade 4 chills and fevers occurred within 1 h of CAR T-cell infusion and required administration of etanercept, which ameliorated the fevers. A marked decrease in the patient's bone marrow blasts was seen after 2 weeks of therapy; however, marked progression occurred 9 weeks after CAR infusion.

CARs targeting CD123 have also been developed. CD123, also known as IL-3 receptor, together with CD131 forms the high-affinity IL-3Rα complex [194].

In contrast to CD33, CD123 is expressed at low to negligible levels on normal hematopoietic stem cells [195]. Antibodies targeting CD123 have already proven safe and possibly effective in clinical trials [196, 197]. CARs targeting CD123 have demonstrated efficacy in preclinical models both in vitro and i*n vivo* [198, 199]. However, a study using xenograft models demonstrated that CD123 directed CARs markedly impaired human hematopoiesis resulting in myeloablation. This suggests that targeting CD123 with CAR T cells may only be feasible if followed by allogeneic stem cell transplantation [200].

LeY is a difucosylated carbohydrate antigen with unknown function and is expressed on a wide range of malignancies including AML [201–204]. An anti-LeY second-generation (CD28/CD3ζ) CAR was evaluated in a small phase I study [204]. Five patients with relapsed AML were enrolled with one patient dying of sepsis prior to receiving the CAR. Of the four patients treated, one achieved a cytogenetic remission, another had a reduction in peripheral blood blasts, and a third had a protracted remission of approximately 23 months. Toxicity was minimal. Interestingly, blasts continued to express LeY in three of the five patients who relapsed, suggesting antigenic escape was not the mechanism of relapse.

CD7, an antigen normally expressed on T and NK cells, is found in approximately 30% of AML cases. A CD7-directed CAR cell has shown efficacy against AML cell lines and spared normal hematopoietic precursors [205]. The hyaluronate receptor (CD44) is expressed ubiquitously on normal tissue [206]. However, the CD44v6 isoform is expressed in AML and multiple myeloma. CARs directed toward this isoform effectively targeted AML blasts in a preclinical model [207]. Other receptors currently being explored as potential targets include folate receptor B [208, 209] and FLT3 [210].

5.7 CAR T-Cell Therapy for Solid Tumors

5.7.1 Introduction

Solid tumors have proven much more difficult to target with CARs than hematologic malignancies. On-target/off-tumor toxicity has been a major obstacle in developing safe and effective CARs in the treatment of solid tumors due to the lower limit of target sensitivity for CARs compared with antibody based therapies [211].

5.7.2 Carcinoembryonic Antigen (CEA)

CEA is a 180 kDa glycoprotein belonging to the immunoglobulin superfamily and is expressed in both normal epithelial cells and malignant epithelial-derived tumors, most notably colorectal cancer [212, 213]. At the National Cancer

Institute, three patients with metastatic colorectal cancer refractory to standard treatments were treated with lymphodepleting chemotherapy followed by administration of a first-generation anti-CEA CAR [213]. All three patients experienced a decrease in the serum CEA, and one patient had regression of their disease in the lung and liver. However, biopsy confirmed inflammatory colitis occurred in all three patients and was dose limiting in two of the patients. A phase I trial has tested a second-generation (CD28/ζ) anti-CEA CAR administered via hepatic arterial infusion in six patients with advanced gastrointestinal cancers with metastases to the liver [214]. Only one patient remained alive at 23 months with stable disease while the rest died of progressive disease. However, biopsies demonstrated an increase in liver metastasis necrosis in four of six patients. Grade 3 colitis only occurred in one patient.

5.7.3 Disialoganglioside (GD2)

GD2 is found normally on neurons, skin melanocytes, and peripheral sensory nerve fibers. It is also overexpressed on numerous malignancies including neuroblastoma, gliomas, retinoblastoma, and sarcomas [215, 216]. Dinutuximab, an anti-GD2 monoclonal antibody, has proven effective in treating children with high-risk neuroblastoma [216]. A first-generation CAR was evaluated in 19 patients with high-risk neuroblastoma (eight in remission and 11 with active disease at the time of CAR infusion) [47, 48]. No dose-limiting toxicity was observed. The persistence of low-level CAR T cells at or beyond 6 weeks was associated with a significant longer time until disease progression. Three of the 11 patients with active disease at the time of CAR infusion achieved a CR. Two of these patients have achieved sustained remissions greater than 21 and 60 months, respectively.

5.7.4 Epidermal Growth Factor Receptor (EGFR)

EGFR is a receptor tyrosine kinase present on many cell types. EGFRvIII, a tumor-specific mutation, is overexpressed on glioblastoma (GBM) and is not present on normal tissues making it an ideal target [217, 218]. EGFRvIII-specific CARs have been shown to cure mice of intracerebral glioma in both mouse-derived and xenografted gliomas [218–221]. A pilot study has evaluated the safety and efficacy of an anti-EGFRvIII CAR T cell in nine patients with EGFRvIII-positive glioblastoma [222]. No CRS was observed; however, one patient developed nonconvulsive status epilepticus 9 days after CAR infusion. All patients showed expansion of the CARs. Pathological specimens obtained from five patients who underwent surgical resection after CAR infusion demonstrated infiltration of the activated CARs.

5.7.5 Interleukin-13 Receptor α2 (IL-13Rα2)

IL-13 is a T-cell-derived cytokine that regulates human monocyte and B-cell function [223]. Pheochromocytomas and paragangliomas and over 50% of glioblastomas (GBMs) overexpress IL-13R [224, 225]. Cytotoxins targeted to the IL-13R have been shown to result in resolution of tumors in GBM animal xenograft models [225]. At City of Hope, intracranial delivery of IL13/ζ "zetakine" (with the IL13 molecule binding the IL13R to give tumor specificity) engineered T cells into three patients with GBM was well tolerated with anti-glioma responses observed in two of the patients [226]. No high-grade therapy side effects were observed. Building on their initial results, an anti-IL-13Rα2 CAR was modified to include a 41BB stimulatory domain and a mutated IgG4-Fc linker receptor to improve potency and reduce off-target Fc-receptor interactions [40, 227]. Results from one patient with GBM treated with this second-generation CAR have been reported [227]. Prior to CAR infusion, the patient underwent resection of three of five intracranial tumors. Regression of all intracranial and spinal tumors was observed, and the response continued for 7.5 months after initiation of therapy. No grade 3 or higher toxicity was observed.

5.7.6 Mesothelin

Mesothelin is overexpressed in numerous tumor types including malignant pleural mesothelioma, pancreatic adenocarcinoma, ovarian cancer, and some lung cancers [228, 229]. Mesothelin has limited expression in normal tissue; however, it is expressed at low levels in the peritoneal, pleural, and pericardial mesothelial surfaces [230]. In a preclinical model, administration of a second-generation anti-mesothelin CAR (CD28/CD3ζ) was found to be more efficacious when injected directly into the pleural as opposed to the intravenous route [231]. Another second-generation CAR (41BB/ CD3ζ)-targeting mesothelin has been evaluated in two patients with advanced cancer (advanced pleural mesothelioma and metastatic pancreatic adenocarcinoma) [230]. The patient with mesothelioma achieved a PR that persisted for 6 months while stable disease was seen in the patient with pancreatic cancer. Biopsy specimens obtained 35 days after infusion of the CARS demonstrated trafficking of cells into the tumor specimens. This CAR has now been evaluated in six patients with metastatic pancreatic adenocarcinoma [232]. Two of the six patients treated experienced stable disease with one patient off therapy for greater than 4 months.

5.7.7 Fibroblast Activation Protein (FAP)

FAP is expressed by activated fibroblasts in approximately 90% of all epithelial cancers including all malignant pleural mesothelioma subtypes (MPM) [233, 234]. A FAP-specific second-generation (CD28/CD3ζ) CAR has been found to lyse

FAP-positive mesothelioma cells and inflammatory fibroblasts in vitro and inhibit the growth of mesothelioma in a xenograft model [234].

5.7.8 HER-2/Neu (ERRB2)

HER-2 is a receptor tyrosine kinase that mediates signaling in normal and malignant breast epithelial cells [235]. Expression has also been identified on epithelial cells in the gastrointestinal, respiratory, reproductive, and urinary tract [236]. Overexpression and amplification of HER-2 is present in approximately 20–25% of breast cancers, and HER-2-directed monoclonal antibodies have proven successful in the treatment of HER-2-positive breast cancers [237]. In addition, HER-2 gene amplification and protein overexpression has been identified in colon, ovarian, and gastric cancer. CARs against HER-2 have been studied extensively and tested in vitro and in animal models [33, 238–240].

A first-generation HER-2-targeted CAR was studied in 14 patients with metastatic ovarian cancer [46]. No responses were seen, and the CARs did not persist in large numbers long term. In an effort to improve responses, the CAR was modified into a third-generation CAR including both 41BB and CD28 co-stimulatory domains [241]. Unfortunately, the first patient treated with this construct died 5 days after cell infusion. Post-mortem analysis revealed high levels of the transfected vector in the patient's lungs. It was hypothesized that the death of this patient was the result of the CAR T cells recognizing low-level expression of HER-2 in normal lung epithelial cells. This case dramatically demonstrated the increased potency and potential risks of CARs compared to monoclonal antibodies.

Finally, a second-generation HER-2-directed CAR (CD28/CD3ζ) was evaluated in 19 patients with HER-2-positive sarcomas (16 osteosarcomas, 1 Ewing sarcoma, 1 primitive neuroectodermal tumor, and 1 desmoplastic small round cell tumor) [242]. CARs persisted for at least 6 weeks in seven of nine evaluable patients; CARs were identified in tumor specimens from two of two patients examined. Four patients had stable disease ranging from 3 to 14 months.

5.7.9 Prostate-Specific Antigen (PSA)

PSA is a type II membrane-bound protein that is expressed normally in the prostate tissue. In addition, it is found in nearly all forms of prostate cancer and in some cases of gastric and colorectal cancers [243, 244]. Reports from two trials suggest that CARs directed toward PSA are safe and have clinical efficacy in advanced prostate cancer [245, 246]. A second-generation CAR (CD28/CD3ζ)-targeting PSA resulted in stable disease in two of three patients treated [246]. Another study using a second-generation CAR (CD28/CD3ζ) reported that two of five patients treated had a decrease in their PSA [245].

5.8 Markers of Response

Currently, there is little information regarding the use of biomarkers to predict efficacy of CAR T-cell therapy. However, it is clear that in vivo expansion and persistence of CARs are attributes of patients who have achieved durable remissions [247]. Furthermore, transcription signatures from patients with durable remissions are associated with early memory T cells. Nonresponders have transcription signatures of terminally differentiated and exhausted T cells [248]. It has been recently demonstrated that high serum levels of IL15 are associated with the effectiveness of CD19-directed CARs in advanced-stage lymphoma patients, and preclinical studies have found that both IL-7 and IL-15 increase the frequency of CD8+, CD45EA+, and CCR7+ T cells during ex vivo expansion of T cells [248, 249].

5.9 Mechanisms of Resistance

5.9.1 Antigen Escape

Antigen escape refers to a relapsed disease that no longer expresses the target antigen and, therefore, remains "invisible" to the antigen-targeted CAR. This phenomenon has been observed in patients with CD19+ B-ALL treated with CD19 targeted CARs [250]. For example, 13 of 20 patients with relapsed/refractory CD19+ B-ALL treated in one study with a second-generation CD19-targeted CAR (41bb/CD3ζ) had CD19-negative disease at the time of relapse [11]. CD19-negative relapse in B-ALL has been seen at all major centers treating patients with CD19 directed CARs [250].

CD19 has conserved extracellular domains critical for mature B-cell function; however, it is unclear what roles these domains play in B-cell differentiation and proliferation [251]. Recently, frameshift mutations and missense mutations in exon 2 of CD19 have been identified in patients with B-ALL who relapsed after receiving CD19-targeted CARs. Furthermore, alternatively spliced CD19 mRNA sequences lacking exon 2 were identified. Loss of exon 2, either by mutations or alternative splicing, leads to the disappearance of a CD19 epitope that is recognized by the FMC63-based antigen-binding moiety of the second-generation CD19-targeted CART19 [250]. Loss of this extracellular epitope appears to result in a truncated CD19 that is no longer susceptible to CART19 and detection by flow cytometry. Recent analysis of six patients with B-ALL suggests that CD19-negative clones exists as a minor subpopulation and may be selected for treatment of CD19-targeted CARs [252].

An alternative mechanism of CD19 escape was identified in patients treated with the BiTE blinatumomab [253]. Molecular analysis of the leukemic blasts from one patient revealed blasts that lacked expression of both CD81 and CD21, two molecules that form the B-cell co-receptor complex with CD19 and CD225 [254]. CD81 belongs to the transmembrane 4 superfamily of proteins and plays an important function in receptor signaling and intracellular protein trafficking [255, 256]. Western blot analysis demonstrated hypoglycosylated immature CD19 precursors; it was hypothesized that lack of CD81 prevented CD19 processing and maturation in the Golgi [253].

5.9.2 Leukemia Phenotype Switching

Rarely, ALL may switch phenotypes when treated with chemotherapy and relapse as AML. However, treatment with CD19-targeted immunotherapies may increase frequency of this phenomenon. A study has reported on two patients with MLL-rearranged B-ALL treated with a CD19-targeted second-generation CAR who relapsed with a CD19-negative myeloid phenotype [257]. After achieving a CR, within 1 month, the two patients relapsed with AML that was clonally related to their B-ALL. Lineage switch was also seen in an infant with MLL-rearranged B-ALL who relapsed with AML 15 days after treatment with blinatumomab [258]. Finally, another study has described a patient with CLL with large cell lymphoma transformation who relapsed with CD19-negative plasmablastic lymphoma following CD19-targeted CAR therapy [259]. Strategies currently being employed and tested to avoid this include co-targeting of multiple tumor antigens, allogeneic HCT following CAR therapy, and a combination therapy with other immunotherapeutics [252, 260, 261].

5.10 Toxicities

CAR T-cell therapy can result in severe and life-threatening toxicities [262, 263]. Toxicity is caused by numerous mechanisms including the gene delivery system, pheresis collection, lymphodepleting chemotherapy, and either on or off-target immune phenomenon [31]. Two severe, common, and potentially fatal toxicities include the cytokine release syndrome (CRS) and neurotoxicity.

5.10.1 On-Target Toxicities

On-target toxicity can be broadly separated into either on-organ or off-organ toxicity [31]. On-target, on-organ toxicity refers to adverse events directly attributable to the CAR T cells engaging their target antigen [31]. The most common example of this is in the treatment of B-cell malignancies with CD19-targeted CARs, which results in B-cell aplasia [264]. Nearly all trials using CD19-targeted CARs report this phenomenon (Table 5.2). CAR induced B-cell aplasia is a highly accurate marker for the pharmacodynamics CAR function [30]. Treatment with immunoglobulin replacement (IVIG) appears to mitigate most infectious complications.

On-target, off-organ toxicity refers to the CAR engaging their target antigen; however, the antigen being engaged is "off organ." [31] For example, targeting CD33 in myeloid malignancies can result in severe hepatotoxicity as CD33 is expressed on the Kupffer cells in the liver [43].

5.10.2 Cytokine Release Syndrome (CRS)

CRS is a non-antigen-specific toxicity that results from overwhelming activation of the immune system [262]. Activation of B and T cells, NK cells, myeloid-derived cells (macrophages, dendritic cells, and monocytes) results in large-scale secretion of numerous inflammatory cytokines including INFγ, IL6, TNFα, IL-2, GM-CSF, IL10, IL8, and IL5 [69, 75, 96, 99]. CRS is not unique to CAR T-cell therapy and has been reported after the administration of alemtuzumab [265], the CD28 superagonist TGN1412 [266], BiTEs [102], and haploidentical mononuclear cells [267]. CRS can occur within minutes to days following drug administration. For example, CRS usually occurs within minutes following administration of the anti-CD20 monoclonal antibody rituximab [268]. However, CRS following CAR T-cell infusions usually occurs days to weeks after product administration, which coincides with maximal in vivo T-cell expansion [262]. Numerous reports indicate that incidence and severity of CRS following CAR T-cell infusion directly correlates with the degree of tumor burden [75, 91, 96, 99].

IL6 has been identified to be a central mediator in the pathogenesis of CRS [262]. IL6 is a pleotropic cytokine that regulates the immune response during inflammation and hematopoiesis [269, 270]. IL6 requires the broadly expressed cell-associated protein gp130 (CD130) for signaling [269]. When IL 6 levels are low, IL6 binds to the IL6 receptor (CD126) present on macrophages, neutrophils, and hepatocytes. However, when levels of IL6 are high, soluble IL6 receptor signaling predominates and initiates *trans* signaling on numerous additional cell types [271]. Two monoclonal antibodies are currently available that block IL6-mediated signaling, the anti-IL6 receptor antibody tocilizumab [272] and the anti-IL6 antibody siltuximab [273].

Symptoms of CRS can range from fevers, chills, and myalgias to frank shock with refractory hypotension and multi-organ failure (Table 5.3). Fevers frequently exceed 40.0 °C [262]. A commonly used grading system for CRS is shown in Table 5.4. In addition to rigorous supportive care, it is now recommended that severe (typically grade 3 or higher) CRS be treated with tocilizumab. Experience at numerous institutions has demonstrated that administration of tocilizumab is an effective therapy for severe and life-threatening CRS [69, 75, 96, 99]. Patients typically respond rapidly to tocilizumab administration. However, for patients who do not respond within 24 h, a second dose of tocilizumab or alternative immunosuppressive agent can be administered [262]. Corticosteroids can be con-

Table 5.3 Symptoms and laboratory findings in CRS [263]

Organ system	Clinical findings
Constitutional	Fevers Rigors Malaise Fatigue Anorexia
Neurologic	Headaches Changes in level of consciousness Delirium Aphasia Apraxia Ataxia Hallucinations Tremor Dysmetria Myoclonus Facial nerve palsy Seizures
Hepatic	Transaminitis Hyperbilirubinemia
Hematologic	Anemia Thrombocytopenia Neutropenia Lymphopenia Elevated D-dimer Prolonged prothrombin time Prolonged activated partial thromboplastin time Hypofibrinogenemia Disseminated intravascular coagulation
Cardiovascular	Tachycardia Hypotension Arrhythmias Decreased left ventricular ejection fraction Troponinemia GT prolongation
Pulmonary	Tachypnea Hypoxia
Renal	Acute kidney injury Hyponatremia Hypokalemia Hypophosphatemia Tumor lysis syndrome
Gastrointestinal	Nausea Emesis Diarrhea
Musculoskeletal	Myalgias Elevated creatine kinase Weakness

Abbreviations: *CRS* cytokine release syndrome

Table 5.4 Cytokine release storm grading system and management [262]

Grade	Toxicity	Management
1	Symptoms are not life threatening and require symptomatic treatment only (fever, nausea, fatigue, headache, myalgias, malaise)	Vigilant supportive care Assess for infection
2	Symptoms require and respond to moderate intervention Oxygen requirement of 40% Hypotension responsive to fluids or low dose of one vasopressor Grade 2 organ toxicity	No extensive comorbidities Vigilant supportive care Extensive comorbidities: Vigilant supportive care Tocilizumab +/− steroids
3	Symptoms require and respond to aggressive intervention Oxygen requirement of 40% Hypotension requiring high-dose or multiple vasopressors Grade 3 organ toxicity or grade 4 transaminitis	Vigilant supportive care Tocilizumab +/− steroids
4	Life-threatening symptoms Requirement for ventilator support Grade 4 organ toxicity (excluding transaminitis)	Vigilant supportive care Tocilizumab +/− steroids
5	Death	

sidered for refractory cases; however, there is emerging evidence that suggests steroids may mediate a greater adverse effect on the antitumor activity of CAR T cells [69, 91].

5.10.3 Neurotoxicity

The neurotoxicity seen in CAR T-cell therapy is similar to what has been reported in patients receiving the BiTE blinatumomab [102]. Reported toxicities include somnolence, global encephalopathy, cranial nerve palsies, seizures, hallucinations, dysphasia, ataxia, and apraxia [11, 69, 89, 91, 96, 263]. Severe neurotoxicity may necessitate mechanical ventilation for airway protection [263]. Several groups have reported anti-CD19-targeted CARs in the cerebrospinal fluid (CSF) of patients [11, 69, 89, 96], and in one study, higher levels of anti-CD19-targeted CARs in the CSF was identified in patients experiencing neurotoxicity versus those who were not [89].

Tocilizumab is generally not recommended for treatment of neurotoxicity as it does not cross the blood-brain barrier [263]. However, IL6 is known to cross the blood-brain barrier and has been shown to mediate neurotoxicity [274]. Administration of tocilizumab can raise serum IL6 levels by saturating IL6 receptors [275]. This theoretically could increase CSF levels of IL6 and worsen toxicity [263]. Many groups currently recommend the CSF-penetrating steroid, dexamethasone, for the treatment of severe neurotoxicity (REF).

5.11 NK Cells for Cancer Therapy

NK cells are CD3⁻CD56⁺ large granular lymphocytes of the innate immune system that were identified in the 1970s based on their ability to kill virally infected cells and tumor cells without prior sensitization and without HLA restriction [276, 277]. Therefore, NK cells are fundamentally different from T cells that are restricted to recognizing self-HLA molecules. This enables use of NK cells as allogeneic anti-cancer cells, in contrast to CAR T cells, are genetically modified autologous cells that must be produced on a patient-specific fashion. While one recent trial has used genetically modified allogeneic CAR-expressing T cells [278], this experience is still limited, and it is unclear whether alloreactive T cells were effectively removed in this system to prevent complications such as graft-versus-host disease. Indeed, as noted, complications such as cytokine release syndrome and neurotoxicity in patients receiving CAR T cells have led to significant morbidity and some deaths [263, 279]. Notably, clinical trials with NK cells from peripheral blood and umbilical cord blood do not show similar toxicities [280–286].

A balance of activating and inhibitory signaling receptors regulate normal NK cell function, allowing for self-tolerance as well as the NK cell effector function including cytotoxicity, cytokine production, and cell proliferation [276]. Inhibitory receptors are utilized to prevent the killing of healthy cells, whereas strong activating signals prompt an immune response against infected or malignant cells. Activating receptors on NK cells that prompt cytotoxicity against tumor cells include NKG2D (or CD314), the natural cytotoxicity receptors (NCRs), DNAM1 (or CD2226), and CD16. When activated by target cell interactions or cytokines in the microenvironment, NK cells produce and secrete interferon-γ (IFNγ), numerous interleukins, tumor necrosis factor (TNF) and growth factors, and chemokines. Secretion of these cytokines activates other components of the immune system, such as MHC class II presentation on antigen-presenting cells, T helper 1 (T_H1) cells, myeloid cells, and angiogenesis. In contrast, inhibitory NK cell receptors detect self-MHC class I ligands on healthy cells and include members of the killer immunoglobulin receptors (KIRs) and the CD94 (or KLRD1)-NKG2 receptor system.

Another important mechanism of NK cell function is antibody-dependent cell-mediated cytotoxicity. This mechanism is activated by CD16 (or FcγRIIIA), which recognizes the constant region (Fc) of IgG antibodies and is responsible for ADCC. Interestingly, CD16 is also expressed by macrophages, and thus both NK cells and macrophages provide therapeutic opportunities that take advantage of their ADCC properties.

5.12 Tumor Immunosurveillance by NK Cells

NK cell deficiencies, marked either by the absence of NK cells or aberrant function, have been implicated in the development of malignancies. For example, patients afflicted by diseases marked by NK cell dysfunction—such as

Chediak-Higashi and X-linked lymphoproliferative syndrome—have a higher risk of developing malignancies, particularly AML (REF).

5.13 NK Cell Clinical Trials

In the past decade, multiple clinical trials have demonstrated that NK cells have the potent ability to treat AML that is refractory or resistant to standard chemotherapy [280–282]. Many recent advances have led to a dramatic increase in NK cell-based clinical trials for AML and other malignancies. Indeed, clinicaltrials.gov currently lists at least 50 different NK cell-based clinical trials recruiting patients for a variety of both hematological malignancies and solid tumors.

While NK cells are known to be a component of TILs used for autologous antitumor therapies as described above, one of the first studies to clearly demonstrate that allogeneic NK cells have direct antitumor activity came from an analysis in patients undergoing allogeneic HCT for AML and ALL [281]. This study demonstrated that a haploidentical HCT that was KIR mismatched in the GVH direction (meaning donor NK cells would not be inhibited by patient HLA class I molecules) lead to long-term CRs in all patients treated for AML. Specifically, KIR- and HLA-C-mismatched NK cells were found to mediate elimination of AML without causing concomitant GVHD. Interestingly, ALL patients did not see good responses by this therapy.

A subsequent study in 2005 augmented this strategy by using adoptive transfer of haploidentical NK cells combined with lymphodepleting regimen prior to NK cell infusion followed by infusions of IL-2. The authors noted a significant rise in endogenous IL-15, a cytokine required for final differentiation of CD34-positive progenitors to NK cells in vitro, among patients who received the more intensive conditioning regimen (high-dose fludarabine and cyclophosphamide). Of note, 5 of 19 of these poor-risk AML patients obtained hematologic remission with this approach [283]. Outside of AML, NK cellular therapy followed by in vivo IL-2 expansion has also been studied in ovarian cancer, breast cancer, and refractory non-Hodgkin lymphoma [287, 288]. In these clinical trials, the persistence and increase in regulatory T cells (Tregs) likely interfered with NK cell expansion and survival. Tregs not only persisted following cytotoxic therapy but also rapidly expanded after the IL-2 course was administered. Tregs directly limit NK cell expansion by competing for IL-2, as Tregs express the high-affinity IL-2 receptor α chain (CD25) and IL-2 provides the strongest proliferative signal for Tregs. An update of this approach used an anti-IL2 diphtheria toxin (IL-2DT)-linked fusion protein to deplete IL2-receptor expressing T regulatory cells. In this study, patients treated with IL2-DT as part of a cyclophosphamide/fludarabine conditioning regimen had increased NK cell expansion and improved rate of remissions [284]. Specifically, 53% (8 of 15) patients whose conditioning included IL2-DT had CRs compared to 21% of patients who did not receive IL2-DT. Several patients who achieved CRs went on to allogeneic hematopoietic cell transplantation to extend the curative potential of this approach.

A recent study describes how novel cytokine-induced memory-like (CIML) NK cells that are pre-activated by IL-12, IL-15, and IL-18 were found to have increased cell proliferation and expression of high-affinity IL-2 receptor αβγ and increased production of interferon-γ, translating to augmented anti-AML activity [285]. A phase 1 clinical trial using the CIML NK cells for patients with relapsed/refractory AML demonstrated responses (either CR or morphologic leukemia-free state) in 5 of 9 (55%) patients, with at least 2 patients remaining in remission over 1 year post-treatment. Again, no GVHD was demonstrated by this NK cell therapy [285].

Umbilical cord blood (UCB) has also been a source of NK cells used for clinical trials against relapsed refractory AML and other hematologic malignancies. One recent study treated older (median age 72) AML patients with lymphodepleting (cyclophosphamide and fludarabine) chemotherapy and UCB-NK cells, though no cytokines were given post-NK cell infusion, as was done in other studies. Here, 4 of 10 patients remained in remission 1–5 years post-NK cell treatment, with at least 2 patients converting from MRD-positive to MRD-negative disease [286]. Another recent trial used UCB-NK cells to treat patients with high-risk or relapsed multiple myeloma [289]. After conditioning with lenalidomide and melphalan, patients received the UCB-NK cells combined with autologous HCT. While difficult to determine the specific role of NK cells in this regimen, 10 of 12 patients did achieve a very good partial response, near CR or CR.

Other NK populations have also been characterized in preclinical and clinical studies. The so-called "adaptive" NK cell has been characterized as $CD56^{dim}$ $CD57^{+}NKG2C^{+}$ cells obtained only from CMV+ individuals [290]. These adaptive NK cell have more potent antitumor activity and will soon be used in clinical trials. An NK cell line termed NK-92 has also been used in clinical trials against diverse refractory malignancies. However, as NK-92 is an aneuploid cell line with malignant potential, these cells must be irradiated before administering to patients, limiting the in vivo expansion potential [291].

5.14 Derivation of NK Cells from Human Pluripotent Stem Cells

These trials of NK cell-based therapy using NK cells isolated from peripheral blood (typically using haploidentical donors) or UCB have generated great interest in expanding the use of NK cells to treat relapsed or refractory cancers. One strategy to increase the supply and access to NK cell-based therapies is to derive NK cells from human pluripotent stem cells. Human pluripotent stem cells consist of both human embryonic stem cells (hESCs) and induced pluripotent stem cells (iPSCs). These cells have the potential to make all the cells in the body, including blood and immune cells [292–294]. Clinical trials using both hESC- and iPSC-derived cells are underway for diseases such as spinal cord injury, diabetes, retinal disease, and cardiac disease [294].

Studies over the past decade demonstrate efficient production of NK cells from human pluripotent stem cells (both hESCs and iPSCs) [295–298]. These hESC- and iPSC-derived NK cells have similar phenotype as PB-NK cells and UCB-NK cells. Moreover, the anti-AML activity of hESC- and iPSC-NK cells is at least as good, if not better, than PB-NK cells and UCB-NK cells [296, 297].

5.15 hESC/iPSC-Based NK Cell Therapy Offers Several Potential Advantages Over Existing Immune Therapies

1. hESC/iPSC-derived NK cells can provide a standardized, "off-the-shelf" homogeneous therapy that is advantageous compared to current patient-specific therapies. As noted, NK cells currently used for clinical trials [193, 296, 299] are typically isolated from peripheral blood of haploidentical donors. Again, this involves significant time and expense. Additionally, the PB-NK cell product is a very heterogeneous cell population that markedly differs between donors. Also, as described, different strategies are used to isolate the NK cells from peripheral blood, making it difficult to compare between products and trials [283–285]. In contrast, hESC/iPSC-derived NK cells provide a standardized cell product that is >97% NK cells [297], and production of hESC-/iPSC-derived NK cells can provide a homogeneous cellular immunotherapy product that can be scaled to potentially treat hundreds, or thousands, of patients [297].
2. *Production of a standardized bank of hESC-/iPSC-derived NK cells enables multiple treatments of the same patient.* The ready availability of hESC-/iPSC-derived NK cells will allow these cells to become part of the standard-of-care treatment for AML. Again, this is in contrast to NK cells isolated from peripheral blood or cord blood that only contain enough NK cells for one treatment dose.
3. *hESC-/iPSC-derived NK cells do not require collecting cells from the patient or donors.* This saves time and expense. Additionally, CAR T cells have been proposed for the treatment of AML (e.g., with an anti-CD123 or anti-CD33 CAR(*23*). However, since these antigens are expressed on normal myeloid cells as well as the leukemic cells, CAR T-cell-based therapy likely needs to be combined with allogeneic hematopoietic cell transplant. This sharply limits patients who would be able to receive CAR T cells for AML. Notably, one test of anti-CD33-CAR T cells for AML did not demonstrate substantial benefit [193].

5.16 Engineering NK Cells for Improved Antitumor Activity

As with T cells, NK cells can be engineered to express CARs to enhance antitumor activity. Much of this work has been done with the NK cell line, NK-92. These cells have been used as they are relatively easy to genetically modify. Additionally, since NK-92 cells have relatively little direct antitumor activity, addition of CARs can provide a significant improvement in the ability to directly kill cancer cells. Preclinical studies have characterized NK-92 cells that target diverse tumor antigens, including CD19 and CD20, ErbB2(HER2), and CD138 [300]. However, none of these CAR-expressing NK-92 cells have yet entered clinical trials.

CARs can also be expressed in peripheral blood NK cells, though the efficiency is typically significantly less than the derivation of CAR-expressing T cells. This difference is likely due to innate immune mechanisms that make NK cells inherently more resistant to foreign DNA. However, multiple studies have clearly demonstrated expression of CAR constructs targeting different tumors and with different intracellular signaling domains [300]. Notably, anti-CD19 CAR-expressing NK cells from haploidentical donors have entered clinical trials for treatment of refractory ALL, though no results have yet been reported [301].

Human pluripotent stem cells (both hESCs and iPSCs) can also be used as a platform for derivation of CAR-expressing NK cells. Here, the undifferentiated hESCs/iPSCs can be genetically modified using viral or non-viral vectors [302]. Then, differentiation of the hESCs/iPSCs leads to the production of stable CAR expression. This strategy offers the advantage of being able to specifically target the insertion to genomic areas that maintain high-level expression, such as the AAVS site. Additionally, the insertion sight can be defined to ensure no untoward effects are likely from the gene modification. This strategy has been used to produce hESC/iPSC-derived NK cells that target both tumor antigens and virally infected cells [300, 303].

One additional strategy to improve NK-cell function is to optimize CD16 expression. CD16 is the Fcγ-receptor that mediates ADCC. However, CD16 expression is downregulated on activated NK cells by the metalloprotease, ADAM17. Notably, the ADAM17 cleavage site has been characterized and mutated to effectively prevent loss of expression. Specifically, substitution of the serine at position 197 in the middle of the CD16 cleavage region for a proline (S197P) effectively blocked CD16a and CD16b cleavage. Importantly, CD16a/S197P was resistant to cleavage when expressed in NK-92 cells and in iPSC-derived NK cells [304]. Therefore, expression of CD16 (S197P) in NK cells provides an important strategy to improve antibody-mediated targeting of NK cells to solid tumors that may be more refractory to NK-cell-mediated killing.

5.17 Conclusion

This chapter highlights the exciting advances in T-cell- and NK-cell-based immunotherapies. However, these therapies remain at an early stage. Clinical trials using HCT to treat hematologic malignancies and immunodeficiencies started in the 1950s and 1960. However, it took decades before HCT demonstrated efficacy and became standard-of-care for many patients with otherwise refractory AML, multiple myeloma, lymphoma, aplastic anemia, and other hematologic diseases so that over 50,000 patients in the United States now receive an allogeneic or autologous

HCT every year. We are at a similarly early stage for T-cell and NK cell-based therapies. Continued advances will certainly make these therapies safer and more effective—eventually leading cell-based therapies to become a routine component of clinical care to better treat and cure otherwise lethal malignancies.

References

1. Jessy T (2011) Immunity over inability: the spontaneous regression of cancer. J Nat Sci Biol Med 2:43–49
2. Dudley ME et al (2002) Cancer regression and autoimmunity in patients after clonal repopulation with antitumor lymphocytes. Science 298:850–854
3. Goff SL et al (2016) Randomized prospective evaluation comparing intensity of lymphodepletion before adoptive transfer of tumor-infiltrating lymphocytes for patients with metastatic melanoma. J Clin Oncol Off J Am Soc Clin Oncol 34:2389–2397
4. Maloney DG (2003) Graft-vs.-lymphoma effect in various histologies of non-Hodgkin's lymphoma. Leuk Lymphoma 44(Suppl 3):S99–105
5. Fenske TS et al (2016) Allogeneic hematopoietic cell transplantation as curative therapy for patients with non-Hodgkin lymphoma: increasingly successful application to older patients. Biol Blood Marrow Transplant 22:1543–1551
6. Chang X, Zang X, Xia C-Q (2016) New strategies of DLI in the management of relapse of hematological malignancies after allogeneic hematopoietic SCT. Bone Marrow Transplant 51:324–332
7. Yee C et al (2002) Adoptive T cell therapy using antigen-specific CD8+ T cell clones for the treatment of patients with metastatic melanoma: in vivo persistence, migration, and antitumor effect of transferred T cells. Proc Natl Acad Sci 99:16168–16173
8. Mackensen A et al (2006) Phase I study of adoptive T-cell therapy using antigen-specific CD8+ T cells for the treatment of patients with metastatic melanoma. J Clin Oncol 24:5060–5069
9. Dudley ME et al (2001) Adoptive transfer of cloned melanoma-reactive T lymphocytes for the treatment of patients with metastatic melanoma. J Immunother Hagerstown Md 1997(24):363–373
10. Fesnak AD, June CH, Levine BL (2016) Engineered T cells: the promise and challenges of cancer immunotherapy. Nat Rev Cancer 16:566–581
11. Maude SL et al (2014) Chimeric antigen receptor T cells for sustained remissions in Leukemia. N Engl J Med 371:1507–1517
12. Porter DL, Levine BL, Kalos M, Bagg A, June CH (2011) Chimeric antigen receptor–modified T cells in chronic lymphoid Leukemia. N Engl J Med 365:725–733
13. Wucherpfennig KW, Gagnon E, Call MJ, Huseby ES, Call ME (2010) Structural biology of the T-cell receptor: insights into receptor assembly, ligand recognition, and initiation of signaling. Cold Spring Harb Perspect Biol 2:a005140
14. Brownlie RJ, Zamoyska R (2013) T cell receptor signalling networks: branched, diversified and bounded. Nat Rev Immunol 13:257–269
15. Voskoboinik I, Whisstock JC, Trapani JA (2015) Perforin and granzymes: function, dysfunction and human pathology. Nat Rev Immunol 15:388–400
16. Chen L, Flies DB (2013) Molecular mechanisms of T cell co-stimulation and co-inhibition. Nat Rev Immunol 13:227–242
17. Schumacher TN, Schreiber RD (2015) Neoantigens in cancer immunotherapy. Science 348:69–74
18. Rosenberg SA, Restifo NP (2015) Adoptive cell transfer as personalized immunotherapy for human cancer. Science 348:62–68

19. Coulie PG, Van den Eynde BJ, van der Bruggen P, Boon T (2014) Tumour antigens recognized by T lymphocytes: at the core of cancer immunotherapy. Nat Rev Cancer 14:135–146
20. Kawashima I et al (1999) Identification of HLA-A3-restricted cytotoxic T lymphocyte epitopes from carcinoembryonic antigen and HER-2/neu by primary in vitro immunization with peptide-pulsed dendritic cells. Cancer Res 59:431–435
21. Simpson AJG, Caballero OL, Jungbluth A, Chen Y-T, Old LJ (2005) Cancer/testis antigens, gametogenesis and cancer. Nat Rev Cancer 5:615–625
22. Mardis ER (2013) Next-generation sequencing platforms. Annu Rev Anal Chem Palo Alto Calif 6:287–303
23. Sette A et al (1994) The relationship between class I binding affinity and immunogenicity of potential cytotoxic T cell epitopes. J Immunol Baltim Md 1950(153):5586–5592
24. Lundegaard C, Lund O, Kesmir C, Brunak S, Nielsen M (2007) Modeling the adaptive immune system: predictions and simulations. Bioinforma Oxf Engl 23:3265–3275
25. Rosenberg SA et al (1988) Use of tumor-infiltrating lymphocytes and interleukin-2 in the immunotherapy of patients with metastatic melanoma. N Engl J Med 319:1676–1680
26. Rosenberg SA et al (1994) Treatment of patients with metastatic melanoma with autologous tumor-infiltrating lymphocytes and interleukin 2. J Natl Cancer Inst 86:1159–1166
27. Dudley ME et al (2005) Adoptive cell transfer therapy following non-myeloablative but lymphodepleting chemotherapy for the treatment of patients with refractory metastatic melanoma. J Clin Oncol Off J Am Soc Clin Oncol 23:2346–2357
28. Greiner J et al (2012) Mutated regions of nucleophosmin 1 elicit both CD4+ and CD8+ T-cell responses in patients with acute myeloid leukemia. Blood 120:1282–1289
29. Comoli P et al (2017) BCR-ABL–specific T-cell therapy in Ph+ ALL patients on tyrosine-kinase inhibitors. Blood 129:582–586
30. Maude SL, Teachey DT, Porter DL, Grupp SA (2015) CD19-targeted chimeric antigen receptor T-cell therapy for acute lymphoblastic leukemia. Blood 125:4017–4023
31. Dotti G, Gottschalk S, Savoldo B, Brenner MK (2014) Design and development of therapies using chimeric antigen receptor-expressing T cells. Immunol Rev 257:107–126
32. Gross G, Waks T, Eshhar Z (1989) Expression of immunoglobulin-T-cell receptor chimeric molecules as functional receptors with antibody-type specificity. Proc Natl Acad Sci U S A 86:10024–10028
33. Stancovski I et al (1993) Targeting of T lymphocytes to Neu/HER2-expressing cells using chimeric single chain Fv receptors. J Immunol 151:6577–6582
34. Chmielewski M, Hombach A, Heuser C, Adams GP, Abken H (2004) T cell activation by antibody-like Immunoreceptors: increase in affinity of the single-chain fragment domain above threshold does not increase T cell activation against antigen-positive target cells but decreases selectivity. J Immunol 173:7647–7653
35. Hombach AA et al (2007) T cell activation by antibody-like Immunoreceptors: the position of the binding epitope within the target molecule determines the efficiency of activation of redirected T cells. J Immunol 178:4650–4657
36. Haso W et al (2013) Anti-CD22–chimeric antigen receptors targeting B-cell precursor acute lymphoblastic leukemia. Blood 121:1165–1174
37. van der Stegen SJC, Hamieh M, Sadelain M (2015) The pharmacology of second-generation chimeric antigen receptors. Nat Rev Drug Discov 14:499–509
38. Hudecek M et al (2015) The Nonsignaling extracellular spacer domain of chimeric antigen receptors is decisive for in vivo antitumor activity. Cancer Immunol Res 3:125–135
39. James SE et al (2008) Antigen sensitivity of CD22-specific chimeric TCR is modulated by target epitope distance from the cell membrane. J Immunol 180:7028–7038
40. Jonnalagadda M et al (2015) Chimeric antigen receptors with mutated IgG4 Fc spacer avoid Fc receptor binding and improve T cell persistence and antitumor efficacy. Mol Ther 23:757–768
41. Bridgeman JS et al (2010) The optimal antigen response of chimeric antigen receptors Harboring the CD3ζ Transmembrane domain is dependent upon incorporation of the receptor into the endogenous TCR/CD3 complex. J Immunol 184:6938–6949

42. Goodman A, Patel SP, Kurzrock R (2016) PD-1-PD-L1 immune-checkpoint blockade in B-cell lymphomas. Nat Rev Clin Oncol, advance online publication 14:203–220 doi:10.1038/nrclinonc.2016.168
43. Jackson HJ, Rafiq S, Brentjens RJ (2016) Driving CAR T-cells forward. Nat Rev Clin Oncol 13:370–383
44. Lamers CHJ et al (2006) Treatment of metastatic renal cell carcinoma with autologous T-lymphocytes genetically retargeted against carbonic anhydrase IX: first clinical experience. J Clin Oncol 24:e20–e22
45. Lamers CH et al (2013) Treatment of metastatic renal cell carcinoma with CAIX CAR-engineered T cells: clinical evaluation and management of on-target toxicity. Mol Ther 21:904–912
46. Kershaw MH et al (2006) A phase I study on adoptive immunotherapy using gene-modified T cells for ovarian cancer. Clin Cancer Res 12:6106–6115
47. Pule MA et al (2008) Virus-specific T cells engineered to coexpress tumor-specific receptors: persistence and antitumor activity in individuals with neuroblastoma. Nat Med 14:1264–1270
48. Louis CU et al (2011) Antitumor activity and long-term fate of chimeric antigen receptor–positive T cells in patients with neuroblastoma. Blood 118:6050–6056
49. Finney HM, Lawson ADG, Bebbington CR, Weir ANC (1998) Chimeric receptors providing both primary and costimulatory signaling in T cells from a single gene product. J Immunol 161:2791–2797
50. Finney HM, Akbar AN, Lawson ADG (2004) Activation of resting human primary T cells with chimeric receptors: costimulation from CD28, inducible costimulator, CD134, and CD137 in series with signals from the TCRζ chain. J Immunol 172:104–113
51. Imai C et al (2004) Chimeric receptors with 4-1BB signaling capacity provoke potent cytotoxicity against acute lymphoblastic leukemia. Leukemia 18:676–684
52. Song D-G et al (2012) CD27 costimulation augments the survival and antitumor activity of redirected human T cells in vivo. Blood 119:696–706
53. Pulè MA et al (2005) A chimeric T cell antigen receptor that augments cytokine release and supports clonal expansion of primary human T cells. Mol Ther 12:933–941
54. Savoldo B et al (2011) CD28 costimulation improves expansion and persistence of chimeric antigen receptor–modified T cells in lymphoma patients. J Clin Invest 121:1822–1826
55. Kochenderfer JN et al (2014) Chemotherapy-refractory diffuse large B-cell lymphoma and indolent B-cell malignancies can be effectively treated with autologous T cells expressing an anti-CD19 chimeric antigen receptor. J Clin Oncol. doi:10.1200/JCO.2014.56.2025
56. Wang J et al (2007) Optimizing adoptive polyclonal T cell immunotherapy of lymphomas, using a chimeric T cell receptor possessing CD28 and CD137 costimulatory domains. Hum Gene Ther 18:712–725
57. Till BG et al (2012) CD20-specific adoptive immunotherapy for lymphoma using a chimeric antigen receptor with both CD28 and 4-1BB domains: pilot clinical trial results. Blood 119:3940–3950
58. Curran KJ et al (2015) Enhancing antitumor efficacy of chimeric antigen receptor T cells through constitutive CD40L expression. Mol Ther 23:769–778
59. Kaiser AD et al (2015) Towards a commercial process for the manufacture of genetically modified T cells for therapy. Cancer Gene Ther 22:72–78
60. Wang X, Rivière I (2016) Clinical manufacturing of CAR T cells: foundation of a promising therapy. Mol Ther Oncolytics 3:16015
61. Powell DJ et al (2009) Efficient clinical-scale enrichment of lymphocytes for use in adoptive immunotherapy using a modified counterflow centrifugal elutriation program. Cytotherapy 11:923–935
62. Singh H, Huls H, Kebriaei P, Cooper LJN (2014) A new approach to gene therapy using sleeping beauty to genetically modify clinical-grade T cells to target CD19. Immunol Rev 257:181–190

63. Levine BL et al (1997) Ex vivo replicative potential of adult human peripheral blood CD4+ T cells. Transplant Proc 29:2028
64. Levine BL et al (1998) Large-scale production of CD4+ T cells from HIV-1-infected donors after CD3/CD28 Costimulation*. J Hematother 7:437–448
65. Jin C et al (2016) Safe engineering of CAR T cells for adoptive cell therapy of cancer using long-term episomal gene transfer. EMBO Mol Med 8:702–711
66. Deichmann A, Schmidt M (2017) Biosafety considerations using gamma-retroviral vectors in gene therapy. http://www.eurekaselect.com. Available at: http://www.eurekaselect.com/117522/article. Accessed: 24 Feb 2017
67. Potter H, Heller R (2003) Transfection by electroporation. Curr Protoc Mol Biol Ed Frederick M Ausubel Al CHAPTER, Unit–9.3
68. Zhao Y et al (2006) High-efficiency transfection of primary human and mouse T lymphocytes using RNA electroporation. Mol Ther 13:151–159
69. Davila ML et al (2014) Efficacy and toxicity management of 19-28z CAR T cell therapy in B cell acute lymphoblastic leukemia. Sci Transl Med 6:224ra25
70. Turtle CJ et al (2016) CD19 CAR–T cells of defined CD4+:CD8+ composition in adult B cell ALL patients. J Clin Invest 126:2123–2138
71. Shah NN et al (2016) Minimal residual disease negative complete remissions following anti-CD22 chimeric antigen receptor (CAR) in children and young adults with relapsed/refractory acute lymphoblastic leukemia (ALL). Blood 128:650–650
72. Lee DW et al (2016) Long-term outcomes following CD19 CAR T cell therapy for B-ALL are superior in patients receiving a fludarabine/cyclophosphamide preparative regimen and post-CAR hematopoietic stem cell transplantation. Blood 128:218–218
73. Deng B et al (2016) Safety and efficacy of low dose CD19 targeted chimeric antigen receptor T (CAR-T) cell immunotherapy in 47 cases with relapsed refractory B-Cell Acute Lymphoblastic Leukemia (B-ALL). Blood 128:649–649
74. Turtle CJ et al (2016) CD19 CAR-T cells are highly effective in Ibrutinib-refractory chronic lymphocytic leukemia. Blood 128:56–56
75. Kochenderfer JN et al (2012) B-cell depletion and remissions of malignancy along with cytokine-associated toxicity in a clinical trial of anti-CD19 chimeric-antigen-receptor–transduced T cells. Blood 119:2709–2720
76. Neelapu SS et al (2016) A phase 2 multicenter trial of KTE-C19 (anti-CD19 CAR T cells) in patients with chemorefractory Primary mediastinal B-Cell Lymphoma (PMBCL) and Transformed Follicular Lymphoma (TFL): interim results from ZUMA-1. Blood 128:998–998
77. Gattinoni L, Powell DJ, Rosenberg SA, Restifo NP (2006) Adoptive immunotherapy for cancer: building on success. Nat Rev Immunol 6:383–393
78. Antony PA et al (2005) CD8+ T cell immunity against a tumor/self-antigen is augmented by CD4+ T helper cells and hindered by naturally occurring T regulatory cells. J Immunol 174:2591–2601
79. North RJ (1982) Cyclophosphamide-facilitated adoptive immunotherapy of an established tumor depends on elimination of tumor-induced suppressor T cells. J Exp Med 155:1063–1074
80. Gattinoni L et al (2005) Removal of homeostatic cytokine sinks by lymphodepletion enhances the efficacy of adoptively transferred tumor-specific CD8+ T cells. J Exp Med 202:907–912
81. Rosenberg SA et al (2011) Durable complete responses in heavily Pretreated patients with metastatic melanoma using T-cell transfer immunotherapy. Clin Cancer Res 17:4550–4557
82. Ninomiya S et al (2015) Tumor indoleamine 2,3-dioxygenase (IDO) inhibits CD19-CAR T cells and is downregulated by lymphodepleting drugs. Blood 125:3905–3916
83. Park JH, Geyer MB, Brentjens RJ (2016) CD19-targeted CAR T-cell therapeutics for hematologic malignancies: interpreting clinical outcomes to date. Blood 127:3312–3320
84. Brentjens RJ et al (2011) Safety and persistence of adoptively transferred autologous CD19-targeted T cells in patients with relapsed or chemotherapy refractory B-cell leukemias. Blood 118:4817–4828
85. Cruz CRY et al (2013) Infusion of donor-derived CD19-redirected virus-specific T cells for B-cell malignancies relapsed after allogeneic stem cell transplant: a phase 1 study. Blood 122:2965–2973

86. Turtle CJ et al (2015) Addition of Fludarabine to cyclophosphamide lymphodepletion improves in vivo expansion of CD19 chimeric antigen receptor-modified T cells and clinical outcome in adults with B cell acute lymphoblastic leukemia. Blood 126:3773–3773
87. Turtle CJ et al (2015) Anti-CD19 chimeric antigen receptor-modified T cell therapy for B cell non-Hodgkin lymphoma and chronic lymphocytic Leukemia: fludarabine and cyclophosphamide lymphodepletion improves in vivo expansion and persistence of CAR-T cells and clinical outcomes. Blood 126:184–184
88. Brudno JN et al (2016) Allogeneic T cells that express an anti-CD19 chimeric antigen receptor induce remissions of B-cell malignancies that progress after allogeneic hematopoietic stem-cell transplantation without causing graft-versus-host disease. J Clin Oncol 34:1112–1121
89. Lee DW et al (2015) T cells expressing CD19 chimeric antigen receptors for acute lymphoblastic leukaemia in children and young adults: a phase 1 dose-escalation trial. Lancet 385:517–528
90. Porter DL et al (2016) Randomized, phase II dose optimization study of chimeric antigen receptor (CAR) modified T cells directed against CD19 in patients (pts) with relapsed, refractory (R/R) CLL. J Clin Oncol 34(5):3009. https://doi.org/10.1200/JCO.2016.34.15_suppl.3009
91. Brentjens R et al (2013) CD19-targeted T cells rapidly induce molecular remissions in adults with chemotherapy-refractory acute lymphoblastic leukemia. Sci Transl Med 5:177ra38
92. Dhédin N et al (2015) Role of allogeneic stem cell transplantation in adult patients with Ph-negative acute lymphoblastic leukemia. Blood 125:2486–2496
93. Topp MS et al (2015) Safety and activity of blinatumomab for adult patients with relapsed or refractory B-precursor acute lymphoblastic leukaemia: a multicentre, single-arm, phase 2 study. Lancet Oncol 16:57–66
94. Topp MS et al (2012) Long-term follow-up of hematologic relapse-free survival in a phase 2 study of blinatumomab in patients with MRD in B-lineage ALL. Blood 120:5185–5187
95. Topp MS et al (2014) Phase II trial of the anti-CD19 bispecific T cell–engager blinatumomab shows hematologic and molecular remissions in patients with relapsed or refractory B-precursor acute lymphoblastic leukemia. J Clin Oncol. doi:10.1200/JCO.2014.56.3247
96. Grupp SA et al (2013) Chimeric antigen receptor–modified T cells for acute lymphoid Leukemia. N Engl J Med 368:1509–1518
97. Maude SL et al (2016) Efficacy of humanized CD19-targeted chimeric antigen receptor (CAR)-modified T cells in children and young adults with relapsed/refractory acute lymphoblastic leukemia. Blood 128:217–217
98. Park JH et al (2015) Efficacy and safety of CD19-targeted 19-28z CAR modified T cells in adult patients with relapsed or refractory B-ALL. J Clin Oncol 33
99. Kalos M et al (2011) T cells with chimeric antigen receptors have potent antitumor effects and can establish memory in patients with advanced leukemia. Sci Transl Med 3:95ra73
100. Porter DL et al (2015) Chimeric antigen receptor T cells persist and induce sustained remissions in relapsed refractory chronic lymphocytic leukemia. Sci Transl Med 7:303ra139
101. Till BG et al (2008) Adoptive immunotherapy for indolent non-Hodgkin lymphoma and mantle cell lymphoma using genetically modified autologous CD20-specific T cells. Blood 112:2261–2271
102. Topp MS et al (2011) Targeted therapy with the T-cell–engaging antibody blinatumomab of chemotherapy-refractory minimal residual disease in B-lineage acute lymphoblastic leukemia patients results in high response rate and prolonged leukemia-free survival. J Clin Oncol. doi:10.1200/JCO.2010.32.7270
103. Pui C-H, Jeha S (2007) New therapeutic strategies for the treatment of acute lymphoblastic leukaemia. Nat Rev Drug Discov 6:149–165
104. Otero DC, Rickert RC (2003) CD19 function in early and late B cell development. II. CD19 facilitates the Pro-B/Pre-B transition. J Immunol 171:5921–5930
105. Kantarjian HM et al (2016) Inotuzumab ozogamicin versus standard therapy for acute lymphoblastic leukemia. N Engl J Med 0, null

106. Wierda WG et al (2010) Ofatumumab as single-agent CD20 immunotherapy in fludarabine-refractory chronic lymphocytic leukemia. J Clin Oncol 28:1749–1755
107. Wierda WG et al (2011) Chemoimmunotherapy with O-FC in previously untreated patients with chronic lymphocytic leukemia. Blood 117:6450–6458
108. Wierda WG et al (2011) Ofatumumab is active in patients with fludarabine-refractory CLL irrespective of prior rituximab: results from the phase 2 international study. Blood 118:5126–5129
109. Goede V et al (2014) Obinutuzumab plus Chlorambucil in patients with CLL and coexisting conditions. N Engl J Med 370:1101–1110
110. Byrd JC et al (2013) Targeting BTK with ibrutinib in relapsed chronic lymphocytic leukemia. N Engl J Med 369:32–42
111. Byrd JC et al (2014) Ibrutinib versus Ofatumumab in previously treated chronic lymphoid leukemia. N Engl J Med 371:213–223
112. Brown JR et al (2014) Idelalisib, an inhibitor of phosphatidylinositol 3-kinase p110δ, for relapsed/refractory chronic lymphocytic leukemia. Blood 123:3390–3397
113. Furman RR et al (2014) Idelalisib and rituximab in relapsed chronic lymphocytic leukemia. N Engl J Med 370:997–1007
114. Woyach JA et al (2014) Resistance mechanisms for the Bruton's tyrosine kinase inhibitor Ibrutinib. N Engl J Med 370:2286–2294
115. Jain P et al (2015) Outcomes of patients with chronic lymphocytic leukemia after discontinuing ibrutinib. Blood 125:2062–2067
116. Roberts AW et al (2015) Targeting BCL2 with venetoclax in relapsed chronic lymphocytic leukemia. N Engl J Med 0, null
117. Zhang S et al (2012) The Onco-embryonic antigen ROR1 is expressed by a variety of human cancers. Am J Pathol 181:1903–1910
118. Al-Shawi R, Ashton SV, Underwood C, Simons JP (2001) Expression of the Ror1 and Ror2 receptor tyrosine kinase genes during mouse development. Dev Genes Evol 211:161–171
119. Hudecek M et al (2010) The B-cell tumor–associated antigen ROR1 can be targeted with T cells modified to express a ROR1-specific chimeric antigen receptor. Blood 116:4532–4541
120. Zegers BJM et al (1976) Kappa-chain deficiency. N Engl J Med 294:1026–1030
121. Vera J et al (2006) T lymphocytes redirected against the κ light chain of human immunoglobulin efficiently kill mature B lymphocyte-derived malignant cells. Blood 108:3890–3897
122. Kahl BS, Yang DT (2016) Follicular lymphoma: evolving therapeutic strategies. Blood 127:2055–2063
123. Korsmeyer SJ (1992) Bcl-2 initiates a new category of oncogenes: regulators of cell death. Blood 80:879–886
124. Salles G et al (2011) Rituximab maintenance for 2 years in patients with high tumour burden follicular lymphoma responding to rituximab plus chemotherapy (PRIMA): a phase 3, randomised controlled trial. Lancet Lond Engl 377:42–51
125. Witzig TE et al (2009) Lenalidomide oral monotherapy produces durable responses in relapsed or refractory indolent non-Hodgkin's lymphoma. J Clin Oncol 27:5404–5409
126. Flinn IW et al (2014) Idelalisib, a selective inhibitor of phosphatidylinositol 3-kinase-δ, as therapy for previously treated indolent non-Hodgkin lymphoma. Blood 123:3406–3413
127. van Besien K et al (2003) Comparison of autologous and allogeneic hematopoietic stem cell transplantation for follicular lymphoma. Blood 102:3521–3529
128. Hainsworth JD et al (2002) Rituximab as first-line and maintenance therapy for patients with indolent non-hodgkin's lymphoma. J Clin Oncol Off J Am Soc Clin Oncol 20:4261–4267
129. Till BG et al (2008) Adoptive immunotherapy for indolent non-Hodgkin lymphoma and mantle cell lymphoma using genetically modified autologous CD20-specific T cells. Blood 112:2261–2271
130. Kochenderfer JN et al (2010) Eradication of B-lineage cells and regression of lymphoma in a patient treated with autologous T cells genetically engineered to recognize CD19. Blood 116:4099–4102

131. Armitage J, How O (2007) I treat patients with diffuse large B-cell lymphoma. Blood 110:29–36
132. Sehn LH, Gascoyne RD (2015) Diffuse large B-cell lymphoma: optimizing outcome in the context of clinical and biologic heterogeneity. Blood 125:22–32
133. Ziepert M et al (2010) Standard international prognostic index remains a valid predictor of outcome for patients with aggressive CD20+ B-cell lymphoma in the rituximab era. J Clin Oncol 28:2373–2380
134. Gisselbrecht C et al (2010) Salvage regimens with autologous transplantation for relapsed large B-cell lymphoma in the rituximab era. J Clin Oncol 28:4184–4190
135. Kochenderfer JN et al (2014) Anti-CD19 CAR T cells administered after low-dose chemotherapy can induce remissions of chemotherapy-refractory diffuse large B-cell lymphoma. Blood 124:550–550
136. Sauter CS et al (2015) Phase I trial of 19-28z chimeric antigen receptor modified T cells (19-28z CAR-T) post-high dose therapy and autologous stem cell transplant (HDT-ASCT) for relapsed and refractory (rel/ref) aggressive B-cell non-Hodgkin lymphoma (B-NHL). J Clin Oncol 33
137. Rajkumar SV (2014) Multiple myeloma: 2014 update on diagnosis, risk-stratification, and management: multiple myeloma. Am J Hematol 89:998–1009
138. Mehta J, Cavo M, Singhal S (2010) How I treat elderly patients with myeloma. Blood 116:2215–2223
139. Stewart AK, Richardson PG, San-Miguel JF (2009) How I treat multiple myeloma in younger patients. Blood 114:5436–5443
140. Rosiñol L et al (2015) Allogeneic hematopoietic SCT in multiple myeloma: long-term results from a single institution. Bone Marrow Transplant 50:658–662
141. Bladé J, Rosiñol L, de Larrea CF (2015) How I treat relapsed myeloma. Blood 125:1532–1540
142. Moreau P, Touzeau C (2015) Multiple myeloma: from front-line to relapsed therapies. Am Soc Clin Oncol Educ Book 35:e504–e511
143. Deaglio S et al (2007) CD38/CD19: a lipid raft–dependent signaling complex in human B cells. Blood 109:5390–5398
144. Lokhorst HM et al (2015) Targeting CD38 with daratumumab monotherapy in multiple myeloma. N Engl J Med 0, null
145. Palumbo A et al (2016) Daratumumab, Bortezomib, and Dexamethasone for multiple myeloma. N Engl J Med 375:754–766
146. Dimopoulos MA et al (2016) Daratumumab, Lenalidomide, and Dexamethasone for multiple myeloma. N Engl J Med 375:1319–1331
147. Krejcik J et al (2016) Daratumumab depletes CD38+ immune-regulatory cells, promotes T-cell expansion, and skews T-cell repertoire in multiple myeloma. Blood. doi:10.1182/blood-2015-12-687749
148. Tai Y-T, Anderson KC (2016) A new era of immune therapy in multiple myeloma. Blood 128:318–319
149. Drent E et al (2016) Pre-clinical evaluation of CD38 chimeric antigen receptor engineered T cells for the treatment of multiple myeloma. Haematologica 101:616–625
150. O'Connor BP et al (2004) BCMA is essential for the survival of long-lived bone marrow plasma cells. J Exp Med 199:91–98
151. Carpenter RO et al (2013) B-cell maturation antigen is a promising target for adoptive T-cell therapy of multiple myeloma. Clin Cancer Res 19:2048–2060
152. Guo B et al (2016) CD138-directed adoptive immunotherapy of chimeric antigen receptor (CAR)-modified T cells for multiple myeloma. J Cell Immunother 2:28–35
153. Hajek R, Okubote SA, Svachova H (2013) Myeloma stem cell concepts, heterogeneity and plasticity of multiple myeloma. Br J Haematol 163:551–564
154. Garfall AL et al (2015) Chimeric antigen receptor T cells against CD19 for multiple myeloma. N Engl J Med 373:1040–1047

155. Yuan J et al (2008) CTLA-4 blockade enhances polyfunctional NY-ESO-1 specific T cell responses in metastatic melanoma patients with clinical benefit. Proc Natl Acad Sci 105:20410–20415
156. Hunder NN et al (2008) Treatment of metastatic melanoma with autologous CD4+ T cells against NY-ESO-1. N Engl J Med 358:2698–2703
157. Jungbluth AA et al (2005) The cancer-testis antigens CT7 (MAGE-C1) and MAGE-A3/6 are commonly expressed in multiple myeloma and correlate with plasma-cell proliferation. Blood 106:167–174
158. Rapoport AP et al (2015) NY-ESO-1-specific TCR-engineered T cells mediate sustained antigen-specific antitumor effects in myeloma. Nat Med 21:914–921
159. Rapoport AP et al (2009) Rapid immune recovery and graft-versus-host disease–like engraftment syndrome following adoptive transfer of Costimulated autologous T cells. Clin Cancer Res 15:4499–4507
160. Juliusson G, Lazarevic V, Hörstedt A-S, Hagberg O, Höglund M (2012) Acute myeloid leukemia in the real world: why population-based registries are needed. Blood 119:3890–3899
161. Ossenkoppele G, Löwenberg B (2015) How I treat the older patient with acute myeloid leukemia. Blood 125:767–774
162. Appelbaum FR et al (2006) Age and acute myeloid leukemia. Blood 107:3481–3485
163. Döhner H et al (2010) Diagnosis and management of acute myeloid leukemia in adults: recommendations from an international expert panel, on behalf of the European LeukemiaNet. Blood 115:453–474
164. Linch DC, Hills RK, Burnett AK, Khwaja A, Gale RE (2014) Impact of FLT3ITD mutant allele level on relapse risk in intermediate-risk acute myeloid leukemia. Blood 124:273–276
165. Taskesen E et al (2011) Prognostic impact, concurrent genetic mutations, and gene expression features of AML with CEBPA mutations in a cohort of 1182 cytogenetically normal AML patients: further evidence for CEBPA double mutant AML as a distinctive disease entity. Blood 117:2469–2475
166. Patel JP et al (2012) Prognostic relevance of integrated genetic profiling in acute myeloid leukemia. N Engl J Med 366:1079–1089
167. Gale RE et al (2008) The impact of FLT3 internal tandem duplication mutant level, number, size, and interaction with NPM1 mutations in a large cohort of young adult patients with acute myeloid leukemia. Blood 111:2776–2784
168. Allen C et al (2013) The importance of relative mutant level for evaluating impact on outcome of KIT, FLT3 and CBL mutations in core-binding factor acute myeloid leukemia. Leukemia 27:1891–1901
169. Preisler HD et al (1983) Therapy of secondary acute nonlymphocytic Leukemia with Cytarabine. N Engl J Med 308:21–23
170. Fernandez HF et al (2009) Anthracycline dose intensification in acute myeloid Leukemia. N Engl J Med 361:1249–1259
171. Burnett AK et al (2015) A randomized comparison of daunorubicin 90 mg/m2 vs 60 mg/m2 in AML induction: results from the UK NCRI AML17 trial in 1206 patients. Blood 125:3878–3885
172. Cassileth PA et al (1988) Maintenance chemotherapy prolongs remission duration in adult acute nonlymphocytic leukemia. J Clin Oncol 6:583–587
173. Koreth J et al (2009) Allogeneic stem cell transplantation for acute myeloid leukemia in first complete remission: a systematic review and meta-analysis of prospective clinical trials. JAMA J Am Med Assoc 301:2349–2361
174. Li D et al (2015) Efficacy of allogeneic hematopoietic stem cell transplantation in intermediate-risk acute myeloid leukemia adult patients in first complete remission: a meta-analysis of prospective studies. PLoS One 10. https://doi.org/10.1371/journal.pone.0132620
175. Wierzbowska A et al (2008) Cladribine combined with high doses of arabinoside cytosine, mitoxantrone, and G-CSF (CLAG-M) is a highly effective salvage regimen in patients with refractory and relapsed acute myeloid leukemia of the poor risk: a final report of the Polish Adult Leukemia Group. Eur J Haematol 80:115–126

176. Montillo M et al (1998) Fludarabine, cytarabine, and G-CSF (FLAG) for the treatment of poor risk acute myeloid leukemia. Am J Hematol 58:105–109
177. Parker JE et al (1997) Fludarabine, cytarabine, G-CSF and idarubicin (FLAG-IDA) for the treatment of poor-risk myelodysplastic syndromes and acute myeloid leukaemia. Br J Haematol 99:939–944
178. Becker PS et al (2011) Clofarabine with high dose cytarabine and granulocyte colony-stimulating factor (G-CSF) priming for relapsed and refractory acute myeloid leukaemia. Br J Haematol 155:182–189
179. Amadori S et al (1991) Mitoxantrone, etoposide, and intermediate-dose cytarabine: an effective and tolerable regimen for the treatment of refractory acute myeloid leukemia. J Clin Oncol Off J Am Soc Clin Oncol 9:1210–1214
180. Fenaux P et al (2009) Efficacy of azacitidine compared with that of conventional care regimens in the treatment of higher-risk myelodysplastic syndromes: a randomised, open-label, phase III study. Lancet Oncol 10:223–232
181. Fenaux P et al (2010) Azacitidine prolongs overall survival compared with conventional care regimens in elderly patients with low bone marrow blast count acute myeloid leukemia. J Clin Oncol 28:562–569
182. Cashen AF, Schiller GJ, O'Donnell MR, DiPersio JF (2010) Multicenter phase II study of Decitabine for the first-line treatment of older patients with acute myeloid leukemia. J Clin Oncol 28:556–561
183. Kantarjian HM et al (2012) Multicenter, randomized, open-label, phase III trial of Decitabine versus patient choice, with physician advice, of either supportive care or low-dose Cytarabine for the treatment of older patients with newly diagnosed acute myeloid leukemia. J Clin Oncol 30:2670–2677
184. Bejanyan N et al (2015) Survival of patients with acute myeloid leukemia relapsing after allogeneic hematopoietic cell transplantation: a Center for International Blood and Marrow Transplant Research Study. Biol Blood Marrow Transplant 21:454–459
185. Soiffer RJ (2008) Donor lymphocyte infusions for acute myeloid leukaemia. Best Pract Res Clin Haematol 21:455–466
186. Dinndorf PA et al (1986) Expression of normal myeloid-associated antigens by acute leukemia cells. Blood 67:1048–1053
187. O'Hear C, Heiber JF, Schubert I, Fey G, Geiger TL (2015) Anti-CD33 chimeric antigen receptor targeting of acute myeloid leukemia. Haematologica 100:336–344
188. Rafiq S, Purdon TJ, Schultz LM, Brentjens RJ (2016) CD33-directed Chimeric Antigen Receptor (CAR) T cells for the treatment of Acute Myeloid Leukemia (AML). Blood 128:2825–2825
189. Kenderian SS et al (2015) CD33-specific chimeric antigen receptor T cells exhibit potent preclinical activity against human acute myeloid leukemia. Leukemia 29:1637–1647
190. Song D et al (2016) Chimeric antigen receptor-modified T cells for the treatment of acute myeloid leukemia expressing CD33. Blood 128:4058–4058
191. Linenberger ML (2004) CD33-directed therapy with gemtuzumab ozogamicin in acute myeloid leukemia: progress in understanding cytotoxicity and potential mechanisms of drug resistance. Leukemia 19:176–182
192. Wadleigh M et al (2003) Prior gemtuzumab ozogamicin exposure significantly increases the risk of veno-occlusive disease in patients who undergo myeloablative allogeneic stem cell transplantation. Blood 102:1578–1582
193. Wang Q et al (2015) Treatment of CD33-directed chimeric antigen receptor-modified T cells in one patient with relapsed and refractory acute myeloid leukemia. Mol Ther 23:184–191
194. Mardiros A, Forman SJ, Budde LE (2015) T cells expressing CD123 chimeric antigen receptors for treatment of acute myeloid leukemia. Curr Opin Hematol 22:484–488
195. Jordan CT et al (2000) The interleukin-3 receptor alpha chain is a unique marker for human acute myelogenous leukemia stem cells. Leukemia 14:1777–1784
196. Roberts AW et al (2008) A phase 1 and correlative biological study of CSL360 (anti-CD123 mAb) in AML. Blood 112:2956–2956

197. Frankel A, Liu J-S, Rizzieri D, Hogge D (2008) Phase I clinical study of diphtheria toxin-interleukin 3 fusion protein in patients with acute myeloid leukemia and myelodysplasia. Leuk Lymphoma 49:543–553
198. Bonifant CL et al (2016) CD123-engager T cells as a novel immunotherapeutic for acute myeloid leukemia. Mol Ther 24:1615–1626
199. Pizzitola I et al (2014) Chimeric antigen receptors against CD33/CD123 antigens efficiently target primary acute myeloid leukemia cells in vivo. Leukemia 28:1596–1605
200. Gill S et al (2014) Preclinical targeting of human acute myeloid leukemia and myeloablation using chimeric antigen receptor–modified T cells. Blood 123:2343–2354
201. Zhang S et al (1997) Selection of tumor antigens as targets for immune attack using immunohistochemistry: II. Blood group-related antigens. Int J Cancer 73:50–56
202. Kobayashi K et al (1993) Lewis blood group-related antigen expression in normal gastric epithelium, intestinal metaplasia, gastric adenoma, and gastric carcinoma. Am J Gastroenterol 88:919–924
203. Sakamoto J et al (1986) Expression of Lewisa, Lewisb, X, and Y blood group antigens in human colonic tumors and normal tissue and in human tumor-derived cell lines. Cancer Res 46:1553–1561
204. Ritchie DS et al (2013) Persistence and efficacy of second generation CAR T cell against the LeY antigen in acute myeloid leukemia. Mol Ther 21:2122–2129
205. Silva D, Tashiro H, Srinivasan M, Brenner MK, Mamonkin M (2016) CD7 CAR for the treatment of acute myeloid and lymphoid leukemia. Blood 128:4555–4555
206. Ponta H, Sherman L, Herrlich PA (2003) CD44: from adhesion molecules to signalling regulators. Nat Rev Mol Cell Biol 4:33–45
207. Casucci M et al (2013) CD44v6-targeted T cells mediate potent antitumor effects against acute myeloid leukemia and multiple myeloma. Blood 122:3461–3472
208. Lynn RC et al (2015) Targeting of folate receptor β on acute myeloid leukemia blasts with chimeric antigen receptor–expressing T cells. Blood 125:3466–3476
209. Lynn RC et al (2016) High-affinity FRβ-specific CAR T cells eradicate AML and normal myeloid lineage without HSC toxicity. Leukemia 30:1355–1364
210. Chien CD et al (2016) Preclinical development of FLT3-redirected chimeric antigen receptor T cell immunotherapy for acute myeloid leukemia. Blood 128:1072–1072
211. Liu X et al (2015) Affinity-tuned ErbB2 or EGFR chimeric antigen receptor T cells exhibit an increased therapeutic index against tumors in mice. Cancer Res 75:3596–3607
212. Hammarström S (1999) The carcinoembryonic antigen (CEA) family: structures, suggested functions and expression in normal and malignant tissues. Semin Cancer Biol 9:67–81
213. Parkhurst MR et al (2011) T cells targeting carcinoembryonic antigen can mediate regression of metastatic colorectal cancer but induce severe transient colitis. Mol Ther 19:620–626
214. Katz SC et al (2015) Phase I hepatic immunotherapy for metastases study of intra-arterial chimeric antigen receptor–modified T-cell therapy for CEA+ liver metastases. Clin Cancer Res 21:3149–3159
215. Suzuki M, Cheung N-KV (2015) Disialoganglioside GD2 as a therapeutic target for human diseases. Expert Opin Ther Targets 19:349–362
216. Yu AL et al (2010) Anti-GD2 antibody with GM-CSF, interleukin-2, and Isotretinoin for Neuroblastoma. N Engl J Med 363:1324–1334
217. Feldkamp MM, Lala P, Lau N, Roncari L, Guha A (1999) Expression of activated epidermal growth factor receptors, Ras-guanosine triphosphate, and mitogen-activated protein kinase in human glioblastoma multiforme specimens. Neurosurgery 45:1442–1453
218. Sampson JH et al (2014) EGFRvIII mCAR-modified T-cell therapy cures mice with established intracerebral glioma and generates host immunity against tumor-antigen loss. Clin Cancer Res Off J Am Assoc Cancer Res 20:972–984
219. Miao H et al (2014) EGFRvIII-specific chimeric antigen receptor T cells migrate to and kill tumor deposits infiltrating the brain parenchyma in an invasive Xenograft model of Glioblastoma. PLoS One 9:e94281

220. Morgan RA et al (2012) Recognition of Glioma stem cells by genetically modified T cells targeting EGFRvIII and development of adoptive cell therapy for Glioma. Hum Gene Ther 23:1043–1053
221. Johnson LA et al (2015) Rational development and characterization of humanized anti–EGFR variant III chimeric antigen receptor T cells for glioblastoma. Sci Transl Med 7:275ra22
222. O'Rourke DM et al (2016) Pilot study of T cells redirected to EGFRvIII with a chimeric antigen receptor in patients with EGFRvIII+ glioblastoma. J Clin Oncol 34
223. McKenzie AN et al (1993) Interleukin 13, a T-cell-derived cytokine that regulates human monocyte and B-cell function. Proc Natl Acad Sci U S A 90:3735–3739
224. Lai EW et al (2009) Overexpression of interleukin-13 receptor-α2 in neuroendocrine malignant pheochromocytoma: a novel target for receptor directed anti-cancer therapy. J Clin Endocrinol Metab 94:2952–2957
225. Debinski W, Gibo DM, Hulet SW, Connor JR, Gillespie GY (1999) Receptor for interleukin 13 is a marker and therapeutic target for human high-grade Gliomas. Clin Cancer Res 5:985–990
226. Brown CE et al (2015) Bioactivity and safety of IL13Rα2-redirected chimeric antigen receptor CD8+ T cells in patients with recurrent Glioblastoma. Clin Cancer Res 21:4062–4072
227. Brown CE et al (2016) Regression of Glioblastoma after chimeric antigen receptor T-cell therapy. N Engl J Med 375:2561–2569
228. Argani P et al (2001) Mesothelin is overexpressed in the vast majority of ductal adenocarcinomas of the pancreas. Clin Cancer Res 7:3862–3868
229. Chang K, Pastan I (1996) Molecular cloning of mesothelin, a differentiation antigen present on mesothelium, mesotheliomas, and ovarian cancers. Proc Natl Acad Sci U S A 93:136–140
230. Beatty GL et al (2014) Mesothelin-specific chimeric antigen receptor mRNA-engineered T cells induce antitumor activity in solid malignancies. Cancer Immunol Res 2:112–120
231. Adusumilli PS et al (2014) Regional delivery of mesothelin-targeted CAR T cell therapy generates potent and long-lasting CD4-dependent tumor immunity. Sci Transl Med 6:261ra151
232. Beatty GL et al (2015) Safety and antitumor activity of chimeric antigen receptor modified T cells in patients with chemotherapy refractory metastatic pancreatic cancer. J Clin Oncol 33
233. Park JE et al (1999) Fibroblast activation protein, a dual specificity serine protease expressed in reactive human tumor stromal fibroblasts. J Biol Chem 274:36505–36512
234. Schuberth PC et al (2013) Treatment of malignant pleural mesothelioma by fibroblast activation protein-specific re-directed T cells. J Transl Med 11:187
235. Yarden Y, Sliwkowski MX (2001) Untangling the ErbB signalling network. Nat Rev Mol Cell Biol 2:127–137
236. Press MF, Cordon-Cardo C, Slamon DJ (1990) Expression of the HER-2/neu proto-oncogene in normal human adult and fetal tissues. Oncogene 5:953–962
237. Slamon D et al (2011) Adjuvant Trastuzumab in HER2-positive breast cancer. N Engl J Med 365:1273–1283
238. Moritz D, Wels W, Mattern J, Groner B (1994) Cytotoxic T lymphocytes with a grafted recognition specificity for ERBB2-expressing tumor cells. Proc Natl Acad Sci U S A 91:4318–4322
239. Kershaw MH et al (2004) Gene-engineered T cells as a superior adjuvant therapy for metastatic cancer. J Immunol 173:2143–2150
240. Zhao Y et al (2009) A Herceptin-based chimeric antigen receptor with modified signaling domains leads to enhanced survival of transduced T lymphocytes and antitumor activity. J Immunol 183:5563–5574
241. Morgan RA et al (2010) Case report of a serious adverse event following the administration of T Cells transduced with a chimeric antigen receptor recognizing ERBB2. Mol Ther 18:843–851
242. Ahmed N et al (2015) Human epidermal growth factor receptor 2 (HER2) –specific chimeric antigen receptor–modified T cells for the immunotherapy of HER2-positive sarcoma. J Clin Oncol 33:1688–1696

243. Chang SS (2004) Overview of prostate-specific membrane antigen. Rev Urol 6:S13–S18
244. Haffner MC et al (2009) Prostate-specific membrane antigen expression in the neovasculature of gastric and colorectal cancers. Hum Pathol 40:1754–1761
245. Junghans RP et al (2016) Phase I trial of anti-PSMA designer CAR-T cells in prostate cancer: possible role for interacting interleukin 2-T cell pharmacodynamics as a determinant of clinical response. Prostate 76:1257–1270
246. Slovin SF et al (2012) Targeting castration resistant prostate cancer (CRPC) with autologous PSMA-directed CAR+ T cells. J Clin Oncol 30:TPS4700–TPS4700
247. Fraietta JA et al (2016) Biomarkers of response to anti-CD19 Chimeric Antigen Receptor (CAR) T-cell therapy in patients with chronic lymphocytic Leukemia. Blood 128:57–57
248. Xu Y et al (2014) Closely related T-memory stem cells correlate with in vivo expansion of CAR.CD19-T cells and are preserved by IL-7 and IL-15. Blood 123:3750–3759
249. Kochenderfer JN et al (2017) Lymphoma remissions caused by Anti-CD19 chimeric antigen receptor T cells are associated with high serum Interleukin-15 levels. J Clin Oncol Off J Am Soc Clin Oncol. doi:10.1200/JCO.2016.71.3024
250. Ruella M, Maus MV (2016) Catch me if you can: leukemia escape after CD19-directed T cell immunotherapies. Comput Struct Biotechnol J 14:357–362
251. Sotillo E et al (2015) Convergence of acquired mutations and alternative splicing of CD19 enables resistance to CART-19 immunotherapy. Cancer Discov. doi:10.1158/2159-8290.CD-15-1020
252. Ruella M et al (2016) Dual CD19 and CD123 targeting prevents antigen-loss relapses after CD19-directed immunotherapies. J Clin Invest 126:3814–3826
253. Braig F et al (2017) Resistance to anti-CD19/CD3 BiTE in acute lymphoblastic leukemia may be mediated by disrupted CD19 membrane trafficking. Blood 129:100–104
254. Velasquez MP, Gottschalk S (2017) Targeting CD19: the good, the bad, and CD81. Blood 129:9–10
255. Levy S (2014) Function of the tetraspanin molecule CD81 in B and T cells. Immunol Res 58:179–185
256. van Zelm MC et al (2010) *CD81* gene defect in humans disrupts CD19 complex formation and leads to antibody deficiency. J Clin Invest 120:1265–1274
257. Gardner R et al (2016) Acquisition of a CD19-negative myeloid phenotype allows immune escape of MLL-rearranged B-ALL from CD19 CAR-T-cell therapy. Blood 127:2406–2410
258. Rayes A, McMasters RL, O'Brien MM (2016) Lineage switch in MLL-rearranged infant leukemia following CD19-directed therapy. Pediatr Blood Cancer 63:1113–1115
259. Evans AG et al (2015) Evolution to plasmablastic lymphoma evades CD19-directed chimeric antigen receptor T cells. Br J Haematol. doi:10.1111/bjh.13562
260. Hegde M et al (2013) Combinational targeting offsets antigen escape and enhances effector functions of adoptively transferred T cells in Glioblastoma. Mol Ther 21:2087–2101
261. Jackson HJ, Brentjens RJ (2015) Overcoming antigen escape with CAR T-cell therapy. Cancer Discov 5:1238–1240
262. Lee DW et al (2014) Current concepts in the diagnosis and management of cytokine release syndrome. Blood 124:188–195
263. Brudno JN, Kochenderfer JN (2016) Toxicities of chimeric antigen receptor T cells: recognition and management. Blood 127:3321–3330
264. Nazimuddin F et al (2013) Long-term functional persistence, B cell aplasia and anti-leukemia efficacy in refractory B cell malignancies following T cell immunotherapy using CAR-redirected T cells targeting CD19. Blood 122:163–163
265. Wing MG et al (1996) Mechanism of first-dose cytokine-release syndrome by CAMPATH 1-H: involvement of CD16 (FcgammaRIII) and CD11a/CD18 (LFA-1) on NK cells. J Clin Invest 98:2819–2826
266. Suntharalingam G et al (2006) Cytokine storm in a phase 1 trial of the anti-CD28 monoclonal antibody TGN1412. N Engl J Med 355:1018–1028
267. Reagan JL et al (2013) Cellular immunotherapy for refractory hematological malignancies. J Transl Med 11:150

268. Winkler U et al (1999) Cytokine-release syndrome in patients with B-cell chronic lymphocytic leukemia and high lymphocyte counts after treatment with an anti-CD20 monoclonal antibody (rituximab, IDEC-C2B8). Blood 94:2217–2224
269. Nishimoto N, Kishimoto T (2006) Interleukin 6: from bench to bedside. Nat Clin Pract Rheumatol 2:619–626
270. Hunter CA, Jones SA (2015) IL-6 as a keystone cytokine in health and disease. Nat Immunol 16:448–457
271. Scheller J, Chalaris A, Schmidt-Arras D, Rose-John S (2011) The pro- and anti-inflammatory properties of the cytokine interleukin-6. Biochim Biophys Acta 1813:878–888
272. De Benedetti F et al (2012) Randomized trial of Tocilizumab in systemic juvenile idiopathic arthritis. N Engl J Med 367:2385–2395
273. Sarosiek S, Shah R, Munshi NC (2016) Review of siltuximab in the treatment of multicentric Castleman's disease. Ther Adv Hematol 7:360–366
274. Weber J et al (1994) A phase I trial of intravenous interleukin-6 in patients with advanced cancer. J Immunother 15:292–302
275. Nishimoto N et al (2008) Mechanisms and pathologic significances in increase in serum interleukin-6 (IL-6) and soluble IL-6 receptor after administration of an anti–IL-6 receptor antibody, tocilizumab, in patients with rheumatoid arthritis and Castleman disease. Blood 112:3959–3964
276. Morvan MG, Lanier LL (2016) NK cells and cancer: you can teach innate cells new tricks. Nat Rev Cancer 16:7–19
277. Caligiuri MA (2008) Human natural killer cells. Blood 112:461–469
278. Qasim W et al (2017) Molecular remission of infant B-ALL after infusion of universal TALEN gene-edited CAR T cells. Sci Transl Med 9:eaaj2013
279. Barrett DM, Singh N, Porter DL, Grupp SA, June CH (2014) Chimeric antigen receptor therapy for cancer. Annu Rev Med 65:333–347
280. Koehl U et al (2016) Advances in clinical NK cell studies: donor selection, manufacturing and quality control. Oncoimmunology 5:e1115178
281. Handgretinger R, Lang P, André MC (2016) Exploitation of natural killer cells for the treatment of acute leukemia. Blood 127:3341–3349
282. Cichocki F et al (2016) The past, present, and future of NK cells in hematopoietic cell transplantation and adoptive transfer. Curr Top Microbiol Immunol 395:225–243
283. Miller JS et al (2005) Successful adoptive transfer and in vivo expansion of human haploidentical NK cells in patients with cancer. Blood 105:3051–3057
284. Bachanova V et al (2014) Clearance of acute myeloid leukemia by haploidentical natural killer cells is improved using IL-2 diphtheria toxin fusion protein. Blood 123:3855–3863
285. Romee R et al (2016) Cytokine-induced memory-like natural killer cells exhibit enhanced responses against myeloid leukemia. Sci Transl Med 8:357ra123
286. Dolstra H et al (2017) Successful transfer of umbilical cord blood CD34+ hematopoietic stem and progenitor-derived NK cells in older acute myeloid leukemia patients. Clin Cancer Res Off J Am Assoc Cancer Res. doi:10.1158/1078-0432.CCR-16-2981
287. Bachanova V et al (2010) Allogeneic natural killer cells for refractory lymphoma. Cancer Immunol Immunother CII 59:1739–1744
288. Geller MA et al (2011) A phase II study of allogeneic natural killer cell therapy to treat patients with recurrent ovarian and breast cancer. Cytotherapy 13:98–107
289. Shah N et al (2017) Phase I study of cord blood-derived natural killer cells combined with autologous stem cell transplantation in multiple myeloma. Br J Haematol. doi:10.1111/bjh.14570
290. Schlums H et al (2015) Cytomegalovirus infection drives adaptive epigenetic diversification of NK cells with altered signaling and effector function. Immunity 42:443–456
291. Suck G et al (2016) NK-92: an 'off-the-shelf therapeutic' for adoptive natural killer cell-based cancer immunotherapy. Cancer Immunol Immunother 65:485–492
292. Thomson JA et al (1998) Embryonic stem cell lines derived from human blastocysts. Science 282:1145–1147

293. Takahashi K et al (2007) Induction of pluripotent stem cells from adult human fibroblasts by defined factors. Cell 131:861–872
294. Angelos MG, Kaufman DS (2015) Pluripotent stem cell applications for regenerative medicine. Curr Opin Organ Transplant 20:663–670
295. Woll PS, Martin CH, Miller JS, Kaufman DS (2005) Human embryonic stem cell-derived NK cells acquire functional receptors and cytolytic activity. J Immunol Baltim Md 1950(175):5095–5103
296. Woll PS et al (2009) Human embryonic stem cells differentiate into a homogeneous population of natural killer cells with potent in vivo antitumor activity. Blood 113:6094–6101
297. Knorr DA et al (2013) Clinical-scale derivation of natural killer cells from human pluripotent stem cells for cancer therapy. Stem Cells Transl Med 2:274–283
298. Hermanson DL et al (2016) Induced pluripotent stem cell-derived natural killer cells for treatment of ovarian cancer. Stem Cells Dayt Ohio 34:93–101
299. Kalos M, June CH (2013) Adoptive T cell transfer for cancer immunotherapy in the era of synthetic biology. Immunity 39:49–60
300. Hermanson DL, Kaufman DS (2015) Utilizing chimeric antigen receptors to direct natural killer cell activity. Front Immunol 6:195. https://doi.org/10.3389/fimmu.2015.00195. eCollection 2015
301. Glienke W et al (2015) Advantages and applications of CAR-expressing natural killer cells. Front Pharmacol 6. https://doi.org/10.3389/fphar.2015.00021
302. Giudice A, Trounson A (2008) Genetic modification of human embryonic stem cells for derivation of target cells. Cell Stem Cell 2:422–433
303. Ni Z, Knorr DA, Bendzick L, Allred J, Kaufman DS (2014) Expression of chimeric receptor CD4ζ by natural killer cells derived from human pluripotent stem cells improves in vitro activity but does not enhance suppression of HIV infection in vivo. Stem Cells Dayt Ohio 32:1021–1031
304. Jing Y et al (2015) Identification of an ADAM17 cleavage region in human CD16 (FcγRIII) and the engineering of a non-cleavable version of the receptor in NK cells. PLoS One 10:e0121788
305. Schuster SJ et al (2015) Phase IIa trial of chimeric antigen receptor modified T cells directed against CD19 (CTL019) in patients with relapsed or refractory CD19+ lymphomas. J Clin Oncol 33

Chapter 6
Combinatorial Checkpoint Blockade Immunotherapy and Radiation

Sangwoo Shawn Kim and Andrew Sharabi

Abstract Radiation therapy plays a critical role in the treatment of a wide variety of cancers. Recent studies have shown that radiation therapy (RT) can modify the adaptive immune response and can work synergistically with checkpoint blockade immunotherapy (CBI) to induce potent endogenous antitumor responses. Preclinical models have demonstrated a potential ability of RT to prime the immune system and augment the efficacy of CBI. Retrospective clinical data has reported a dramatic improvement in overall survival and response rates when radiation is combined with immunotherapy in patients with metastatic melanoma. Case reports have also documented evidence of enhanced responses outside of the radiation field, also termed "abscopal effects." The immunologic mechanism of the abscopal effect, however, has not been fully characterized. Prospective clinical trials are currently ongoing to uncover the details of the abscopal effect and demonstrate the clinical efficacy of combined RT and CBI in treating cancer in both the definitive and metastatic setting. Here we review select preclinical and clinical data on radiation checkpoint blockade combinations.

Keywords Radiation • Immunotherapy • Abscopal • Checkpoint blockade • PD-1 • CTLA-4 • Stereotactic

S.S. Kim (✉)
School of Medicine, University of California San Diego, San Diego, CA, USA
e-mail: ssk050@ucsd.edu

A. Sharabi
Department of Radiation Medicine and Applied Sciences, University of California San Diego Moores Cancer Center, San Diego, CA, USA
e-mail: sharabi@ucsd.edu

S.P. Patel, R. Kurzrock (eds.), *Early Phase Cancer Immunotherapy*, Current Cancer Research, DOI 10.1007/978-3-319-63757-0_6

6.1 Radiation Therapy and the Abscopal Effect: Preclinical Data

Radiation therapy (RT) remains one of the pillars of cancer therapy. Recently advances in RT have made it possible to deliver focused radiation to tumor sites within the body with millimeter accuracy by using advanced patient immobilization systems, onboard real-time imaging, respiratory management, and stereotactic patient localization. This technique is known as stereotactic body radiation therapy (SBRT) for sites outside the CNS and stereotactic radiosurgery (SRS) for sites within the CNS, although the overall techniques are fairly equivalent. SBRT has given clinicians the ability to deliver high doses of radiation to a specific site in one to five total treatments while minimizing radiation to surrounding tissues. Furthermore, using the same technological advances, radiation oncologists can now deliver image-guided intensity-modulated radiation therapy (IG-IMRT) with conventional daily fractionation that allows for rapid dose gradients and the ability to exquisitely control where dose is deposited to allow for dose escalation while sparing nearby critical structures and limiting toxicity. These technological advances call for a reevaluation of the use of radiation therapy in combination with novel immunologic anticancer agents.

Traditionally, RT is known to kill cancer cells by inducing significant DNA damage by directly breaking DNA strands and creating free radical induced oxidation, leading to apoptosis or mitotic catastrophy [1]. However, RT has been shown to elicit a wider, more systemic effect, as it can drastically alter the expression of cell surface molecules and shape the adaptive immune response [2–7]. In a seminal study, Reits et al. showed that high-dose RT increases not only the expression of major histocompatibility complex (MHC) class I molecules but also the diversity of peptides presented [2]. Burnette et al. then illustrated the importance of RT in stimulating type I IFN production and its critical role in initiating a local antitumor response [3]. Using CT26 and MC38 colon tumors, Filatenkov et al. additionally demonstrated the role high-dose radiation can play in shifting the immunogenic landscape of the tumor microenvironment by increasing infiltration of CD8+ T cells and decreasing the population of myeloid-derived suppressor cells. This effect ultimately stimulated long-term remission in a type I IFN-dependent manner [4]. However, T-regulatory cells (Treg) seem preferentially resistant to RT and may induce other molecules that contribute to tumor-mediated immunosuppression [5–7].

The role that RT plays in shifting the adaptive immune response has inspired efforts to seek ways to combine RT with other methods that augment the endogenous antitumor response. One such method is checkpoint blockade immunotherapy (CBI), which targets molecules including CTLA-4 and PD-1/PD-L1. It has been observed that RT combined with CBI can elicit an antitumor response within and outside the field of radiation—this has been termed the "abscopal effect" [8, 9]. The immunologic mechanisms of this effect, however, have not been fully elucidated.

6.1.1 Combined Radiation Therapy and Anti-CTLA-4 Immunotherapy

Cytotoxic T-lymphocyte antigen-4 (CTLA-4) plays a key role in modulating the adaptive immune response. For proper T-cell activation and proliferation, CD28 on the T cell must bind the B7 ligands present on an antigen-presenting cell (APC), an interaction that can be outcompeted by CTLA-4 due to its significantly increased binding affinity [10, 11]. In fact, CTLA-4 has been shown to play a key role in controlling Tregs' abilities to suppress activity of other T cells [12, 13]. Therefore, it represents an ideal drug target to study in combination with radiation therapy to enhance antitumor responses.

Combined RT and anti-CTLA-4 IT has then been tested in various metastatic cancer models. In a study by Demaria et al., a poorly immunogenic metastatic breast carcinoma (4 T1 cell line) in mice was best controlled by a combination of RT and anti-CTLA-4 IT—an effect that was mediated by CD8+ T cells [14]. The fractionation pattern or total number of radiation treatments may also influence resultant antitumor immune responses. Dewan et al. demonstrated that fractionated RT (8 Gy × 3 fractions or 6 Gy × 5 fractions) combined with anti-CTLA-4 IT could prompt an abscopal effect in both metastatic breast carcinoma and colon carcinoma (MCA38 cell line), an effect that correlated with increased frequency of infiltration by tumor-specific CD8+ T cells [15].

Filatenkov et al. further characterized the critical importance of dose and sequencing on CD8+ T-cell infiltration [4]. Using a dose of 30 Gy, either in a single fraction or ten fractions, the authors examined the mechanisms that contribute to complete remissions in murine colorectal tumor models (CT26 and MC38). They reported that high-dose radiation modified the tumor microenvironment and induced a robust CD8+ T-cell infiltrate with a synchronous loss of myeloid-derived suppressor cells (MDSC) [4]. These changes depend on dendritic cells as well as CD4+ T-helper cells. Interestingly the single-fraction radiation therapy was more effective than the extended fractionated radiation therapy [4]. Furthermore, adding additional radiation doses after a single large fraction of radiation abrogated responses. The time course of these events were also examined with absolute numbers of T cells decreasing immediately within 1–2 days after radiation but then increasing significantly above baseline at 7 and 14 days after radiation therapy [4]. These findings support the concept that radiation can rapidly induce T-cell apoptosis, but that the downstream immunologic effects of radiation can result in enhanced immune responses.

Importantly, tumors have been demonstrated to activate resistance mechanisms to single-agent anti-CTLA-4 IT. In a high-profile study in *Nature* by Twyman-Saint Victor et al., the authors demonstrated that while melanoma mouse models can be successfully treated using a combined RT and anti-CTLA-4 IT approach, resistance is common with one mechanism operating via upregulation of PD-L1 and T-cell exhaustion. These findings highlight the potential critical importance of combined dual-agent checkpoint blockade [16]. Another fascinating finding the authors reported is that radiation and checkpoint blockade can increase the T-cell receptor diversity [16], suggesting that radiation can induce a more broad array of tumor antigen presentation by APCs and contribute to epitope spreading. Taken together, this study characterized both preclinical and clinical immune correlates, and emphasized the importance of targeting resistance mechanisms with dual-agent checkpoint blockade combined with radiation therapy. Along these lines, other cell-mediated resistance mechanisms, including natural killer T cells, have been implicated in modulating responses to RT and anti-CTLA-4 IT [17], highlighting the importance of addressing both direct and indirect mechanisms by which tumors can evade immune responses.

6.1.2 Combined Radiation Therapy and Anti-PD-1 Immunotherapy

The programmed death-1 (PD-1)/programmed death ligand-1 (PD-L1) axis is critically important in dampening and controlling the adaptive immune response [18]. PD-1 is highly expressed on activated T cells among other cell types, while PD-L1 is normally expressed at low levels on various cells but is upregulated by APCs and various solid tumors, the latter of which may do so after exposure to RT [7, 19]. Tumor cells are able to hijack the PD-1/PD-L1 system to evade the endogenous antitumor response by inactivating tumor-specific T cells and creating a subset of Tregs and myeloid-derived suppressor cells (MDSC) [6, 20]. Preclinical models have demonstrated that RT may serve to prime the immune system and, when used in conjunction with anti-PD-1 IT, can generate endogenous antigen-specific immune responses.

A study by Dovedi et al. illustrated that type I IFN produced by CD8+ T cells was one key mechanism which causes tumor cells to upregulate PD-L1 expression. However, by using concomitant anti-PD-1/PD-L1 IT, it was possible to circumvent that checkpoint and induce a powerful antitumor response [21]. Additionally, tumors that are resistant to earlier therapies and upregulate PD-1 can be successfully treated with additional anti-PD-1 IT by preventing decreases in CD8+ T cells and further promoting mature T-cell proliferation [16].

The combination of RT and anti-PD-1 IT has shown survival benefits in both tumors that have widely metastasized and primary brain tumors [22–24]. In a study by Zeng et al., mice with glioma had a nearly twofold increase in survival when treated with both RT and anti-PD-1 IT, with control mice surviving 25 days, mice with RT only and PD-1 IT only surviving 27 days and 28 days, respectively, and mice with the combination therapy surviving 53 days. The survival benefit was shown to correlate with an increase in CD8+ T cells and a concomitant decrease in Treg cells [22]. Similarly, mice with melanoma that had metastasized to the brain demonstrated a greater than threefold increase in survival (from 15 to 58 days) when treated with high-dose RT and anti-PD-1 IT; interestingly, this combination treatment may additionally lengthen tumor dormancy [23]. These studies demonstrate the ability for stereotactic radiation therapy to better reach tumors in locations that were previously difficult to treat.

Recently a novel combination of dual-agent anti-PD-1 and anti-T-cell immunoglobulin mucin-3 (TIM-3) with radiation therapy was reported in a murine glioma model [25]. TIM-3 is a negative immune regulator which the authors demonstrate can be present in human glioblastoma multiforme. Using a murine glioma model, the authors demonstrated that anti-TIM-3 combined with SRS or dual-agent anti-TIM-3 and anti-PD-1 improved survival compared to anti-TIM-3 antibody alone. Furthermore the triple combination of SRS + anti-TIM-3 + anti-PD-1 resulted in complete response and long-term survival which was associated with immune cell infiltration and development of memory responses [25]. These findings provide additional evidence that dual-agent checkpoint blockade combined with radiation therapy may be synergistic and help to improve locoregional and distant tumor control.

6.2 Combined Radiation Therapy and Checkpoint Blockade Immunotherapy: Clinical Data

With the success of combined RT with CBI in preclinical models, clinical translation was rapidly initiated. While the use of combined RT and checkpoint blockade IT to treat cancers has remained largely investigational, here, we will provide an overview of select studies and case reports that have applied combination therapy in treating melanoma, non-small cell lung cancer (NSCLC), prostate cancer, and head and neck cancers.

6.2.1 Melanoma

A majority of published studies investigating the combined use of RT and checkpoint blockade IT have featured metastatic melanoma, primarily as that disease was the first histology to have an FDA-approved indication for checkpoint blockade [26–32]. A case report published by Postow et al. first demonstrated the efficacy of combined RT and anti-CTLA-4 IT in treating metastatic melanoma. This patient received a total of 28.5 Gy RT over three fractions in 1 week along with 10 mg/kg body weight anti-CTLA-4 IT every 3 weeks for three total doses and responded with significant tumor regression [26]. An early study of combination therapy for melanoma with brain metastases by Silk et al. demonstrated a significant increase in the proportion of patients who responded to RT when previously receiving anti-CTLA-4 IT (40% when given RT, 9.1% without RT) [27]. A retrospective analysis by Kiess et al. then revealed that not only can RT and anti-CTLA-4 be safely administered to patients, but it is also correlated with improved tumor control and longer survival, especially when radiation was given concurrently with anti-CTLA-4 [28]. Another analysis by Qian et al. of patients with melanoma that had metastasized to the brain exhibited a significantly increased reduction in tumor volume when treated with concurrent (as defined by administration within 4 weeks of each other) RT and CBI. Seventy-five patients received both RT and CBI, and at 6 months, these patients exhibited a 94.9% decrease in tumor volume, compared to a 66.2% decrease for patients who received nonconcurrent therapy ($P < 0.0001$). This study additionally demonstrated a superior efficacy of anti-PD-1 IT compared to anti-CTLA-4 IT [30].

A recent retrospective analysis of 127 patients with metastatic melanoma by Theurich et al. reported that combined local radiation therapy and anti-CTLA-4 IT resulted in a significant increase in the proportion of patients who had either a complete response, partial remission, or stable disease compared to anti-CTLA-4 alone (from 38.8% in anti-CTLA-4 IT only to 57.7% in RT + anti-CTLA-4 IT; $P = 0.05$). Furthermore, the combination therapy significantly increased patient survival compared to anti-CTLA-4 alone irrespective of other clinical characteristics of the tumor, such as BRAF status, stage, grade, and presence of metastases [29]. Although retrospective, this is strong clinical evidence of the efficacy and benefit of radiation combined with checkpoint blockade immunotherapy.

Recent data from a second group corroborates the findings by Theurich et al. In an independent retrospective analysis by Koller, K. M. et al., 101 patients that received anti-CTLA-4 alone or anti-CTLA-4 combined with radiation therapy were analyzed. Median overall survival significantly increased from 10 to 19 months in patients that received concurrent anti-CTLA-4 and radiation therapy. Similarly, the rates of complete responses were significantly increased in the anti-CTLA-4 plus radiation group (6.5% vs. 25.7%, $P = 0.04$) [33]. The overall response rates (19.4% vs. 37.1%) were also increased in the combined treatment group compared to anti-CTLA-4 alone group [33]. Importantly the authors reported no significant increase in toxicities in the combined group, providing further safety data regarding radiation combined with checkpoint blockade. These two studies on over 200 patients with metastatic melanoma who received radiation combined with anti-CTLA-4 provide strong evidence for the clinical efficacy of this combined treatment in improving complete response rates and overall survival. Prospective studies are currently underway to further address these findings.

6.2.2 Non-Small Cell Lung Cancer

A case report by Golden et al. featured a patient with metastatic NSCLC that continued to spread after treatment with traditional chemotherapy. The patient received a total of 30 Gy RT over five fractions in 10 days followed by 3 mg/kg body weight anti-CTLA-4 IT every 3 weeks for four total doses. The patient responded with significantly decreased tumor metabolic activity at sites both inside and outside the radiation field, consistent with an abscopal effect [34]. There have been few other published reports on using combined RT and CBI for treating NSCLC; however, ongoing trials have indicated that there is likely no significant increase in additional adverse effects associated with RT when given alongside anti-PD-1 IT [35]. Numerous trials are active in this space, and we eagerly await the results of the ongoing studies.

6.2.3 Prostate Cancer

A large randomized double-blinded placebo-controlled phase III trial by Kwon et al. compared anti-CTLA-4 IT with placebo after administration of RT to assess both efficacy and safety of anti-CTLA-4 IT for treating metastatic castration-resistant prostate cancer (mCRPC). A total of 799 patients were enrolled and were given a single dose (8 Gy) of RT followed by 10 mg/kg anti-CTLA-4 IT (399 patients) or placebo (400 patients) every 3 weeks. Patients who were given anti-CTLA-4 IT experienced significantly more "immune-related" adverse effects—the most common being diarrhea, fatigue, anemia, and colitis—and experienced a modest increase in median overall survival from 10.0 months with placebo to 11.2 months with anti-CTLA-4 IT (hazard ratio = 0.85, $P = 0.053$) [36]. While this study did not meet its primary endpoint, the P value of 0.053 was close to significance, and in an exploratory subset analysis, patients with advanced visceral disease may have contributed to excess deaths in the treatment arms. However, further studies must be done to further evaluate the efficacy of combination therapy in treating prostate cancer.

One such ongoing phase I/II study by Slovin et al. explored the use of RT combined with anti-CTLA-4 IT to treat mCRPC. Patients received either anti-CTLA-4 monotherapy every 3 weeks for four total doses or IT combined with 8 Gy/lesion RT. The most common adverse effects were colitis and rash, which were managed with a course of corticosteroids. While this trial is ongoing, RT in combination with anti-CTLA-4 IT seems to demonstrate antitumor activity with a manageable side effect profile [37].

While previous data did not show significant activity of anti-PD-1 agents in mCRPC, recent early data has challenged that observation, with a number of men with mCRPC experiencing a rapid drop in PSA on an anti-PD-1 agent, suggesting that the activity of anti-PD-1/PD-L1 agents in mCRPC could be reexamined [38].

6.2.4 *Head and Neck Cancer*

While no large series of radiation checkpoint blockade combinations have been reported in head and neck cancer at this time, a case report submitted by Nagasaka et al. presented a patient with squamous cell carcinoma in the floor of her mouth that advanced after successive treatments with carboplatin and paclitaxel, and then methotrexate and cetuximab. Although the patient initially demonstrated a partial response and stable disease for a few months, the disease ultimately progressed locally, and the patient was started on anti-PD-1 IT. After six cycles of stable disease, the disease again progressed locally, and the patient was treated with 30 Gy RT, after which the patient demonstrated a significant clinical response, demonstrating a potential role of checkpoint blockade IT as a radiosensitizer [39]. A number of clinical trials combining radiation with checkpoint blockade in head and neck cancer have been proposed, and we will await the results of these studies to determine the safety and efficacy of this combination in this disease site.

6.3 Select Clinical Trials Featuring Combined Radiation Therapy and Checkpoint Blockade Immunotherapy

RT and checkpoint blockade IT can work synergistically to induce a potent antitumor response. However, many details concerning the precise immunologic mechanism of the abscopal effect have yet to be revealed. In sum, numerous clinical trials seek to treat various cancers, both metastatic and nonmetastatic, with RT and CBI with the goal of elucidating the mechanistic details of their synergistic relationship (Table 6.1).

6.4 Conclusion

In summary, there is now an established body of preclinical evidence that radiation therapy can synergize with single- and dual-agent checkpoint blockade immunotherapy in many different tumor types. Published clinical series including large phase III studies have demonstrated the relative safety of this combination with low palliative doses of radiation in the metastatic setting. Recent retrospective clinical data has demonstrated striking increases in overall survival and complete responses rates when radiation therapy is combined with checkpoint blockade in patients with metastatic melanoma. This clinical data supports the safety and efficacy of radiation combined with checkpoint blockade. Ongoing prospective clinical trials will further elucidate and define the effect of radiation combined with checkpoint blockade in both the metastatic and definitive setting.

Table 6.1 Selected active clinical trials studying combination radiation therapy and checkpoint blockade immunotherapy

Title (trial number)	Phase	Intervention	Cancer	Institution
Chemoradiation therapy and Ipilimumab in treating patients with locally advanced cervical cancer *(NCT01711515)*	1	Anti-CTLA-4 + cisplatin + EBRT + IRT	Cervical	National Cancer Institute
Nivolumab with or without stereotactic radiosurgery in treating patients with recurrent, advanced, or metastatic chordoma *(NCT02989636)*	1	Anti-PD-1 + SBRT	Chordoma	Sidney Kimmel Comprehensive Cancer Center and National Cancer Institute
PI Pembro in combination with stereotactic body radiotherapy for liver metastatic colorectal cancer *(NCT02837263)*	1	Anti-PD-1 + SBRT	Colorectal	University of Wisconsin, Madison and Merck Sharp & Dohme Corp.
Nivolumab or Nivolumab /Ipilimumab prior to Chemoradiation plus Nivolumab with II/III Gastro/ Esophageal Cancer *(NCT02044613)*	1	Anti-PD-1 + carboplatin/ paclitaxel + SBRT	Gastric, esophageal, gastroesophageal	Sidney Kimmel Comprehensive Cancer Center
Checkpoint blockade immunotherapy combined with stereotactic body radiation in advanced metastatic disease *(NCT02843165)*	1	Anti-PD-1/PD-L1 + SBRT	Metastatic cancer	University of California San Diego
MPDL3280A and stereotactic ablative radiotherapy in patients with non-small cell lung cancer *(NCT02400814)*	1	Anti-PD-1 + SBRT	NSCLC	University of California, Davis, National Cancer Institute, and Genentech, Inc.
Study of PD1 blockade by Pembrolizumab with stereotactic body radiotherapy in advanced solid tumors *(NCT02608385)*	1	Anti-PD-1 + SBRT	NSCLC	University of Chicago
Immune checkpoint inhibition (Tremelimumab and/ or MEDI4736) in combination with radiation therapy in patients with unresectable pancreatic cancer *(NCT02311361)*	1	Anti-CTLA-4 and/or anti-PD-L1 + SBRT	Pancreatic	National Cancer Institute

(continued)

Table 6.1 (continued)

Title (trial number)	Phase	Intervention	Cancer	Institution
Study of immune checkpoint inhibition with radiation therapy in unresectable, non-metastatic pancreatic cancer *(NCT02868632)*	1	Anti-CTLA-4 + SBRT	Pancreatic	New York University School of Medicine and AstraZeneca
A study of Chemoradiation plus Pembrolizumab for locally advanced laryngeal squamous cell carcinoma *(NCT02759575)*	1 | 2	Anti-PD-1 + RT	Head and neck	University of Cincinnati and Merck Sharp & Dohme Corp.
Evaluating the combination of MK-3475 and stereotactic body radiotherapy in patients with metastatic melanoma or NSCLC *(NCT02407171)*	1 | 2	Anti-PD-1 + SBRT	Melanoma, NSCLC	Yale University
Avelumab with Hypofractionated radiation therapy in adults with Isocitrate Dehydrogenase (IDH) Mutant Glioblastoma *(NCT02968940)*	2	Anti-PD-L1 + HFRT	Glioblastoma	New York University School of Medicine and EMD Serono
Stereotactic radiation therapy and Ipilimumab in treating patients with metastatic melanoma *(NCT02107755)*	2	Anti-CTLA-4 + SBRT	Melanoma	Ohio State University and Bristol-Myers Squibb
Phase II trial of stereotactic body radiotherapy followed by Ipilimumab in treating patients with stage iv melanoma *(NCT01970527)*	2	Anti-CTLA-4 + SBRT	Melanoma	University of Washington and National Cancer Institute
Combination radiation and PD-1 inhibition in metastatic or recurrent renal cell carcinoma *(NCT02962804)*	2	Anti-PD-1 + RT	Renal cell	University of Kansas Medical Center
Tremelimumab and Durvalumab with or without radiation therapy in patients with relapsed small cell lung cancer *(NCT02701400)*	2	Anti-CTLA-4 + anti-PD-1 + SBRT	SCLC	Emory University and AstraZeneca

EBRT External beam radiation therapy, *HFRT* hypofractionated radiation therapy, *IRT* internal radiation therapy, *RT* radiation therapy, *SBRT* stereotactic body radiation therapy, *NSCLC* non-small cell lung cancer, *SCLC* small cell lung cancer

References

1. Prise KM, Schettino G, Folkard M, Held KD (2005) New insights on cell death from radiation exposure. Lancet Oncol 6(7):520–528
2. Reits EA, Hodge JW, Herberts CA, Groothuis TA, Chakraborty M, Wansley EK, Camphausen K, Luiten RM, de Ru AH, Neijssen J, Griekspoor A, Mesman E, Verreck FA, Spits H, Schlom J, van Veelen P, Neefjes JJ (2006) Radiation modulates the peptide repertoire, enhances MHC class I expression, and induces successful antitumor immunotherapy. J Exp Med 203(5):1259–1271
3. Burnette BC, Liang H, Lee Y, Chlewicki L, Khodarev NN, Weichselbaum RR, Fu YX, Auh SL (2011) The efficacy of radiotherapy relies upon induction of type i interferon-dependent innate and adaptive immunity. Cancer Res 71(7):2488–2496
4. Filatenkov A, Baker J, Mueller AM, Kenkel J, Ahn GO, Dutt S, Zhang N, Kohrt H, Jensen K, Dejbakhsh-Jones S, Shizuru JA, Negrin RN, Engleman EG, Strober S (2015) Ablative tumor radiation can change the tumor immune cell microenvironment to induce durable complete remissions. Clin Cancer Res 21(16):3727–3739
5. Kachikwu EL, Iwamoto KS, Liao YP, DeMarco JJ, Agazaryan N, Economou JS, McBride WH, Schaue D (2011) Radiation enhances regulatory T cell representation. Int J Radiat Oncol Biol Phys 81(4):1128–1135
6. Deng L, Liang H, Burnette B, Beckett M, Darga T, Weichselbaum RR, Fu YX (2014) Irradiation and anti-PD-L1 treatment synergistically promote antitumor immunity in mice. J Clin Invest 124(2):687–695
7. Deng L, Liang H, Burnette B, Weicheslbaum RR, Fu YX (2014) Radiation and anti-PD-L1 antibody combinatorial therapy induces T cell-mediated depletion of myeloid-derived suppressor cells and tumor regression. Oncoimmunology 3:e28499
8. Demaria S, Ng B, Devitt ML, Babb JS, Kawashima N, Liebes L, Formenti SC (2004) Ionizing radiation inhibition of distant untreated tumors (abscopal effect) is immune mediated. Int J Radiat Oncol Biol Phys 58(3):862–870
9. Park SS, Dong H, Liu X, Harrington SM, Krco CJ, Grams MP, Mansfield AS, Furutani KM, Olivier KR, Kwon ED (2015) PD-1 restrains radiotherapy-induced abscopal effect. Cancer Immunol Res 3(6):610–619
10. van der Merwe PA, Bodian DL, Daenke S, Linsley P, Davis SJ (1997) CD80 (B7-1) binds both CD28 and CTLA-4 with a low affinity and very fast kinetics. J Exp Med 185(3):393–403
11. Linsley PS, Brady W, Urnes M, Grosmaire LS, Damle NK, Ledbetter JA (1991) CTLA-4 is a second receptor for the B cell activation antigen B7. J Exp Med 174(3):561–569
12. Wing K, Onishi Y, Prieto-Martin P, Yamaguchi T, Miyara M, Fehervari Z, Nomura T, Sakaguchi S (2008) CTLA-4 control over Foxp3+ regulatory T cell function. Science 322(5899):271–275
13. Egen JG, Kuhns MS, Allison JP (2002) CTLA-4: new insights into its biological function and use in tumor immunotherapy. Nat Immunol 3(7):611–618
14. Demaria S, Kawashima N, Yang AM, Devitt ML, Babb JS, Allison JP, Formenti SC (2005) Immune-mediated inhibition of metastases after treatment with local radiation and CTLA-4 blockade in a mouse model of breast cancer. Clin Cancer Res 11(2 Pt 1):728–734
15. Dewan MZ, Galloway AE, Kawashima N, Dewyngaert JK, Babb JS, Formenti SC, Demaria S (2009) Fractionated but not single-dose radiotherapy induces an immune-mediated abscopal effect when combined with anti-CTLA-4 antibody. Clin Cancer Res 15(17):5379–5388
16. Twyman-Saint Victor C, Rech AJ, Maity A, Rengan R, Pauken KE, Stelekati E, Benci JL, Xu B, Dada H, Odorizzi PM, Herati RS, Mansfield KD, Patsch D, Amaravadi RK, Schuchter LM, Ishwaran H, Mick R, Pryma DA, Xu X, Feldman MD, Gangadhar TC, Hahn SM, Wherry EJ, Vonderheide RH, Minn AJ (2015) Radiation and dual checkpoint blockade activate non-redundant immune mechanisms in cancer. Nature 520(7547):373–377
17. Grosso JF, Jure-Kunkel MN (2013) CTLA-4 blockade in tumor models: an overview of preclinical and translational research. Cancer Immun 13:5

18. Pardoll DM (2012) The blockade of immune checkpoints in cancer immunotherapy. Nat Rev Cancer 12(4):252–264
19. Śledzińska A, Menger L, Bergerhoff K, Peggs KS, Quezada SA (2015) Negative immune checkpoints on T lymphocytes and their relevance to cancer immunotherapy. Mol Oncol 9(10):1936–1965
20. Spranger S, Spaapen RM, Zha Y, Williams J, Meng Y, Ha TT, Gajewski TF (2013) Up-regulation of PD-L1, IDO, and T(regs) in the melanoma tumor microenvironment is driven by CD8(+) T cells. Sci Transl Med 5(200):200ra116
21. Dovedi SJ, Adlard AL, Lipowska-Bhalla G, McKenna C, Jones S, Cheadle EJ, Stratford IJ, Poon E, Morrow M, Stewart R, Jones H, Wilkinson RW, Honeychurch J, Illidge TM (2014) Acquired resistance to fractionated radiotherapy can be overcome by concurrent PD-L1 blockade. Cancer Res 74(19):5458–5468
22. Zeng J, See AP, Phallen J, Jackson CM, Belcaid Z, Ruzevick J, Durham N, Meyer C, Harris TJ, Albesiano E, Pradilla G, Ford E, Wong J, Hammers HJ, Mathios D, Tyler B, Brem H, Tran PT, Pardoll D, Drake CG, Lim M (2013) Anti-PD-1 blockade and stereotactic radiation produce long-term survival in mice with intracranial gliomas. Int J Radiat Oncol Biol Phys 86(2):343–349
23. Smilowitz HM, Micca PL, Sasso D, Wu Q, Dyment N, Xue C, Kuo L (2016) Increasing radiation dose improves immunotherapy outcome and prolongation of tumor dormancy in a subgroup of mice treated for advanced intracerebral melanoma. Cancer Immunol Immunother 65(2):127–139
24. D'Souza NM, Fang P, Logan J, Yang J, Jiang W, Li J (2016) Combining radiation therapy with immune checkpoint blockade for central nervous system malignancies. Front Oncol 6:212
25. Kim JE, Patel MA, Mangraviti A, Kim ES, Theodros D, Velarde E, Liu A, Sankey EW, Tam A, Xu H, Mathios D, Jackson CM, Harris-Bookman S, Garzon-Muvdi T, Sheu M, Martin AM, Tyler BM, Tran PT, Ye X, Olivi A, Taube JM, Burger PC, Drake CG, Brem H, Pardoll DM, Lim M (2017) Combination therapy with anti-PD-1, anti-TIM-3, and focal radiation results in regression of murine Gliomas. Clin Cancer Res 23(1):124–136
26. Postow MA, Callahan MK, Barker CA, Yamada Y, Yuan J, Kitano S, Mu Z, Rasalan T, Adamow M, Ritter E, Sedrak C, Jungbluth AA, Chua R, Yang AS, Roman RA, Rosner S, Benson B, Allison JP, Lesokhin AM, Gnjatic S, Wolchok JD (2012) Immunologic correlates of the abscopal effect in a patient with melanoma. N Engl J Med 366(10):925–931
27. Silk AW, Bassetti MF, West BT, Tsien CI, Lao CD (2013) Ipilimumab and radiation therapy for melanoma brain metastases. Cancer Med 2(6):899–906
28. Kiess AP, Wolchok JD, Barker CA, Postow MA, Tabar V, Huse JT, Chan TA, Yamada Y, Beal K (2015) Stereotactic radiosurgery for melanoma brain metastases in patients receiving ipilimumab: safety profile and efficacy of combined treatment. Int J Radiat Oncol Biol Phys 92(2):368–375
29. Theurich S, Rothschild SI, Hoffmann M, Fabri M, Sommer A, Garcia-Marquez M, Thelen M, Schill C, Merki R, Schmid T, Koeberle D, Zippelius A, Baues C, Mauch C, Tigges C, Kreuter A, Borggrefe J, von Bergwelt-Baildon M, Schlaak M (2016) Local tumor treatment in combination with systemic Ipilimumab immunotherapy prolongs overall survival in patients with advanced malignant melanoma. Cancer Immunol Res 4(9):744–754
30. Qian JM, Yu JB, Kluger HM, Chiang VL (2016) Timing and type of immune checkpoint therapy affect the early radiographic response of melanoma brain metastases to stereotactic radiosurgery. Cancer 122(19):3051–3058
31. Stamell EF, Wolchok JD, Gnjatic S, Lee NY, Brownell I (2013) The abscopal effect associated with a systemic anti-melanoma immune response. Int J Radiat Oncol Biol Phys 85(2):293–295
32. Grimaldi AM, Simeone E, Giannarelli D, Muto P, Falivene S, Borzillo V, Giugliano FM, Sandomenico F, Petrillo A, Curvietto M, Esposito A, Paone M, Palla M, Palmieri G, Caracò C, Ciliberto G, Mozzillo N, Ascierto PA (2014) Abscopal effects of radiotherapy on advanced melanoma patients who progressed after ipilimumab immunotherapy. Oncoimmunology 3:e28780

33. Koller KM, Mackley HB, Liu J, Wagner H, Talamo G, Schell TD, Pameijer C, Neves RI, Anderson B, Kokolus KM, Mallon CA, Drabick JJ (2017) Improved survival and complete response rates in patients with advanced melanoma treated with concurrent ipilimumab and radiotherapy versus ipilimumab alone. Cancer Biol Ther 18(1):36–42
34. Golden EB, Demaria S, Schiff PB, Chachoua A, Formenti SC (2013) An abscopal response to radiation and ipilimumab in a patient with metastatic non-small cell lung cancer. Cancer Immunol Res 1(6):365–372
35. Gerber DE, Urbanic JJ, Langer C, Hu C, Chang IF, Lu B, Movsas B, Jeraj R, Curran WJ, Bradley JD (2016) Treatment design and rationale for a randomized trial of cisplatin and etoposide plus thoracic radiotherapy followed by nivolumab or placebo for locally advanced non-small-cell lung cancer (RTOG 3505). Clin Lung Cancer 18(3):333–339
36. Kwon ED, Drake CG, Scher HI, Fizazi K, Bossi A, van den Eertwegh AJ, Krainer M, Houede N, Santos R, Mahammedi H, Ng S, Maio M, Franke FA, Sundar S, Agarwal N, Bergman AM, Ciuleanu TE, Korbenfeld E, Sengeløv L, Hansen S, Logothetis C, Beer TM, McHenry MB, Gagnier P, Liu D, Gerritsen WR, Investigators C (2014) Ipilimumab versus placebo after radiotherapy in patients with metastatic castration-resistant prostate cancer that had progressed after docetaxel chemotherapy (CA184-043): a multicentre, randomised, double-blind, phase 3 trial. Lancet Oncol 15(7):700–712
37. Slovin SF, Higano CS, Hamid O, Tejwani S, Harzstark A, Alumkal JJ, Scher HI, Chin K, Gagnier P, McHenry MB, Beer TM (2013) Ipilimumab alone or in combination with radiotherapy in metastatic castration-resistant prostate cancer: results from an open-label, multicenter phase I/II study. Ann Oncol 24(7):1813–1821
38. Graff JN, Alumkal JJ, Drake CG, Thomas GV, Redmond WL, Farhad M, Cetnar JP, Ey FS, Bergan RC, Slottke R, Beer TM (2016) Early evidence of anti-PD-1 activity in enzalutamide-resistant prostate cancer. Oncotarget 7(33):52810–52817
39. Nagasaka M, Zaki M, Kim H, Raza SN, Yoo G, Lin HS, Sukari A (2016) PD1/PD-L1 inhibition as a potential radiosensitizer in head and neck squamous cell carcinoma: a case report. J Immunother Cancer 4:83

Chapter 7
Combinatorial Immunotherapy and Chemotherapy

Christin B. DeStefano and Stephen V. Liu

Abstract Immunotherapy has emerged as an effective strategy in several cancer types that, unlike most conventional therapies, can deliver durable disease control with a favorable toxicity profile. In an unselected population, however, the majority of patients will not respond. Combining immunotherapy with other treatment modalities may increase the likelihood and potentially the depth of response. One approach is to combine immunotherapy with cytotoxic chemotherapy. There are both potential benefits and limitations to this approach, and while early data are encouraging, more work is needed to optimize these combinations and clearly define their role in the therapeutic landscape.

Keywords Chemotherapy • Immunotherapy • Combination • Checkpoint inhibitors • Chemoimmunotherapy

7.1 Introduction

There have been few therapeutic advances in oncology that have garnered as much attention as immunotherapy, specifically, the development of checkpoint inhibitors. Their appeal is in large part tied to the potential for durable responses, an outcome not characteristic of other systemic treatments. Initially, with immunotherapy agents such as interleukin (IL)-2 and interferon (IFN)-gamma, the likelihood of durable disease control was quite low and offset by an unfavorable toxicity profile [1]. With the development of checkpoint inhibitors, both efficacy and safety improved, and with experience, adverse effects could be better managed and anticipated.

C.B. DeStefano, MD
Division of Hematology-Oncology, Washington Cancer Institute, Washington, DC, USA
e-mail: Christin.B.Destefano@medstar.net

S.V. Liu, MD (✉)
Division of Medical Oncology, Georgetown University School of Medicine, Washington, DC, USA
e-mail: stephen.v.liu@gunet.georgetown.edu

S.P. Patel, R. Kurzrock (eds.), *Early Phase Cancer Immunotherapy*, Current Cancer Research, DOI 10.1007/978-3-319-63757-0_7

Immunotherapy has evolved from an academic pursuit for relatively uncommon malignancies to the standard of care for a steadily increasing number of common cancers. When compared to cytotoxic chemotherapy in the right populations, checkpoint inhibitors have often proven better tolerated and more effective, offering some patients an opportunity for long-lasting benefit. In their current form, however, checkpoint inhibitors offer only a minority of patients this transformative benefit and current efforts are focused on optimization of this treatment strategy.

Development of more potent immunotherapy agents is underway and the search for predictive biomarkers to properly deliver these agents is a global priority. Meanwhile, an inviting strategy is to combine checkpoint inhibitors with other agents to improve the quantity and quality of responses. While the field is young, there have been promising results when combining checkpoint inhibitors with chemotherapy, radiation, surgery, targeted agents, biologics, and other molecules that manipulate the immune response. This chapter will focus on combinations of immune checkpoint inhibitors with cytotoxic chemotherapy in solid tumors, reviewing the rationale of these combinations and summarizing selected studies.

7.2 Benefits of Combining Immunotherapy and Chemotherapy

The relationship between cytotoxic chemotherapy and the immune system is complex and despite many preconceptions, not necessarily antagonistic [2]. It has become clear that chemotherapy has the potential to enhance an antitumor immune response, though its immunomodulatory role is incompletely understood. Similarly, an immune response can be critical to the efficacy of chemotherapy, previously thought to exert its antitumor effects independently. For example, doxorubicin has an antitumor effect in several cancer models including colorectal cancer and sarcoma. In mice, the antitumor effect was seen in immunocompetent mice but not seen in immunodeficient mice treated under the same conditions [3]. The nature of the relationship between cytotoxic therapy and the immune system will vary with each specific agent and circumstance, ensuring challenges in optimization of combinatorial strategies [4]. One preclinical study demonstrated in vivo synergy between blockade of cytotoxic T-lymphocyte-associated protein 4 (CTLA-4) and use of various cytotoxic agents including paclitaxel, ixabepilone, gemcitabine, and etoposide, but the effect of each agent was slightly different [5]. There is scientific rationale to combine cytotoxic agents with immunotherapy, and though much of the existing evidence is preclinical, there are several potential mechanisms supporting the use of combination strategies. Ongoing clinical studies exploring various combinations will strengthen our understanding of the multifaceted and dynamic relationship between cytotoxic chemotherapy, immunotherapy, the tumor, and the host.

7.2.1 Depletion of Immunosuppressive Cells

Myeloid-derived suppressor cells (MDSCs) play a critical role in the development or prevention of an antitumor immune response. MDSCs include a variety of myeloid-derived cells that suppress effector cells via cell-cell interactions and soluble mediators [6]. MDSCs and T-regulatory cells (Tregs) have emerged as contributors to the pathogenesis of cancer, and with the development of immunotherapy, they remain central to any discussion of primary or acquired resistance. Elimination or reduction of these suppressor cells may facilitate a more robust response to immunotherapy. While novel immunotherapy agents are in development to target the immunosuppressive microenvironment, cytotoxic chemotherapy can also play a role in the depletion of immunosuppressive cells.

Gemcitabine, a widely used cytotoxic agent, was found to potentiate responses to a novel breast cancer vaccine in mice [7]. In these studies, tumor-bearing mice were treated with adenoviral vaccination followed by an anti-GITR agonist antibody, and while treatment promoted cytotoxic T lymphocyte activity, it was insufficient to generate an antitumor response. Addition of gemcitabine promptly led to an antitumor response and after a subsequent tumor rechallenge, mice remained tumor free, suggesting establishment of memory. Gemcitabine significantly reduced the number of splenic MDSCs, potentially explaining the observed benefit. This reduction of splenic MDSCs was also seen following gemcitabine treatment in mice bearing mesothelioma or non-small cell lung cancer (NSCLC) tumors [8]. While not limited to gemcitabine, this effect is far from universal among cytotoxic agents. In an illustrative experiment, mice bearing thymoma tumors were treated with gemcitabine, cyclophosphamide, doxorubicin, oxaliplatin, paclitaxel, and 5-fluorouracil (5-FU) [9]. In these mice, MDSCs were abundant within the spleen prior to therapy. Following treatment, MDSCs were depleted only in the mice that received gemcitabine or 5-FU. The effect was seen on both granulocytic and monocytic MDSCs and was more pronounced with 5-FU than with gemcitabine. In these studies, the MDSCs underwent apoptotic cell death and the low expression of thymidylate synthase in MDSCs may have contributed to their selective sensitivity. Cisplatin has also been associated with a reduction in MDSCs [10].

Other suppressive cells in the microenvironment can also be depleted with cytotoxic chemotherapy. Administration of paclitaxel can reduce the fraction of Treg cells with no notable change in the T effector cell percentage [11]. Cyclophosphamide, when given at a low dose or in a metronomic schedule, also selectively depletes Treg cells in several models [12–14]. Gemcitabine can also affect differentiation, promoting a shift from protumorigenic M2 macrophages to antitumorigenic M1 macrophages [15].

7.2.2 Activation of Immune Effectors

Equally important is the effect of chemotherapy on effector cells, though the activation of effectors and inhibition of suppressors often occur together. Early observation of the cytotoxic agent melphalan showed that high doses induced cell death but lower, subtherapeutic doses had a unique impact on the tumor microenvironment, shifting the cytokine milieu by reducing suppressive T cells and promoting CD8+ T cell immunity [16]. In murine models, administration of anti-CTLA-4 monoclonal antibodies had no effect on growth of some tumors, but pretreatment with low doses of melphalan led to a permissive environment and left the tumor susceptible to anti-CTLA-4 therapy [17].

Cytotoxic T cells are often absent from tumors, which may limit efficacy of immunotherapy efforts. In mice bearing AB1-HA mesothelioma tumors, tumor growth was associated with a depletion of intratumoral CD8 T cells [18]. Gemcitabine treatment reversed this T cell depletion and increased intratumoral infiltration of CD8+ T cells. In another study, gemcitabine reduced total lymphocyte numbers, but the impact was far more pronounced on B-lymphocytes, as gemcitabine administration actually enhanced CD8+ T cell recall responses [19]. In a similar fashion, cisplatin also promotes intratumoral T cell infiltration in murine models [20]. Tumor infiltration of antigen-presenting cells is also noted after treatment with anthracyclines including mitoxantrone and doxorubicin [21].

In addition to migration and tumor infiltration, chemotherapy can promote effector cell function. Monocyte-derived dendritic cells exposed to carboplatin, cisplatin, or oxaliplatin enhanced T cell proliferation in a dose-dependent manner [22]. These T cells produced higher levels of IFN-γ and IL-2 compared to untreated dendritic cells. Treatment with paclitaxel, methotrexate, doxorubicin, or vinblastine leads to upregulation of MHC class I antigen processing machinery. This facilitates antigen presentation and tumor recognition [23]. MHC class I upregulation has also been seen following treatment with cisplatin plus vinorelbine [24] and cisplatin plus 5-FU [25], as well as cisplatin alone [26].

7.2.3 Sensitization of Tumor Cells to Lysis

Immune-mediated cell apoptosis is regulated by many factors including members of the tumor necrosis factor (TNF) receptor family such as Fas and DR4/DR5. The ligands for these receptors (Fas-L and TRAIL) are expressed by CD8+ T cells and NK lymphocytes. Response to these cytokines can be enhanced with several cytotoxic agents including cisplatin, doxorubicin, mitomycin C, 5-FU, and camptothecin [27].

Conventional chemotherapy may also increase sensitivity to cytotoxic T cell perforin and granzyme B mediated cell death [28]. This can occur through upregulation of mannose-6-phosphate receptors on tumor surfaces, demonstrated in murine models exposed to taxane, platinum, or anthracycline therapy [29]. Traditional chemotherapy can also put stress on the endoplasmic reticulum in tumor cells, which leads to exposure of its luminal protein, calreticulin, on the tumor cell surface. Calreticulin serves as an engulfment signal for essential antigen-presenting cells, thus further enhancing immune recognition [29].

7.2.4 Exploiting Chemosensitive Tumors

There is also a practical consideration, particularly in the treatment of aggressive cancers where standard therapy is at least initially effective, such as small-cell lung cancer (SCLC). If immunotherapy alone is administered, patients may be spared the toxicity of chemotherapy and achieve a high-quality response. If, however, treatment is ineffective, the natural history of some aggressive cancers may render a patient ineligible for subsequent therapy. For immunotherapy agents with a relatively low response rate, use of immunotherapy alone could come at the cost of forfeiting potentially effective cytotoxic treatment. In these circumstances, combining cytotoxic chemotherapy with immunotherapy would ensure that all patients receive the benefit of chemotherapy while a subset could also receive a more durable benefit from immunotherapy. Reduction of tumor burden with chemotherapy, particularly in a symptomatic patient, is appealing and in many cases, more reliable.

Cytotoxic chemotherapy has the potential to facilitate a favorable response to immunotherapy and combination strategies may prove superior to either chemotherapy or immunotherapy alone. It is certainly possible, however, that combinations may be ultimately prove to be detrimental, as outlined below.

7.3 Limitations of Combining Immunotherapy and Chemotherapy

While the immunomodulatory properties of cytotoxic chemotherapy are intriguing, cytotoxic therapy has the potential to be detrimental to inducing an immune response. Many cytotoxic agents can induce lymphopenia and that effect of chemotherapy on T cells may limit immune responses. In fact, several cytotoxic agents are used clinically for the treatment of autoimmune conditions, including cyclophosphamide and methotrexate, though the dosing schedules are different in this capacity [30].

While both gemcitabine and 5-FU have been shown to reduce MDSCs, studies have also shown the potential for an immunosuppressive effect [31]. Treatment of MDSCs with gemcitabine or 5-FU led to activation of the Nlrp3-dependent caspace-1 activation complex. This activation prompts release of IL-1β, a cytokine that promotes T cell immunoregulation and can suppress an immune response. In addition to possibly blunting an immune response, combinations of chemotherapy and immunotherapy may be more toxic. Several early clinical studies have shown relatively high rates of adverse events.

Clearly, the effect of cytotoxic chemotherapy on the immune system is highly variable. While the potential for a positive partnership between chemotherapy and immunotherapy exists, details regarding specific agents used, doses, schedule, and sequence are likely to have dramatic consequences. Empiric combinations of chemotherapy and immunotherapy must be properly studied before routine implementation. A relatively minor variable may make the difference between a beneficial and a detrimental partnership.

7.4 Clinical Experience Combining Immunotherapy and Chemotherapy

In light of the potential benefit, while acknowledging the potential limitations, studies combining cytotoxic chemotherapy and immunotherapy rapidly emerged. When combined with vaccine therapy, chemotherapy was primarily given to target MDSCs and Tregs. Though well tolerated, efficacy was modest. The most promising combinations have involved checkpoint inhibitors targeting CTLA-4, anti-programmed death receptor-1 (PD-1), and anti-programmed death receptor-1 ligand (anti-PD-L1). While the experience is relatively limited, combinations between checkpoint inhibitors and cytotoxic chemotherapy do appear to be tolerable and signals of efficacy are intriguing. We will focus this chapter on some of the early experience with these combinations. There are a large number of variables between these studies, and direct comparisons between trials are not appropriate. With a growing body of experience, it is likely that combination therapy will find a place in the management of specific cancer types but the specific clinical circumstances are not yet defined.

7.4.1 NSCLC

Use of checkpoint inhibitors has become the standard of care for the treatment of advanced NSCLC. The PD-1 inhibitors pembrolizumab and nivolumab and the PD-L1 inhibitor atezolizumab were all shown in separate phase III studies to improve outcomes compared to standard chemotherapy in the salvage setting [32–35]. Pembrolizumab was also superior to chemotherapy in the first-line setting, for tumors that have a high expression of PD-1 (at least 50% of cells positive using the Dako 22C3 immunohistochemistry assay) [36]. Due to the clear activity of checkpoint inhibitors in NSCLC and the consistent benefit with platinum-based chemotherapy, combinatorial chemotherapy and immunotherapy have been of particular interest in this disease (Table 7.1).

Table 7.1 Immunotherapy plus chemotherapy combination studies in NSCLC

References	Immunotherapy	Chemotherapy	Response rate	mPFS	mOS	Grade 3 or 4 AEs	Grade 3 or 4 irAEs
Lynch et al. [37]	Ipilimumab	Carboplatin plus paclitaxel phased	32%	5.7	12.2	15%	39%
	Ipilimumab	Carboplatin plus paclitaxel concurrent	21%	5.5	9.7	20%	41%
		Carboplatin plus paclitaxel	18%	4.6	8.3	6%	37%
Gadgeel et al. [38]	Pembrolizumab	Carboplatin plus paclitaxel	52%	10.3	NR	16%	56%
	Pembrolizumab	Carboplatin plus paclitaxel plus bevacizumab	48%	NR	NR	38%	71%
	Pembrolizumab	Carboplatin plus pemetrexed	71%	10.2	NR	29%	67%
Langer et al. [39]	Pembrolizumab	Carboplatin plus paclitaxel	55%	13.0	NR	22%	40%
		Carboplatin plus paclitaxel	29%	8.9	NR	12%	25%
Rizvi et al. [40]	Nivolumab	Cisplatin plus gemcitabine	33%	5.7	11.6	NR	25%
	Nivolumab	Cisplatin plus pemetrexed	47%	6.8	19.2	NR	47%
	Nivolumab	Carboplatin plus paclitaxel	47%	4.8	14.9	NR	73%
	Nivolumab[a]	Carboplatin plus paclitaxel	43%	7.1	NR	NR	29%
Liu et al. [41]	Atezolizumab	Carboplatin plus paclitaxel	50.%	NR	NR	NR	71%
	Atezolizumab	Carboplatin plus pemetrexed	77%	NR	NR	NR	54%
	Atezolizumab	Carboplatin plus nab-paclitaxel	56%	NR	NR	NR	85%

Abbreviations: *AE* adverse event, *irAE* immune-related adverse event, *mOS* median overall survival, *mPFS* median progression-free survival, *NR* not reported
[a]Nivolumab was given at a lower dose in this arm

7.4.1.1 Ipilimumab plus Carboplatin and Paclitaxel

Ipilimumab is an anti-CTLA-4 antibody currently approved for the treatment of advanced melanoma. An important phase II study combined ipilimumab with the commonly used chemotherapy doublet of carboplatin plus paclitaxel in chemotherapy-naïve NSCLC [37]. This trial randomized patients to one of three arms. Patients in the control arm received carboplatin AUC 6 plus paclitaxel 175 mg/m^2 with placebo every 3 weeks for six cycles. Patients in the concurrent arm received carboplatin plus paclitaxel with ipilimumab 10 mg/kg for four cycles followed by carboplatin plus paclitaxel with placebo for two cycles. Patients in the phased arm received carboplatin plus paclitaxel with placebo for two cycles followed by carboplatin plus paclitaxel with ipilimumab for four cycles. Patients could then continue to receive ipilimumab or placebo once every 12 weeks. The primary outcome was immune-related progression-free survival (irPFS).

This study randomized 204 patients with chemotherapy-naïve NSCLC to one of the three arms. As expected, the addition of ipilimumab increased the rate of immune-related adverse events (control 6%, concurrent 20%, phased 15%), but the overall incidence of treatment-related grade 3 and 4 adverse events was similar across the arms (control 37%, concurrent 41%, phased 39%). There were two cases of grade 3 colitis in the phased arm, one case of grade 3 hypophysitis in the concurrent arm and one case of grade 3 hypopituitarism in the concurrent arm. Grade 3 elevation in liver function tests was noted in one patient in each of the three arms. Discontinuation due to drug-related toxicity occurred in 5% of patients in the control arm, 10% in the concurrent arm, and 6% in the phased arm. There were two treatment-related deaths, one in the control arm and one in the concurrent arm.

The study met its primary endpoint of improved irPFS in the phased arm versus the control arm (HR 0.72, $p = 0.05$) but not for the concurrent arm versus control (HR 0.81, $p = 0.13$). The median irPFS was 4.6 months in the control arm, 5.5 months in the concurrent arm and 5.7 months in the phased arm. Median overall survival (OS) numerically favored the phased arm though there was no statistically significant difference noted (control 8.3 months, concurrent 9.7 months, phased 12.2 months).

While the absolute improvement was modest, this phase II trial did show superior outcomes with the addition of ipilimumab to chemotherapy. Importantly, the benefit was dependent on the sequence. Concurrent administration did not improve irPFS but when chemotherapy was given alone for two cycles before the addition of ipilimumab, there was a significant improvement. The precise mechanism is not clear, but carboplatin and paclitaxel may have facilitated subsequent T cell activation.

7.4.1.2 Pembrolizumab plus Platinum-Based Chemotherapy

The KEYNOTE-021 study was a multicohort phase I/II trial that included several cohorts of patients with treatment-naïve NSCLC treated with pembrolizumab and platinum-based chemotherapy [38]. Patients received pembrolizumab (randomized 1:1 to 2 or 10 mg/kg) with carboplatin AUC 6 plus paclitaxel 200 mg/m^2 (cohort A, $n = 25$); carboplatin AUC 6, paclitaxel 200 mg/m^2, and bevacizumab 15 mg/kg (cohort B, $n = 25$); or carboplatin AUC 5 plus pemetrexed 500 mg/m^2 (cohort C, $n = 24$). Immune-related adverse events were seen in 16% of patients in cohort A,

38% of patients in cohort B, and 29% of patients in cohort C. There was one dose-limiting toxicity of toxic epidermal necrolysis in cohort C (pembrolizumab 10 mg/kg), accounting for the only treatment-related drug discontinuation in that cohort. Discontinuation due to drug-related adverse event occurred in three patients in cohort B (one grade 3 pneumonitis, one grade 3 drug hypersensitivity, and one grade 3 autoimmune colitis), while there were none in cohort A.

The objective response rate for the three cohorts was 52% in cohort A, 48% in cohort B, and 71% in cohort C including one complete response. Median PFS was 10.3 months in cohort A, not reached in cohort B, and 10.2 months in cohort C. Though the study was not designed to compare across arms, toxicity seemed to be higher in cohort B.

Based on these data and the high response rate seen in cohort C, a randomized cohort was opened to further explore the addition of pembrolizumab to first-line carboplatin plus pemetrexed [39]. Patients with advanced non-squamous NSCLC received carboplatin AUC 5 plus pemetrexed 500 mg/m^2 every 3 weeks for four cycles followed by pemetrexed maintenance therapy every 3 weeks thereafter. Patients randomized to the experimental arm (1:1) also received pembrolizumab 200 mg every 3 weeks for up to 24 months.

In this phase II cohort, 123 patients were randomized to treatment. Grade 3 or 4 treatment-related adverse events were seen in 26% of patients in the chemotherapy arm and 39% of patients in the chemotherapy plus pembrolizumab arm. Among the adverse events more common in the pembrolizumab combination arm were fatigue (all grade, 64% vs. 40%), nausea (all grade, 58% vs. 44%), anemia (all grade, 53% vs. 32%), rash (all grade, 27% vs. 15%), and immune-related adverse events (23% vs. 12%). The most common immune-related adverse events in the pembrolizumab arm were hypothyroidism (15%, all grade 1 or 2) and hyperthyroidism (8%, all grade 1 or 2), with three cases of pneumonitis, including one grade 2 pneumonitis. There were also two cases of infusion reaction, including one grade 4 event. Overall, tolerability was similar in the two arms. Treatment discontinuation due to drug-related toxicity occurred in 13% of patients in the chemotherapy arm and 10% of patients in the chemotherapy plus pembrolizumab arm. There were two deaths in the chemotherapy alone arm (one attributed to pancytopenia and one attributed to sepsis) and one death in the chemotherapy plus pembrolizumab arm (attributed to sepsis).

After a median follow-up of 10.6 months, progression-free survival (PFS) favored the pembrolizumab combination (HR 0.53, $p = 0.010$) with a median PFS of 13.0 months compared to 8.9 months with chemotherapy alone. The estimated 6 months PFS rate was 77% with pembrolizumab and 63% with only chemotherapy. The response rate was higher with pembrolizumab (55% vs. 29%) with a shorter median time to best response of 1.5 months compared to 2.7 months. Duration of response also favored the pembrolizumab arm (8.0 months vs. 4.9 months). There was no difference in survival between the two groups, though there was a high rate of censoring in this early analysis and 32% of patients in the chemotherapy alone arm crossed over to receive pembrolizumab.

Current use of pembrolizumab monotherapy in the front-line and salvage settings is limited to patients whose tumors express PD-L1 by immunohistochemistry using the Dako 22C3 assay. In this combination study, efficacy was seen regardless of PD-L1 status. Among patients whose tumors had no PD-L1 expression (<1%), the response rate was 57% (12 of 21); when PD-L1 expression was present (≥1%), the response rate was 54% (21 of 39), though it was highest among patients with the highest expression (≥50%), where responses were seen in 16 of 20 patients (80%). While pembrolizumab monotherapy is standard for patients whose tumors highly express PD-L1 (≥50%), combination strategies are appealing for those with lower or no PD-L1 expression and may be superior to monotherapy alone. Larger studies are underway exploring carboplatin and paclitaxel with or without pembrolizumab (KEYNOTE-407, NCT02775435) and carboplatin and pemetrexed with or without pembrolizumab (KEYNOTE-189, NCT02578680).

7.4.1.3 Nivolumab plus Platinum-Based Chemotherapy

Checkmate 012 was a phase I multicohort trial that included 56 patients with advanced, treatment-naïve NSCLC treated with nivolumab and platinum-based chemotherapy [40]. Patients received nivolumab concurrently with chemotherapy every 3 weeks for four cycles followed by nivolumab monotherapy until progression or unacceptable toxicity. To reflect different practices, several platinum-based regimens were explored. One arm, limited to squamous histology, combined gemcitabine 1250 mg/m^2 plus cisplatin 75 mg/m^2 with nivolumab 10 mg/kg. One arm, restricted to non-squamous NSCLC, combined pemetrexed 500 mg/m^2 plus cisplatin 75 mg/m^2 with nivolumab 10 mg/kg. One arm, open to any histology, combined paclitaxel 200 mg/m^2 plus carboplatin AUC 6 with nivolumab 10 mg/kg. The final arm, also open to any histology, combined paclitaxel 200 mg/m^2 plus carboplatin AUC 6 with nivolumab 5 mg/kg. There was no randomization; each arm enrolled independently and the study was not designed to compare across the arms.

Grade 3 and 4 treatment-related adverse events were observed in 45% of patients and adverse events were much more likely during the combination treatment period (95% all grade, 38% grade 3 and 4) than in the nivolumab monotherapy period (61% and 16%, respectively). Hypersensitivity infusion reactions occurred in 23% of patients. Colitis was seen in two patients with one case of grade 3 or 4 colitis. Pneumonitis was seen in seven patients (13%) and four cases (7%) were grade 3 or 4. Endocrine adverse events were noted in four patients (7%), and there were no cases of grade 3 or 4 liver function test elevation. Treatment discontinuation due to drug toxicity occurred in 21% of patients, specifically 8% in the gemcitabine plus cisplatin with nivolumab arm, 33% in the pemetrexed plus cisplatin with nivolumab arm, 13% in the paclitaxel plus carboplatin with nivolumab 10 mg/kg arm, and 29% in the paclitaxel plus carboplatin with nivolumab 5 mg/kg arm. The most common reasons for discontinuation due to treatment-related adverse events were pneumonitis and acute renal failure (three patients each). There were no treatment-related deaths.

Response rates were promising: 33% in the gemcitabine plus cisplatin with nivolumab arm, 47% in the pemetrexed plus cisplatin with nivolumab arm, 47% in the paclitaxel plus carboplatin with nivolumab 10 mg/kg arm, and 43% in the paclitaxel plus carboplatin with nivolumab 5 mg/kg arm. Median duration of response was 10.3, 5.8, 5.5, and 19.6 months, respectively. Two-year survival rates were 25%, 33%, 27%, and 62%, respectively.

It is challenging to draw meaningful conclusions in a relatively small study with no comparator arms. While the combinations were tolerable, toxicity was not insignificant, and the rate of discontinuation due to treatment toxicity was higher than that seen in ipilimumab studies. The efficacy also appeared to be greater, though, with an impressive duration of response. A phase III trial is underway comparing nivolumab with or without ipilimumab to carboplatin plus gemcitabine or pemetrexed (Checkmate 227, NCT02477826).

7.4.1.4 Atezolizumab plus Platinum-Based Chemotherapy

GP28328 was a phase Ib multicohort trial exploring atezolizumab with chemotherapy that included three cohorts of patients with treatment-naïve NSCLC [41, 42]. Patients in Arm C received carboplatin AUC 6 with paclitaxel 200 mg/m^2 every 3 weeks. Patients in Arm D received carboplatin AUC 6 with pemetrexed 500 mg/m^2 every 3 weeks and, at the investigator's discretion, maintenance pemetrexed every 3 weeks. Patients in Arm E received carboplatin AUC 6 with every 3 weeks with nab-paclitaxel 100 mg/m^2 given weekly. Patients could receive four to six cycles of chemotherapy. All patients received atezolizumab 15 mg/kg (later amended to a flat dose of 1200 mg) given every 3 weeks with chemotherapy and continued every 3 weeks thereafter.

The incidence of treatment-related grade 3 and 4 adverse events was 69% (71% in Arm C, 54% in Arm D, and 85% in Arm E) including one treatment-related death in Arm D due to prolonged neutropenia. Grade 3 or 4 elevation in the liver function tests alanine aminotransferase (ALT) and aspartate aminotransferase (AST) was uncommon, with two events in Arm D (ALT 4.2%, AST 4.2%) and four events in Arm E (ALT 10.0%, AST 10.0%) but none in Arm C (overall ALT 5.2%, AST 5.2%). The rate of discontinuation due to adverse event was 3.4%. Early assessment revealed promising response rates: 50% in Arm C, 76.5% in Arm D, and 56.3% in Arm E, including a 25% complete response rate.

As above, more data is needed to draw conclusions regarding these combinations. In the presented preliminary analyses, there was a low rate of discontinuation due to toxicity with encouraging response rates including numerous complete responses. While we await final results, randomized trials are already underway assessing the benefit of adding atezolizumab to carboplatin plus nab-paclitaxel (IMpower130, NCT02367781), atezolizumab to carboplatin plus paclitaxel or nab-paclitaxel (IMpower131, NCT02367794), atezolizumab to carboplatin or cisplatin plus pemetrexed (IMPower132, NCT02657434), and atezolizumab to carboplatin and paclitaxel with or without bevacizumab (IMpower150, NCT02366143).

7.4.2 *SCLC*

Early studies of immunotherapy in previously treated SCLC have been promising, with responses seen in the phase I/II Checkmate 032 study of nivolumab alone or in combination with ipilimumab [43]. SCLC is particularly responsive to chemotherapy, though responses are transient. As a result, combination approaches have been appealing in this disease.

7.4.2.1 Ipilimumab plus Carboplatin and Paclitaxel

A phase II study combined ipilimumab with carboplatin plus paclitaxel in chemotherapy-naïve SCLC [44]. As with the NSCLC study described above, this study randomized patients to one of three arms: a control arm of carboplatin AUC 6 plus paclitaxel 175 mg/m^2 with placebo every 3 weeks for six cycles, a concurrent arm with carboplatin plus paclitaxel with ipilimumab 10 mg/kg for four cycles followed by carboplatin plus paclitaxel with placebo for two cycles, or a phased arm of carboplatin plus paclitaxel with placebo for two cycles followed by carboplatin plus paclitaxel with ipilimumab for four cycles. The primary outcome was irPFS.

This study randomized 130 patients with SCLC 1:1:1 to one of the three arms. In this patient population, there was more toxicity seen with the addition of ipilimumab. The incidence of treatment-related grade 3 and 4 adverse events was 30% in the control arm, 43% in the concurrent arm and 50% in the phased arm. The incidence of grade 3 and 4 immune-related adverse events was higher with ipilimumab (control 9%, concurrent 21%, phased 17%). Grade 3 or 4 elevation in liver function tests was noted in the concurrent arm (ALT 18%, AST 13%) and the phased arm (ALT 4%, AST 7%) but not in the control arm. The one treatment-related death was in the concurrent arm and attributed to hepatotoxicity. There was one case of grade 3 colitis (in the phased arm) and four cases of grade 3 arthralgias (in the phased arm) but no cases of hypophysitis reported. While the toxicity profile was different among the three arms, the rate of discontinuation due to drug-related toxicity was similar across the study (control 9%, concurrent 7%, phased 5%).

As with the NSCLC study, this trial met its primary endpoint of improved irPFS versus control in the phased arm (HR 0.64, $p = 0.03$) but not in the concurrent arm (HR 0.75, $p = 0.11$). Median irPFS was 5.3 months in the control arm, 5.7 months in the concurrent arm, and 6.4 months in the phased arm, and the median OS was 9.9 months, 9.1 months, and 12.9 months, respectively.

7.4.2.2 Ipilimumab plus Carboplatin and Etoposide

Based on the encouraging phase II results of ipilimumab with carboplatin and paclitaxel, a phase III study combined ipilimumab with platinum plus etoposide, the standard first-line regimen for chemotherapy-naïve SCLC [45]. All patients received etoposide 100 mg/m^2 on days 1–3 with carboplatin AUC 5 or cisplatin 75 mg/m^2 (investigator's choice) on day 1 in a 3-week cycle for four cycles. Patients were randomized to receive ipilimumab 10 mg/kg or placebo in a phased approach, with chemotherapy alone for two cycles then the addition of ipilimumab or placebo every 3 weeks with cycle 3 and maintenance therapy every 12 weeks. The primary endpoint of this phase III trial was overall survival.

This trial randomized 1132 patients and 954 patients received at least one dose of ipilimumab or placebo. This study did show a difference in tolerability. Grade 3 and 4 treatment-related adverse events were noted in 48% of patients in the ipilimumab arm and 44% in the control arm. Immune-related adverse events were more common with ipilimumab and included diarrhea (25% in the ipilimumab arm vs. 10% in the control arm), rash (19% vs. 3%), colitis (6% vs. 1%), and endocrine events (10% vs. 2%). The endocrine events included hypothyroidism (3%), hyperthyroidism (2%), hypophysitis (1%), and adrenal insufficiency (1%). There were five treatment-related deaths in the ipilimumab arm, attributed to colitis (2), sepsis (2), and hepatotoxicity (1). The two treatment-related deaths in the control arm were attributed to sepsis (1) and bone marrow suppression (1). Drug-related treatment discontinuation was higher in the ipilimumab arm (18% vs. 2%).

The study did not meet its primary endpoint. No difference in median OS was observed: 10.9 months in the control arm and 11.0 months in the experimental arm (HR 0.94, $p = 0.3775$). There was also no difference in PFS or response rate.

With activity seen in studies of PD-1 and PD-L1 inhibitors in SCLC, combination studies featuring these agents are underway. Studies of atezolizumab with carboplatin plus etoposide in treatment-naïve, extensive stage SCLC are ongoing (NCT02748889; IMpower 133, NCT02763579).

7.4.3 *Breast Cancer*

The role of immunotherapy in the treatment of advanced breast cancer remains unclear, but modest success has been seen in triple negative breast cancer (TNBC). Lymphocyte infiltration is highest in the TNBC subset of breast cancer, and high degrees of lymphocyte infiltration have been associated with better response to treatment and improved survival [46]. Much of the focus on immunotherapy combinations is in this subset.

7.4.3.1 Atezolizumab + nab-paclitaxel

The phase Ib GP28328 multicohort trial discussed above included a cohort of patients with metastatic TNBC (Arm E) [47]. Patients received atezolizumab 800 mg every 2 weeks with nab-paclitaxel 125 mg/m^2 given on days 1, 8, and 5 in a 4-week schedule. Treatment-related adverse events were seen in 34% of patients. There was only one discontinuation due to atezolizumab-related toxicity (grade 2

AST elevation), and there were no study treatment-related deaths. Responses were seen in 46% of the 13 patients treated in the first-line setting, 22% of the 9 patients treated in the second-line setting, and 40% of the 10 patients treated in the third-line setting. A randomized phase III study comparing nab-paclitaxel with placebo or with atezolizumab (IMpassion 130, NCT02425891) is underway.

7.4.4 Colorectal Cancer

Colorectal cancer remains one of the most common and lethal cancers for both men and women. When microsatellite instability is present (MSI-H), immunotherapy has proven to be very effective but this accounts for less than 5% of colorectal cancer [48]. New strategies are needed to expand the benefit of immunotherapy beyond MSI-H cases.

7.4.4.1 Atezolizumab plus FOLFOX Chemotherapy

The phase Ib GP28328 multicohort trial discussed above also included a cohort of patients (Arm B) with colorectal cancer who received FOLFOX plus bevacizumab given with atezolizumab [49]. Patients received modified FOLFOX6 with bevacizumab 10 mg/kg every 2 weeks and atezolizumab 14 mg/kg given with chemotherapy. The incidence of atezolizumab-related grade 3 or 4 adverse events was 20%. Preliminary results showed a response rate of 36% with an unconfirmed response rate of 44% for treatment-naïve patients.

7.4.5 Pancreatic Cancer

Immunotherapy strategies have been explored as a means to improve the poor outcomes with standard therapy in pancreatic cancer. Vaccine studies have been initially encouraging but have failed to enter practice [50]. Early use of checkpoint inhibitor monotherapy has not shown a strong signal of activity. Combinations may be necessary to evoke an immune response in pancreatic cancer.

7.4.5.1 Tremelimumab plus Gemcitabine

A phase I study explored the combination of standard gemcitabine (given at a dose of 1000 mg/m^2 on days 1, 8, and 15 of a 28-day cycle) with escalating doses of tremelimumab, an anti-CTLA-4 antibody [51]. The study enrolled 34 patients and escalated to the maximum planned dose of tremelimumab (15 mg/kg). No dose-limiting toxicities were noted, and the most common grade 3 or 4 adverse events were asthenia (11.8%) and nausea (8.8%). Median survival was 7.4 months, and 2 of the 28 evaluable patients, both at the 15 mg/kg dose of tremelimumab, achieved a partial response.

7.4.6 *Gastric Cancer*

PD-1 inhibition has shown some efficacy in gastric cancer [52] and the need for new treatment options persists. Combination studies in this disease type are just underway.

7.4.6.1 Pembrolizumab plus 5-FU and Cisplatin

KEYNOTE-059 was an open-label phase II study of pembrolizumab monotherapy and combination therapy in gastric and gastroesophageal carcinoma [53]. Patients received pembrolizumab 200 mg every 3 weeks either alone or with cisplatin 80 mg/m^2 on day 1 plus 5-FU 800 mg/m^2 on days 1–5 given every 3 weeks for up to 2 years. In a preliminary analysis, the combination was tolerable with the most frequent grade 3 or 4 treatment-related adverse events hematologic in nature (40% decreased neutrophils) and only one case of pneumonitis (grade 1). There were three treatment-related discontinuations (12%), all attributed to chemotherapy, and no treatment-related deaths.

7.4.7 *Melanoma*

Malignant melanoma has been one of the most immunogenic cancers, consistently showing the potential for durable response to cytokine therapy (IFN-α-2b, high dose IL-2), vaccine therapy and more recently, checkpoint inhibitors [54, 55]. Combinations of chemotherapy and cytokine therapy have provided inconsistent benefit and toxicity has been significant [56]. Combinations of chemotherapy and checkpoint inhibitors are being explored but due to the high efficacy of immunotherapy combinations, the bar is much higher than that seen in other tumors [57].

7.4.7.1 Ipilimumab plus Dacarbazine

A phase II study randomized 72 patients with advanced melanoma to receive ipilimumab 3 mg/kg every 4 weeks for four doses as monotherapy or in combination with dacarbazine (DTIC), an approved cytotoxic agent, at a dose of 250 mg/m^2/day for 5 days every 3 weeks (up to six cycles) [58]. The response rate favored the combination (14.3% vs. 5.4%) with a 36-month survival rate of 20% compared to 9% with monotherapy.

This prompted a larger randomized phase III study of 502 patients with advanced melanoma in the untreated, first-line setting [59]. All patients received dacarbazine 850 mg/m^2 every 3 weeks for up to eight cycles and were randomized to receive either ipilimumab or placebo. Ipilimumab was given at a dose of 10 mg/kg every 3 weeks for four doses followed by a maintenance phase, with dosing every 12 weeks starting at week 24. The addition of ipilimumab to dacarbazine increased the rate of specific adverse events compared to dacarbazine alone including elevation of ALT (33.2% vs. 5.6%), elevation of AST (29.1% vs. 5.6%), diarrhea (36.4% vs. 24.7%), and rash (24.7% vs. 6.8%). Grade 3 or 4 immune-mediated colitis was seen in 4.9% of patients receiving the combination and none of the patients receiving only dacarbazine.

The increased toxicity was offset by superior outcomes in the combination arm. The primary endpoint of overall survival was met, with a median OS of 11.2 months in the dacarbazine-ipilimumab arm and 9.1 months in the dacarbazine-placebo arm ($p < 0.001$). Three-year survival rate was 20.8% with the combination, compared to 12.2% with monotherapy, and response rates also favored the combination arm (15.2% vs. 10.3%).

7.4.7.2 Ipilimumab plus Temozolomide

Temozolomide is an oral alternative to dacarbazine often used in the treatment of melanoma. A nonrandomized study explored the combination of ipilimumab 10 mg/kg with temozolomide 200 mg/m^2 on days 1–4 every 3 weeks for four doses [60]. While final results have not been released, preliminary analysis revealed a response rate of 22% with another 44% achieving stable disease, and in this early report, the combination was well tolerated.

7.4.7.3 Ipilimumab plus Either Dacarbazine or Carboplatin plus Paclitaxel

Designed primarily to explore pharmacokinetic consequences, a phase I study explored ipilimumab monotherapy (10 mg/kg every 3 weeks for four doses), ipilimumab with dacarbazine 850 mg/m^2 every 3 weeks for eight doses, or ipilimumab with carboplatin AUC 6 plus paclitaxel 175 mg/m^2 every 3 weeks for eight doses in patients with advanced melanoma [61]. The study randomized 99 patients in a 1:1:1 fashion to one of the three arms. There were no major pharmacokinetic interactions observed.

Toxicity varied in the three arms. Elevation of liver function tests was more frequent in the dacarbazine combination (ALT 47.4%, AST 42.6%) than the monotherapy arm (15.0%, 15.0%) or the carboplatin plus paclitaxel combination (25.0%, 25.0%). Treatment-related grade 3 or 4 adverse events were seen in 50% of patients receiving monotherapy, 73.7% of patients receiving dacarbazine, and 75% of patients receiving carboplatin plus paclitaxel. Discontinuation due to toxicity was noted in 25% of patients with monotherapy, 36.8% of patients with dacarbazine plus ipilimumab, and 30% of patients receiving carboplatin, paclitaxel and ipilimumab. Efficacy favored monotherapy over dacarbazine and carboplatin plus paclitaxel combinations in this study, with response rates of 29.4%, 27.8%, and 11.1%, respectively, though the study was not designed to compare efficacy of the three regimens.

7.5 Conclusions

The addition of immunotherapy into our therapeutic arsenal is dramatically altering cancer treatment, offering patients with incurable cancers the opportunity to achieve meaningful, durable responses. In many studies of checkpoint inhibitors, the duration of response approaches or exceeds the median survival duration, suggesting that these durable benefits are limited to a subset of patients. It is critical to identify those patients that will achieve a durable response with immunotherapy alone. Other patients may still derive benefit from checkpoint inhibitors, but they will require an alternative approach. Combining chemotherapy with immunotherapy will be an appropriate strategy for some of these patients. As we refine these combinations, it is important that we develop the necessary biomarkers that will help implement these combinations for patients where the added toxicity and risk provides the greatest opportunity for added benefit.

References

1. Floros T, Tarhini AA (2015) Anticancer cytokines: biology and clinical effects of interferon-a2, interleukin (IL)-2, IL-15, IL-21, and IL-12. Semin Oncol 42(4):539–548
2. Antonia SJ, Larkin J, Ascierto PA (2014) Immuno-oncology combinations: a review of clinical experience and future prospects. Clin Cancer Res 20(24):6258–6268
3. Apetoh L, Ghiringhelli F, Tesniere A et al (2007) Toll-like receptor 4-dependent contribution of the immune system to anticancer chemotherapy and radiotherapy. Nat Med 13(9):1050–1059
4. Kershaw MH, Devaud C, John LB et al (2013) Enhancing immunotherapy using chemotherapy and radiation to modify the tumor microenvironment. Oncoimmunology 2(9):e25962
5. Jure-Kunkel M, Masters G, Girit E et al (2013) Synergy between chemotherapeutic agents and CTLA-4 blockade in preclinical tumor models. Cancer Immunol Immunother 62(9):1533–1545
6. Su Z, Ni P, Zhou C et al (2016) Myeloid-derived suppressor cells in cancers and inflammatory diseases: angel or demon? Scand J Immunol 84(5):25–61
7. Ko HJ, Kim YJ, Kim YS et al (2007) A combination of chemoimmunotherapies can efficiently break self-tolerance and induce antitumor immunity in a tolerogenic murine tumor model. Cancer Res 67(15):7477–7486
8. Suzuki E, Kapoor V, Jassar AS et al (2005) Gemcitabine selectively eliminates splenic Gr-1+/CD11b+ myeloid suppressor cells in tumor-bearing animals and enhances antitumor immune activity. Clin Cancer Res 11(18):6713–6721

9. Vincent J, Mignot G, Calmin F et al (2010) 5-fluorouracil selectively kills tumor-associated myeloid-derived suppressor cells resulting in enhanced T cell-dependent antitumor immunity. Cancer Res 70(8):52–61
10. Tseng CW, Hung CF, Alvarez RD et al (2008) Pretreatment with cisplatin enhances E7-specific CD8+ T-cell-mediated antitumor immunity induced by DNA vaccination. Clin Cancer Res 14:3185–3192
11. Zhu Y, Liu N, Xiong SD et al (2011) CD4+Foxp3+ regulatory t-cell impairment by paclitaxel is independent of Toll-like receptor 4. Scand J Immunol 73(4):301–308
12. Ghiringhelli F, Larmonier N, Schmitt E et al (2004) CD4+CD25+ regulatory T cells suppress tumor immunity but are sensitive to cyclophosphamide which allows immunotherapy of established tumors to be curative. Eur J Immunol 34:336–344
13. Brode S, Raine T, Zaccone P et al (2006) Cyclophosphamide-induced type-1 diabetes in the NOD mouse is associated with a reduction of CD4+ CD25+ Foxp3+ regulatory T cells. J Immunol 177:6603–6612
14. Ghiringhelli F, Menard C, Puig PE et al (2007) Metronomic cyclophosphamide regimen selectively depletes CD4+CD25+ regulatory T cells and restores T and NK effector functions in end stage cancer patients. Cancer Immunol Immunother 56:641–648
15. Fridlender ZG, Sun J, Singhal S et al (2010) Chemotherapy delivered after viral immunogene therapy augments antitumor efficacy via multiple immune-mediated mechanisms. Mol Ther 18(11):1947–1959
16. Takesue BY, Pyle JM, Mokyr MB (1990) Importance of tumor-specific cytotoxic CD8+ T-cells in eradication of a large subcutaneous MOPC-315 tumor following low-dose melphalan therapy. Cancer Res 50:7641–7649
17. Mokyr MB, Kalinichenko T, Gorelik L et al (1998) Realization of the therapeutic potential of CTLA-4 blockade in low-dose chemotherapy-treated tumor-bearing mice. Cancer Res 58:5301–5304
18. Nowak AK, Robinson BW, Lake RA (2003) Synergy between chemotherapy and immunotherapy in the treatment of established murine solid tumors. Cancer Res 63:4490–4496
19. Nowak AK, Robinson BW, Lake RA (2002) Gemcitabine exerts a selective effect on the humoral immune response. Cancer Res 62(8):2353–2358
20. Wu L, Yun Z, Tagawa T et al (2012) CTLA-4 blockade expands infiltrating T cells and inhibits cancer cell repopulation during the intervals of chemotherapy in murine mesothelioma. Mol Cancer Ther 11:1809–1819
21. Ma Y, Adjemian S, Mattarollo SR et al (2013) Anticancer chemotherapy-induced intratumoral recruitment and differentiation of antigen-presenting cells. Immunity 38:729–741
22. Lesterhuis WJ, Punt CJ, Hato SV et al (2011) Platinum-based drugs disrupt STAT6-mediated suppression of immune responses against cancer in humans and mice. J Clin Invest 121(8):3100–3108
23. Shurin GV, Tourkova IL, Kaneno R, Shurin MR (2009) Chemotherapeutic agents in noncytotoxic concentrations increase antigen presentation by dendritic cells via an IL-12 dependent mechanism. J Immunol 183:137–144
24. Gameiro SR, Caballero JA, Hodge JW (2012) Defining the molecular signature of chemotherapy-mediated lung tumor phenotype modulation and increased susceptibility to T –cell killing. Cancer Biother Radiopharm 27:23–35
25. Gelbard A, Garnett CT, Abrams SI et al (2006) Combination chemotherapy and radiation of human squamous cell carcinoma of the head and neck augments CTL-mediated lysis. Clin Cancer Res 12:1897–1905
26. Wan S, Pestka S, Jubin RG et al (2012) Chemotherapeutics and radiation stimulate MHC class I expression through elevated interferon-beta signaling in breast cancer cells. PLoS One 7:e32542
27. Menard C, Martin F, Apetoh L et al (2008) Cancer chemotherapy: not only a direct cytotoxic effect, but also an adjuvant for antitumor immunity. Cancer Immunol Immunother 57:1579–1587

28. de Biasi AR, Villena-Vargas J, Adusumilli PS (2014) Cisplatin-induced antitumor immunomodulation: a review of preclinical and clinical evidence. Clin Cancer Res 20(21):5384–5391
29. Zitvogel L, Kepp O, Kroemer G (2011) Immune parameters affecting the efficacy of chemotherapeutic regimens. Nat Rev Clin Oncol 8:151–160
30. Negrei C, Bojinca V, Balanescu A et al (2016) Management of rheumatoid arthritis: impact and risks of various therapeutic approaches. Exp Ther Med 11(4):1177–1183
31. Bruchard M, Mignot G, Derangere V et al (2013) Chemotherapy-triggered cathepsin B release in myeloid-derived suppressor cells activates the Nlrp3 inflammasome and promotes tumor growth. Nat Med 19(1):57–64
32. Borghaei H, Paz-Ares L, Horn L et al (2015) Nivolumab versus docetaxel in advanced nonsquamous non-small-cell lung cancer. N Engl J Med 373(17):1627–1639
33. Brahmer J, Reckamp KL, Baas P et al (2015) Nivolumab versus docetaxel in advanced squamous-cell non-small-cell lung cancer. N Engl J Med 373(2):123–135
34. Garon EB, Rizvi NA, Hui R et al (2015) Pembrolizumab for the treatment of non-small-cell lung cancer. N Engl J Med 372(21):2018–2028
35. Rittmeyer A, Barlesi F, Waterkamp D et al (2017) Atezolizumab versus Docetaxel in patients with previously treated non-small-cell lung cancer (OAK): a phase 3, open-label, multicentre randomised controlled trial. Lancet 389(10066):255–265
36. Reck M, Rodriguez-Abreu D, Robinson AG et al (2016) Pembrolizumab versus chemotherapy for PD-L1-positive non-small-cell lung cancer. N Engl J Med 375(19):1823–1833
37. Lynch TJ, Bondarenko I, Luft A et al (2012) Ipilimumab in combination with paclitaxel and carboplatin as first-line treatment in stage IIIB/IV non-small-cell lung cancer: results from a randomized, double-blind multicenter phase II study. Ann Oncol 30(17):2046–2064
38. Gadgeel SM, Stevenson J, Langer CJ et al (2016) Pembrolizumab (pembro) plus chemotherapy as front-line therapy for advanced NSCLC: KEYNOTE-021 cohorts A-C. Proc Am Soc Clin Oncol 34:Abstr 9016
39. Langer CJ, Gadgeel SM, Borghaei H et al (2016) Carboplatin and pemetrexed with or without pembrolizumab for advanced, non-squamous non-small-cell lung cancer: a randomised, phase 2 cohort of the open-label KEYNOTE-021 study. Lancet Oncol 17:1497–1508
40. Rizvi NA, Hellmann MD, Brahmer JR et al (2016) Nivolumab in combination with platinum-based doublet chemotherapy for first-line treatment of advanced non-small-cell lung cancer. JCO 34(25):2969–2979
41. Liu SV, Powderly J, Camidge DR et al (2015) Safety and efficacy of atezolizumab (anti-PDL1) in combination with platinum-based doublet chemotherapy in patients with advanced non-small cell lung cancer (NSCLC). Proc Am Soc Clin Oncol 33:Abstr 8030
42. Camidge DR, Liu SV, Powderly JD et al (2015) Atezolizumab (MPDL3280A) combined with platinum-based chemotherapy in non-small cell lung cancer (NSCLC): a phase 1b study. J Thorac Oncol 10:Abstr 02.7
43. Antonia SJ, Lopez-Martin JA, Bendell J et al (2016) Nivolumab alone and nivolumab plus ipilimumab in recurrent small cell lung cancer (Checkmate 032): a multicenter, open-label, phase 1/2 trial. Lancet Oncol 17(7):883–895
44. Reck M, Bondarenko I, Luft A et al (2013) Ipilimumab in combination with paclitaxel and carboplatin as first-line therapy in extensive-disease-small-cell lung cancer: results from a randomized, double-blind, multicenter phase 2 trial. Ann Oncol 24:75–83
45. Reck M, Luft A, Szczesna A et al (2016) Phase III randomized trial of ipilimumab plus etoposide and platinum versus placebo plus etoposide and platinum in extensive-stage small-cell lung cancer. J Clin Oncol 34(31):3740–3748
46. Ono M, Tsuda H, Shimizu C et al (2012) Tumor-infiltrating lymphocytes are correlated with response to neoadjuvant chemotherapy in triple negative breast cancer. Breast Cancer Res Treat 132(3):793–805
47. Adams S, Diamond JR, Hamilton EP et al (2016) Phase Ib trial of atezolizumab in combination with nab-paclitaxel in patients with metastatic triple-negative breast cancer (mTNBC). Proc Am Soc Clin Oncol 34:Abstr 1009

48. Le DT, Uram JN, Wang H et al (2015) PD-1 blockade in tumors with mismatch-repair deficiency. N Engl J Med 372(26):2509–2520
49. Bendell JC, Powderly JD, Lieu CH et al (2015) Safety and efficacy of MPDL3280A (anti-PDL1) in combination with bevacizumab (bev) and/or FOLFOX in patients (pts) with metastatic colorectal cancer (mCRC). Proc Am Soc Clin Oncol 33:Abstr 704
50. Kunk PR, Bauer TW, Slingluff CL, Rahma OE (2016) From bench to bedside a comprehensive review of pancreatic cancer immunotherapy. J Immunother Cancer 4:14
51. Aglietta M, Barone C, Sawyer MB et al (2014) A phase I dose escalation trial of tremelimumab (CP-675,206) in combination with gemcitabine in chemotherapy-naïve patients with metastatic pancreatic cancer. Ann Oncol 25(9):1750–1755
52. Bang YJ, Chung HC, Shankaran V et al (2015) Relationship between PD-L1 expression and clinical outcomes in patients with advanced gastric cancer treated with the anti-PD-1 monoclonal antibody pembrolizumab (MK-3475) in KEYNOTE-012. Proc Am Soc Clin Oncol 33:Abstr 4001
53. Fuchs CS, Ohtsu A, Tabernero J et al (2016) Preliminary safety data from KEYNOTE-059: pembrolizumab plus 5-fluorouracil and cisplatin for first-line treatment of advanced gastric cancer. Proc Am Soc Clin Oncol 34:Abstr 4037
54. Redman JM, Gibney GT, Atkins MB (2016) Advances in immunotherapy for melanoma. BMC Med 14:20
55. George DD, Armenio VA, Katz SC (2017) Combinatorial immunotherapy for melanoma. Cancer Gene Ther 24(3):141–147
56. Hamm C, Verma S, Petrella T et al (2008) Biochemotherapy for the treatment of metastatic malignant melanoma: a systematic review. Cancer Treat Rev 34(2):145–156
57. Hodi FS, Chesney J, Pavlick AC et al (2016) Combined nivolumab and ipilimumab versus ipilimumab alone in patients with advanced melanoma: 2-year overall survival outcomes in a multicentre, randomised, controlled, phase 2 trial. Lancet Oncol 17(11):1558–1568
58. Hersh EM, O'Day SJ, Powderly J et al (2011) A phase II multicenter study of ipilimumab with or without dacarbazine in chemotherapy-naïve patients with advanced melanoma. Investig New Drugs 29:489–498
59. Robert C, Thomas L, Bondarenko I et al (2011) Ipilimumab plus Dacarbazine for previously untreated metastatic melanoma. N Engl J Med 364(26):2517–2526
60. Patel SP, Bedikian AY, Papadopoulos NE et al (2011) Ipilimumab plus temozolomide in metastatic melanoma. Proc Am Soc Clin Oncol 29:Abstr 8579
61. Weber J, Hamid O, Amin A et al (2013) Randomized phase I pharmacokinetic study of ipilimumab with or without one of two different chemotherapy regimens in patients with untreated advanced melanoma. Cancer Immun 13:7

Chapter 8
Immune Checkpoint Combinations with Inflammatory Pathway Modulators

N. DeVito, M.A. Morse, B. Hanks, and J.M. Clarke

Abstract Immune checkpoint inhibition of program death protein-1 (PD-1) and its ligands PD-L1 and PD-L2 is an established therapeutic modality in melanoma, non-small cell lung cancer, renal cell carcinoma, and other tumor types. Unfortunately, 60 to 80% of all patients experience disease progression and become refractory to immune checkpoint therapies. Broadly, mechanisms of immune checkpoint inhibitor resistance can be categorized as presence of oncogenic driver mutations, severe T cell exhaustion, neoantigen burden, epigenetic alterations, or mutations involved in critical pathways including PTEN, JAK, or Wnt signaling. The dysregulation of inflammatory signaling pathways (namely, genes involved in angiogenesis, chemotaxis, matrix remodeling, wound healing, and mesenchymal transition) is of critical importance to response to immune checkpoint therapies. Inflammatory cytokine signaling pathways exert downstream effects on immunosuppressive elements such as regulatory T cells (Tregs) and myeloid-derived suppressor cells (MDSCs) which inhibit the function of effector T cells, NK cells, and dendritic cells, promoting immune tolerance and tumor growth. We herein review three targets for inflammatory pathway modulation: indoleamine 2,3-dioxygenase (IDO), transforming growth factor β (TGFβ), and adenosine. Targeting these pathways may address the unmet need to develop novel therapeutic approaches to increase response rates to immune checkpoint inhibitors and improve clinical outcomes.

Keywords PD-1 • PD-L1 • Immune checkpoint inhibitor • Indoleamine 2,3-dioxygenase (IDO) • Transforming growth factor β (TGFβ) • Adenosine receptor (CD73) • Immune checkpoint inhibitor resistance • T regulatory cell (Treg) • Myeloid-derived suppressor cells (MDSCs)

N. DeVito (✉) • M.A. Morse • B. Hanks • J.M. Clarke
Duke Cancer Institute, Duke University Medical Center, Durham, NC, USA
e-mail: Nicholas.DeVito@Duke.edu; Michael.Morse@Duke.edu; Brent.Hanks@Duke.edu; Jeffrey.Clarke@Duke.edu

S.P. Patel, R. Kurzrock (eds.), *Early Phase Cancer Immunotherapy*,
Current Cancer Research, DOI 10.1007/978-3-319-63757-0_8

8.1 Introduction

The targeted inhibition of program death protein-1 (PD-1) and its ligands PD-L1 and PD-L2 is an established modality of anticancer therapy. These proteins are aberrantly expressed in the tumor microenvironment and mediate T cell exhaustion and immune tolerance. Monoclonal antibody-mediated inhibition of their interaction has demonstrated substantial clinical efficacy in a growing list of tumor types including melanoma, non-small cell lung cancer, renal cell carcinoma, and head and neck cancer among others [1–3]. While many patients derive durable clinical benefit from these therapies, approximately 60 to 80% of all patients will experience disease progression and become refractory to immune checkpoint therapies. Therefore, there is currently an urgent unmet need to develop novel therapeutic approaches to increase response rates to immune therapy and augment current clinical activity.

A variety of mechanisms have been described governing both primary and acquired resistance to immune checkpoint therapies in human malignancy. Broadly, these can be categorized by mechanisms such as the presence of oncogenic driver mutations, severe T cell exhaustion, neoantigen burden, epigenetic alterations, or mutations involved in critical pathways including PTEN, JAK, or Wnt signaling [4]. In particular, dysregulation of inflammatory signaling pathways in the tumor microenvironment is of critical importance to mediating tumor immunity and ultimately response to immune checkpoint therapies. For example, in metastatic melanoma with innate resistance to anti-PD-1 therapy, compared with sensitive tumors, there is upregulated gene expression of multiple key inflammatory genes involved in angiogenesis, chemotaxis, matrix remodeling, wound healing, and mesenchymal transition [5]. Additionally, PD-L1 is upregulated by multiple inflammatory cytokines including IFN-γ contributing to T cell dysfunction [6]. Inflammatory cytokine signaling pathways exert broad downstream effects on various immunosuppressive elements in cancer such as regulatory T cells (Tregs) and myeloid-derived suppressor cells (MDSCs) among others. Intratumoral recruitment and expansion of Tregs and MDSCs are known to inhibit differentiation and function of effector T cells, NK cells, and dendritic cells, promoting immune tolerance and ultimately tumor growth [7, 8]. Therefore, combinatorial approaches targeting tumor inflammation are urgently needed to overcome both primary and acquired resistance mechanisms to improve clinical outcomes with immune checkpoint agents.

We herein review three targets for inflammatory pathway modulation: indoleamine 2,3-dioxygenase (IDO), transforming growth factor β (TGFβ), and adenosine. Other targets with a growing amount of evidence supporting combination with immunotherapies include vascular endothelial growth factor inhibitors, which have been recently reviewed by others [9]. Novel therapeutic strategies targeting IDO, TGFβ, and molecules involved in generating adenosine in the tumor microenvironment such as CD73 have been developed in recent years and have compelling rationale for use in combination with immune checkpoint agents to improve clinical outcomes.

8.2 IDO

8.2.1 Overview

IDO is an evolutionarily conserved enzyme expressed predominantly in lymphoid and placental tissues that converts the amino acid substrate tryptophan (Trp) into a series of metabolic by-products known as the kynurenines via a catalytic reaction that facilitates cleavage of the 2,3-double bond of the Trp indole ring [10, 11]. This 45 kDa enzyme expressed by the *INDO* gene located at human chromosome 8p12 was initially identified in 1963 [12]. More recent biochemical structural studies have revealed IDO to be comprised of two α-helical domains and a central heme prosthetic group that serves as a superoxide anion donor capable of driving its catalytic activity [13].

It was not until 1998 that the immunoregulatory role of IDO was recognized when studies demonstrated this enzyme to prevent allogeneic rejection of the mouse fetus by suppressing the maternal T cell response [14]. A variety of studies have described several IDO-dependent mechanisms that contribute to the regulation of effector T cell activity. The initial and more direct mechanism of T cell suppression was demonstrated to be a local depletion of the essential amino acid Trp, leading to inhibition of T cell proliferation. This inhibitory effect arrests T cells within the mid-G1 phase of the cell cycle due to the phosphorylation of the stress response kinase GCN2 which functionally inhibits the α-subunit of eukaryotic translation initiation factor 2 (eIF2α) [15]. Additional studies have shown IDO to also suppress mTOR and subsequently promote T cell autophagy [16]. Perhaps the most critical underlying mechanism of immune tolerance is the simultaneous generation of the downstream kynurenine by-products that promote the differentiation of naïve $CD4^+$ T cells into the highly immunosuppressive $CD4^+FoxP3^+$ regulatory Treg population by signaling through the aryl hydrocarbon receptor [17, 18]. While genetic ablation of IDO in mouse models does not have the widespread impact observed in CTLA-4-deficient mice, studies have shown that the development of acquired peripheral tolerance is significantly impaired in IDO null hosts and that IDO is critical for the development of immune tolerance to apoptotic cells, including those generated by dying tumor cells [19, 20].

8.2.2 IDO in Cancer

It is clear that tumors continue to develop despite expressing immunogenic antigens, suggesting that these malignant tissues acquire a strategy for evading detection and destruction by the host immune system. IDO is thought to contribute significantly to this process [21, 22]. Expression studies have documented IDO in several tissues including various tumors, dendritic cells (DCs), macrophages, and endothelial cells. A role for IDO in carcinogenesis began with early studies in the

1950s noting elevated levels of kynurenine in the blood and urine specimens of cancer patients relative to healthy control subjects [23, 24]. Additional reports demonstrated an association between IDO expression levels and/or enzymatic activity with inferior prognosis in a plethora of tumor types, including breast, colon, non-small cell lung cancer, ovarian, and melanoma [25]. Overall, these studies have implicated IDO as an important contributor to the phenomenon of tumor-mediated immunosuppression [26].

Despite these growing insights into the biological role of IDO in cancer, our understanding of the cell type of origin that exhibits the most potent and clinically relevant IDO activity within the tumor microenvironment still remains elusive. Certainly cell-specific posttranslational modulation of IDO could potentially lead to differential function and disparate downstream immunologic effects. Early studies utilizing an IDO1-selective inhibitor have shown persistent antitumor efficacy in transplant tumor models in IDO1$^{-/-}$ hosts suggesting that tumor expression of IDO1 is important. This has been supported by other bone marrow transplant experiments demonstrating that non-hematopoietic cell IDO expression is essential for inflammatory-related malignancies. However, there is also a large body of evidence implicating DC expression of IDO within the tumor microenvironment as a particularly potent contributor to the generation of local immune tolerance [27]. As opposed to the PD-1 and CTLA-4 checkpoints that undergo upregulation following T cell activation, the DC-expressed IDO enzyme is capable of suppressing several other more proximal mechanisms important for the induction of cell-mediated immunity. This includes the ability of IDO activity to inhibit DC expression of the pro-inflammatory cytokines IL-12 and IL-6 which, in turn, promotes the stabilization and prevents the proteosomal degradation of IDO [20, 28, 29]. This positive “feed-forward loop” along with the intrinsic ability of each DC to interact with multiple T cells and subsequently inhibit their proliferative expansion and/or drive their differentiation into Tregs serves to generate a potent state of immune tolerance that enables cancers to progress and metastasize [30]. Indeed, DC IDO expression within tumor-draining lymph node tissues has been shown to correlate with inferior survival in different forms of cancer [31]. Whether the cell type of origin or tissue expressing IDO is a critical contributor to its modulation of the tumor immune microenvironment remains unclear and is in need of further investigation.

Several transcriptional and posttranslational mechanisms that modulate the expression and enzymatic activity of IDO have been previously described. These regulatory mechanisms likely differ dependent upon the cellular origin of the IDO enzyme. In DCs, several stimuli have been found to induce the upregulation of IDO including Toll-like receptor agonists, CD40, CD200, and the type I and type II interferons (IFNs) [32]. One of the primary roles of IDO in the immune system is to serve as a negative regulator of acute inflammation. As such, IDO expression is upregulated both rapidly and transiently by IFN-γ [33]. This is opposed to the more durable stimulation of IDO expression by TGFβ in DCs [34]. In this case, the IDO enzyme can be converted into a phosphorylated signaling mediator that drives the expression of further IDO and TGFβ and contributes to the establishment of long-term immune tolerance [35]. More recent work has revealed that this alternative signaling function of IDO is dependent on arginase I-generated polyamines which can be supplied in the tumor microenvironment by myeloid-derived suppressor cells [36].

Other pathways that regulate IDO in a posttranslational manner also modulate its catalytic activity and play an important role in driving IDO-dependent immune tolerance. These pathways often regulate IDO activity by manipulating the heme prosthetic group either by direct binding to this moiety by nitrous oxide or by heme depletion via the enzyme, heme oxygenase-1 [37].

8.2.3 Preclinical IDO Inhibitor Studies

The realization that cancers hijack IDO to establish a site of immune privilege made it clear that IDO activity was capable of compromising immunotherapy efficacy. Indeed, recent studies have implicated IDO as a contributor to anti-CTLA-4 antibody immunotherapy resistance [38]. This has further supported the concept of IDO inhibition as a strategy to stimulate tumor immunity. The absence of spontaneous autoimmunity in the $IDO^{-/-}$ mouse model as well as in mice treated for prolonged periods with the 1-methyltryptophan (1-MT) IDO inhibitor also supported the safety of IDO inhibition as a viable therapeutic strategy.

Early preclinical tumor model studies were utilized to demonstrate the ability of the 1-MT IDO inhibitor to promote the development of an effective antitumor T cell response and suppress the progression of various in vivo tumor models [39]. These studies demonstrated no evidence of antitumor activity when either the 1-MT inhibitor or more traditional therapies including chemotherapy were administered alone in transplant models of both B16 melanoma and 4T1 breast cancer. However, the addition of the 1-MT inhibitor to chemotherapy agents, such as cyclophosphamide and paclitaxel, induced a synergistic antitumor response that was ablated in immunodeficient hosts. These effects were also seen in the MMTV-neu autochthonous breast cancer model and favored the D-1-MT stereoisomer for further phase I clinical trial development that began in 2007.

A separate group of investigators conducted a high-throughput screen revealing a hydroxyamidine small-molecule competitive inhibitor that bound to the heme active site of IDO1 [40]. INCB024360 was found to increase the $CD8^+$ T cell/Treg ratio while showing efficacy in both the CT26 colon cancer model and the PAN02 pancreatic tumor model [41, 42]. This therapeutic effect correlated with diminished kynurenine levels in the tumor and tumor-draining lymph node tissues of treated mice and was absent in both immunodeficient and $IDO1^{-/-}$ hosts. After transitioning to phase I trials in 2010, several clinical studies are now beginning to investigate the ability of INCB024360 to augment the efficacy of other checkpoint inhibitor therapies.

8.2.4 Clinical Development of IDO Inhibitor Therapies

The two agents most advanced in the clinical development pipeline currently include epacadostat (INCB024360, Incyte), an oral small-molecule selective inhibitor of IDO1, and the oral D-1-MT inhibitor, indoximod (NLG-8189, NewLink Genetics), which has been described as an IDO pathway modulator. GDC-0919, currently in co-development by NewLink Genetics and Genentech, is also an oral selective IDO1 inhibitor that recently entered phase I trials. A separate peptide vaccine approach developed from fragments of the IDO1 protein remains in early stages of development (IO Biotech and others).

As previously noted, early studies have shown that IDO inhibition is therapeutically relevant only in combination with other therapeutics, namely chemotherapy, vaccines, or other forms of immunotherapy [43, 44]. Table 8.1 describes the select active, combinatorial trials investigating solid tumor malignancies with available IDO inhibitors.

While combinatorial immune checkpoint blockade with anti-CTLA-4 and anti-PD-1 agents is highly effective in patients with metastatic melanoma and potentially other malignancies, the propensity for side effects from the combination regimen is significant. Although their efficacy has been limited, phase I IDO inhibitor monotherapy studies have demonstrated safety with relatively modest side effects, effectively validating preclinical studies in $IDO^{-/-}$ mice suggesting that these agents would be well tolerated. Indeed, in the 52-patient phase I dose escalation study of epacadostat (NCT01195311), grade 3/4 adverse events including abdominal pain, hypokalemia, and fatigue occurred in 9.6% of participating patients [45]. In a trial of epacadostat with ipilimumab in patients with stage IV melanoma (NCT01604889), transaminitis leads to cessation of drug therapy in five of seven patients in the 300 mg BID cohort, triggering a dose reduction to 50 mg BID. This combination then yielded a well-tolerated treatment regimen with only 4/18 patients experiencing Grade 3/4 toxicity and an overall response rate of 31.3% along with a disease control rate of 62.5% in immunotherapy-naïve metastatic melanoma patients [46].

In the Keynote 037 trial (NCT02178722), which combined epacadostat dose escalation with pembrolizumab, there were six grade 3 and no grade 4 AEs of the 56 patients treated. Of the 36 patients with metastatic melanoma, overall response rate was 53% with a disease control rate of 74%, resembling response data from the Checkmate 067 trial of nivolumab and ipilimumab but without the side effect profile [1, 47]. Whether these responses are similarly durable will likely be answered by the phase III trial (NCT02752074).

Indoximod was also demonstrated to be safe without significant side effects in its phase I study (NCT00567931), and five of the seven patients who received 200 mg per day had either objective responses or disease stabilization. When combined with docetaxel (NCT01191216), 4 of 22 evaluable patients had partial responses, and the most frequent adverse events were fatigue, anemia, nausea, and infections. This will be expanded into a phase II trial in breast cancer patients. A phase II of indoximod with gemcitabine/nab-paclitaxel in treatment-naïve metastatic pancreatic cancer

Table 8.1 Select active, combinatorial trials investigating solid tumor malignancies with available IDO inhibitors

Agent	Indication(s)	Phase	Combination	Status	Identifier[a]
Indoximod	NSCLC	I/II	Docetaxel and tergenpumatucel	Enrolling	NCT02460367
	Breast	II	Taxane	Completed	NCT01792050
	Breast	I/II	Vaccine	Ongoing, not recruiting	NCT01042535
	Melanoma	I/II	Ipilimumab, pembrolizumab, nivolumab	Enrolling	NCT02073123
	Pancreatic	I/II	Gemcitabine and nab-paclitaxel	Enrolling	NCT02077881
	Prostate	II	Sipuleucel-T	Ongoing, not recruiting	NCT01560923
	Advanced solid tumors	I	Docetaxel	Completed	NCT01191216
Epacadostat	Melanoma	I/II	Vaccine	Ongoing, not recruiting	NCT01961115
	Melanoma	I/II	Ipilimumab	Ongoing not recruiting	NCT01604889
	Advanced solid tumors	I	PI3K-delta inhibitor	Recruiting	NCT02559492
	Advanced solid tumors	II	Pembrolizumab and azacitidine	Recruiting	NCT02959437
	Pancreatic	I/II	Pembrolizumab, CRS-207, +/− CY GVAX	Recruiting	NCT03006302
	Advanced solid tumors	I/II	Chemotherapy or anti-PD-1	Not yet recruiting	NCT03085914
GDC-099	Advanced solid tumors	I	Atezolizumab	Recruiting	NCT02471846
Vaccine	NSCLC	I	n/a	Completed	NCT01219348
	Melanoma	I/II	Nivolumab	Not yet recruiting	NCT03047928
	Melanoma	I	Vemurafenib or ipilimumab	Completed	NCT02077114

[a]Trials from clinicaltrials.gov as of 4/17/2017

(NCT02077881) has so far demonstrated 11 objective responses in 30 patients, with 1 event of colitis requiring study withdrawal [48]. Indoximod is currently being evaluated in metastatic melanoma patients in combination with investigator's choice of immune checkpoint inhibitor (NCT02073123). As of March 2017, 94 patients had received indoximod with pembrolizumab, and of 60 evaluable patients, 87% of which had stage IV disease, there were 3 grade 3 adverse events, and the overall response rate was 52% [49]. This trial will likely move into phase III given these impressive results and safety profiles.

Another approach to modulating IDO activity involves a synthetic HLA-A2-restricted IDO peptide vaccine that was administered to 15 patients with metastatic non-small cell lung cancer in phase I study (NCT01219348). This vaccine approach was deemed to be safe with six patients exhibiting disease stabilization and one having a significant response durable over 2 years. Median OS was 25.9 months in the treated population compared to 7.7 months in the intention to treat group [50]. When an IDO peptide vaccine was combined with ipilimumab in ten metastatic melanoma patients, it was well tolerated with one response and four patients with stable disease [51].

8.2.5 IDO and Biomarker Development

One of the challenges sure to be faced in the field of IDO inhibitor therapies is the lack of validated biomarkers capable of determining if a patient can benefit from the addition of an IDO inhibitor. While many of the above trials have measured serum tryptophan and kynurenine levels as a pharmacokinetic parameter of IDO inhibition or examined IDO expression levels in tumor tissue, these have yet to consistently determine patients that are responding or to predict those that will respond to this treatment approach. Potentially measuring IDO in select immune cell populations such as DCs within the tumor microenvironment, including the tumor bed or perhaps the tumor-draining lymph node tissues may generate more useful markers of response to IDO inhibition. In addition, an improved understanding of the manner in which IDO is regulated within the tumor microenvironment is also likely to lead to the development of improved predictive markers in future clinical trial protocols.

Earlier studies showed that IL-10 within melanoma conditioned media results in sustained IDO expression by local DCs [52]. More recently, the β-catenin signaling pathway stimulated by melanoma-derived Wnt5a ligand has been shown to promote the transcriptional expression of IDO in DCs [53]. Additional intrinsic and extrinsic regulatory pathways of IDO have also been described in a series of different cancers [54]. These have included enhanced IDO transcription by the downregulation of the *Bin* tumor suppressor in several cancers as well as enhanced paracrine TGFβ-mediated upregulation of IDO by local plasmacytoid DCs following the downregulation of the soluble type III TGFβ receptor in models of both breast cancer and melanoma [55, 56]. Finally, tumor cell apoptosis has been demonstrated to induce IDO activity in tumor-draining lymph node DCs and whole tumor tissues via the stimulator of interferon genes (STING) and type I IFN pathway [57, 58]. Each of these mechanisms contribute to tumor progression and do not necessarily occur in the setting of an inflamed tumor microenvironment, arguing against the perception that the effectiveness of IDO inhibition would be restricted to those tumors exhibiting an inflamed phenotype. Therefore, the inducers of each of these regulatory pathways may serve as superior markers of IDO inhibition. We can speculate that those pathways capable of modulating both the expression of IDO as well as its enzymatic activity would be the most effective predictive markers of IDO inhibitor efficacy. One candidate for this dual control mechanism would be the Wnt5a-β-catenin signaling pathway in DCs which has recently been shown to not only induce DC expression of IDO but also to regulate the enzymatic activity of DC IDO via a post-translational mechanism [59]. Studies are currently underway to determine whether the activation status of this pathway may indicate those tumors which would be more susceptible to IDO inhibitor therapy. Additional studies are also needed to determine the relative importance of these regulatory pathways and to decipher which of these mechanisms may be dominating IDO control in any one tumor.

8.2.6 *Novel IDO Targeting Strategies*

Alternative upstream inhibitory pathways of IDO expression, including those that involve JAK/STAT signaling, PGE2, and c-kit, have been studied as potential strategies to manipulate IDO activity to a more limited degree [60, 61]. It has been postulated, however, that pharmacologically targeting the IDO enzyme itself is the preferred therapeutic strategy due to its many upstream regulatory pathways [62]. This selective IDO targeting approach may, however, prove to be inferior if this enzyme is found to be a component of a broader immunotolerization program in DCs. Indeed, early findings in DC immunometabolism research suggest that this may be the case, opening up specific metabolic pathways as targets capable of regulating both DC IDO activity and pro-inflammatory cytokine expression [59]. In particular, findings linking paracrine Wnt signaling and the regulation of IDO activity via DC metabolic alterations have implicated this pathway as a promising pharmacologic target worthy of further investigation [63].

8.3 TGFβ

8.3.1 *Overview*

The targeted inhibition of TGFβ in the tumor microenvironment is an appealing strategy to modulate the effect of immune checkpoint therapy for human malignancies. TGFβ is upregulated in most human malignancies and has been shown to correlate with worse clinical outcomes in multiple tumor types, including lung, breast, colon, and pancreatic cancers [64]. TGFβ has dual cancer growth-suppressing and growth-promoting effects; however, later in the course of the disease, its dysregulation is intimately involved in tumor cell stemness, survival, invasion, and proliferation, while modulating stroma formation and tumor angiogenesis [65]. While the TGFβ superfamily of cytokines exerts pleiotropic, context-dependent effects on tumor cells and surrounding stroma, TGFβ promotes broad immunosuppression on multiple immune and inflammatory cell subsets [66].

The TGFβ superfamily is composed of 33 proteins encompassing TGFβ, activins, and bone morphogenic proteins (BMP), NODAL, growth and differentiation factor, and anti-Mullerian hormone [67]. TGFβ signaling is primarily dependent on ligand binding type I and type II serine kinase receptors, including activin receptor like kinase 5 (ALK5, TGFβRI), TGFβRII, and TGFβRIII. Initial binding of TGFβ ligand by type II receptors leads to heterotetrameric complex formation between type I and type II receptors and results in subsequent serine/threonine kinase activation. The serine/threonine kinase activity is responsible for downstream phosphorylation and activation of the canonical pathway through SMAD2/3 [68]. SMAD2/3 proteins complex with SMAD4 allowing for nuclear translocation and transcriptional regulation. Noncanonical signaling can also occur through MAPK, PI3K, NF-κB, and other pathways upon binding of TGFβ to the receptor complex. The pleiotropic effects of TGFβ are mediated by the relative promiscuity of receptor-ligand interactions within TGFβ superfamily, phosphorylation of other downstream SMAD proteins (i.e., SMAD5/8, 6/7), noncanonical signaling pathways, and signaling pathway cross talk, among other mechanisms [69].

8.3.2 TGFβ and the Immune System in Malignancy

TGFβ is recognized as among the most immunosuppressive cytokines and plays a critical role in regulation of both innate and adaptive tumor immunity [70]. Deletion of TGFβRII in mice, as an example, results in the development of lethal autoimmune inflammation of multiple organs as a result of overwhelming T cell activation, maturation, and loss of T cell tolerance [71]. Furthermore, TGFβ is known to promote Treg proliferation in the thymus while supporting maintenance of peripheral Treg populations [71, 72]. The differentiation and function of multiple immune cell subsets are inhibited by TGFβ including tumor specific cytotoxic T cells and NK cells. Additional immunosuppressive effects are mediated by promoting opposing Th17 cells, Treg, and MDSC [66, 73–76]. The professional antigen presentation and immunogenic function of dendritic cells are also altered by the presence of TGFβ resulting in a variety of important immunosuppressive effects [77]. Specifically, TGFβ inhibits the activation, differentiation, and migration of dendritic cells and can decrease antigen presentation as well as promote presence of MDSC in the tumor microenvironment [76, 78, 79]. Immature dendritic cells are known to result in antigen tolerance of T cells and promote proliferation of Tregs [75, 80]. Collectively, these lines of evidence demonstrate the wide impact of TGFβ on tumor immunity through suppression of effector T cell subsets and support of immunosuppressive cells including MDSC and Tregs.

The natural role of TGFβ in maintaining homeostasis by regulating inflammation and reducing autoimmunity is exploited in malignancy resulting in immune evasion and tumor growth. The downstream broad immunologic effects of TGFβ are likely driven by increased expression of certain transcriptional regulators, namely, inhibitor of differentiation 1 (Id1), which promotes immunosuppression through affecting dendritic cell maturation, T cell proliferation, and MDSC accumulation [81]. TGFβ-mediated Id1 upregulation ultimately results in tumor growth and metastasis. Importantly, TGFβ also promotes antigen-induced expression of PD-1 on tumor-infiltrating T cells in vivo through a SMAD3-dependent pathway, providing a mechanism for T cell exhaustion and immunosuppression within the tumor micro-environment [82]. Elevated intratumoral T cell expression of PD-1, reflecting exhaustion, is known to mediate primary resistance to anti-PD-1 therapies in murine tumor models [83]. Thus, combinational therapeutic strategies directed at blocking PD-1 overexpression while reducing cellular immunosuppressive elements in the tumor microenvironment through blockade of TGFβ may improve the efficacy over standard anti-PD-1/PD-L1 monotherapy approaches.

8.3.3 *Inhibition of TGFβ in Preclinical Models*

Based on the compelling rationale that TGFβ is intimately tied to multifaceted mechanisms of immunosuppression in the tumor microenvironment, a variety of targeted therapies have been developed and leveraged over the past decade to selectively inhibit TGFβ-mediated signaling. Several recent publications have reviewed these therapies in detail [84, 85]. In general, over the past decade, these strategies have included small-molecule kinase inhibitors, neutralizing monoclonal antibodies, and antisense oligonucleotides targeting TGFβ-related genes.

Preclinically, multiple strategies have been employed to assess the impact of inhibition of TGFβ on immune cell subsets and tumor biology. For example, use of a TGFβR1-specific receptor kinase inhibitor (SM16) in conjunction with an adenovirus expressing interferon-β in LKR murine mouse tumor model resulted in increased intratumoral leukocytes, activation of T cells, and increased tumor growth and survival compared with either treatment alone [86]. When SM16 was used in combination with an antibody targeting the OX40 receptor in murine models, there was a synergistic effect on tumor regression of established tumors with increase activated CD8+ T cells [87]. Other approaches, such as neutralization of TGFβ isoforms in the tumor microenvironment by monoclonal antibodies (1D11), have been demonstrated to synergistically improve tumor growth inhibition in combination with an antitumor peptide vaccination [88, 89]. Furthermore, gene silencing with anti-TGFβ siRNA improves tumor growth delay in combination with TLR-activated antigen-pulsed dendritic cell vaccine in a murine model using B16 melanoma cells, while suppressing Tregs and enhancing tumor-infiltrating lymphocytes [90]. Monoclonal antibody blockade of TGFβRII also results in enhanced CTL and NK antitumor activity, inhibition of Treg and MDSCs, and increased growth inhibition in murine tumor models [91]. Finally, our group has demonstrated that loss of expression of the type III TGFβ receptor upregulated indoleamine 2,3-dioxygenase (IDO) in plasmacytoid DCs and the CCL22 chemokine in myeloid DCs in animal models, resulting in increased Treg recruitment and an immunotolerant tumor microenvironment [56]. These strategies demonstrate that selective blockade of TGFβ promotes a favorable tumor microenvironment enabling antitumor immunogenicity and complement immune therapy activity.

8.3.4 Clinical Strategies Targeting TGFβ

Galunisertib *(LY2157299)* is a potent small-molecule inhibitor with a pyrazole structure and specificity for ALK5 (TGFβ type I receptor) [92]. In murine tumor models, galunisertib demonstrated inhibition of SMAD phosphorylation and reduction in tumor growth, as well as hepatocellular carcinoma cell SMAD2 phosphorylation, migration, cell growth, and VEGF expression [92, 93]. Hanks et al. showed that galunisertib in combination with an anti-CTLA-4 monoclonal antibody synergistically inhibited tumor growth of both primary and metastatic melanoma in a murine model and increased the ratio of intratumoral CD8+/Tregs [94]. Additionally, the combination galunisertib plus anti-PD-L1 therapy was demonstrated to generate stronger immune responses than either therapy alone in a CT26 murine carcinoma model, resulting in a response rate of approximately 50% and improved growth inhibition compared with controls [95]. Galunisertib monotherapy has been studied in multiple early-phase clinical trials [96]. Combination approaches utilizing galunisertib with immune checkpoint inhibitors are currently being evaluated in multiple clinical trials. A phase I/II study evaluating galunisertib with nivolumab is currently enrolling patients and will include expansion cohorts evaluating activity in hepatocellular carcinoma and non-small cell lung cancer (NCT02423343). Galunisertib is also being combined with durvalumab in patients with metastatic refractory pancreatic cancer in a phase Ib clinical trial (NCT02734160). These studies will be instrumental in determining proof of concept and effects of adding targeted TGFβ inhibition to standard immune checkpoint therapies.

TEW-7197 is another highly potent ALK5-specific small-molecule serine/threonine kinase inhibitor with oral bioavailability [97]. TEW-7197 has been shown to effectively inhibit TGFβ-induced SMAD signaling; inhibit cell migration, invasion, and lung metastasis; and improve survival of 4T1 orthotopic breast tumor-bearing mice [98]. Importantly, TEW-7197 has recently been shown to promote cytotoxic T lymphocyte mediated immune responses and suppress progression of melanoma in vivo [99]. TEW-7197 monotherapy is currently being evaluated in a multisite phase I trial in patients with advanced-stage solid tumors (NCT02160106).

Fresolimumab (GC1008) is a fully human, monoclonal antibody which binds TGFβ isoforms with high affinity. Fresolimumab has been evaluated in a single phase I clinical trial and found to be well tolerated without dose limiting toxicity up to a dose of 15 mg/kg in patients with mesothelioma and renal cell carcinoma [100]. Treatment in patients with mesothelioma resulted in uniform, marked reduction in circulating plasma TGFβ levels. While no effects were seen on NK, CD4+, or CD8+ cell subsets, multiple patients developed new antibodies to mesothelioma tumor lysates suggesting treatment with fresolimumab resulted in immunomodulation [101]. Published data is currently limited regarding combination approaches utilizing TGFβ-neutralizing antibodies with immune checkpoint agents; however, agents such as fresolimumab may effectively modulate inflammation and ultimately improve antitumor immunity.

M7824 (MSB0011359C) is a novel, bifunctional fusion protein consisting of a fully human IgG1, antibody targeting PD-L1 linked to the extracellular domain of TGFβRII [102]. The TGFβRII domain on M7824 functions as a ligand trap for TGFβ isoforms. Treatment with M7824 in preclinical murine models with breast and colon carcinomas results in depletion of TGFβ, improved tumor growth delay, survival, and durable antitumor immunity. Interestingly, in treated tumor-bearing mice, M7824 resulted in increased frequency of CD8+ T cells and NK cells with decreased MDSCs and tumor-associated macrophages [103]. Preliminary data from a phase I clinical trial demonstrates the agent to be well tolerated and results in suppression of circulating all TGFβ isoforms. Currently two phase I clinical trials are ongoing in patients with advanced solid tumors (NCT02699515 and NCT02517398).

Finally, FANG (Vigil) is a unique autologous tumor cell vaccine which is electroporated with a plasmid resulting in co-expression of granulocyte-macrophage colony-stimulating factor and a bifunctional short hairpin RNAi (bi-shRNAi) targeting furin, a proprotein convertase responsible for activation of TGFβ1 and 2 [104]. The furin bi-shRNAi/GMCSF DNA/autologous tumor cell vaccine is being studied in multiple clinical trials in combination with immune checkpoint inhibitors. In the initial phase I clinical trial, FANG monotherapy resulted in effective knockdown of TGFβ1 and 2 levels and generated T cell response in 50% of patients which correlated with survival. FANG is currently being evaluated in multiple early-phase clinical trials in combination with nivolumab for metastatic non-small cell lung cancer (NCT02639234) and with pembrolizumab in patients with metastatic melanoma (NCT02574533). FANG is also being studied in combination with durvalumab in patients with advanced breast cancer (NCT02725489) and atezolizumab in gynecologic malignancies (NCT03073525).

8.4 Adenosine

8.4.1 Adenosine in the Tumor Microenvironment

Although well known as components of DNA and RNA and participants in intracellular signaling, nucleosides and nucleotides have also been implicated in extracellular signaling in processes such as inflammation and malignancy (recently reviewed by di Virgilio) [105]. Hypoxic, metabolically stressed or inflamed tissues undergoing immunogenic cell death release ATP, in addition to exposing calreticulin at the cell membrane and secreting HMGB1 [106]. The released ATP acts as a danger signal [107], recruiting innate immune cells and priming antitumor immune responses; however, in the tumor microenvironment, extracellular ATP is rapidly converted to adenosine by the ectonucleotidases CD39 (ENTPD1) and CD73 (ecto-5'-nucleotidase) which act in tandem to convert ATP to AMP and then AMP to adenosine, respectively [108]. Therefore, adenosine accumulates in the tumor microenvironment in conditions associated with tissue damage such as hypoxia

[109, 110]. The generated adenosine subsequently signals through the G-protein-coupled cell surface receptors A1, A2A, A2B, and A3. Notably, signaling through the A2A receptor stimulates adenylyl cyclase resulting in increased intracellular cAMP, an immunosuppressive mediator [111]. Adenosine has widespread immunosuppressive effects because of the wide array of cell types expressing its receptors. Adenosine reduces T helper cells and increases Tregs [112], increases myeloid-derived suppressor cells and their immunosuppressive function [113], reduces dendritic cell antigen presentation [114], causes macrophages to differentiate toward the M2 phenotype [115], and inhibits cytolytic function of NK cells [116]. In aggregate these immunosuppressive activities of adenosine inhibit antitumor immunity.

8.4.1.1 Ectonucleotidases and Adenosine Receptors in Antitumor Immune Response

As critical (and accessible) components of the adenosine generation and signaling pathways, the CD39 and CD73 ectonucleotidases and the adenosine receptors have been understandably the focus of studies seeking to document their expression in murine and human tumors, their prognostic significance, and their utility as targets for immune modulation strategies.

CD39, anchored to the cell membrane by two transmembrane domains, is expressed widely in solid tumors, lymphomas, and some leukemias and tumor-infiltrating immune and stromal cells including endothelium, activated and exhausted T cells, $FoxP3^+$ Tregs, Tr1, $FoxP3^-$ memory T cells, Th17, $\gamma\delta$ T cells, B cells, NK and NKT cells, macrophages, neutrophils, and MDSC [117]. Its expression is upregulated by hypoxia. Prognostic significance, in general a poor prognosis, has been demonstrated for CD39 expression by tumor cells and the infiltrating cells of human malignancies [118–123]. More rapid tumor growth has been observed in CD39 expressing transgenic models, while CD39 knockout models demonstrate greater immune-mediated antitumor responses [124] and treatment with the CD39 inhibitor POM1 limited tumor growth.

CD73, a glycosylphosphatidylinositol (GPI)-anchored cell surface enzyme, is expressed on the endothelium and epithelium, stromal cells, naive/memory $CD8^+$ T cells, $ICOS^+$ Tregs, Th17, $\gamma\delta$ T cells, B cells, some NK cells, neutrophils, MDSC, solid tumors, and certain leukemias [117]. Its expression is driven by hypoxia, Wnt and TGFβ signaling, and the process of epithelial to mesenchymal transformation [110, 125–127]. CD73 expression has been related to poor clinical outcome in diverse malignancies including triple negative breast cancer; head and neck cancers; glioblastoma; pancreatic, colorectal, prostate, gastric, bladder, kidney, ovarian, and endometrial cancer; and CLL (reviewed in Antonioli 2016) [128], although some studies have paradoxically found a good prognosis with CD73 expression. CD73-deficient mice experience slower tumor growth in several models [111, 129]. In addition to its role in the generation of adenosine, CD73 may also mediate signaling pathways and tumor adhesion and invasion through non-adenosine mediated pathways [130].

The adenosine receptors A2a and A2b when stimulated lead to activation of adenylyl cyclases which hydrolyze intracellular ATP into cyclic AMP (cAMP) which in turn activates protein kinase A (PKA), which has a role in inhibiting T cell receptor signaling [117]. Tumor rejection has been reported in A2a-deficient mice [131, 132].

The forgoing suggests that CD39, CD73, and A2a and A2b receptors may be targets for enhancing antitumor immunity. Indeed, in preclinical models, drugs and antibodies targeting these molecules have demonstrated proof of principal. The A2a antagonist SCH58261 enhanced the antitumor efficacy of adoptively transferred tumor-antigen-specific T cells [133] and could potentiate the immunogenic cell death induced by anthracyclines [134]. Similar enhancement of adoptively transferred T cells by the dual A2a and A2b receptor antagonist (ZM241,385) was reported [112]. Because it was noted that A2A receptor expression on tumor-infiltrating CD8+ T cells occurs with PD-1 blockade, it is gratifying to note that dual blockade of PD-1 and A2A significantly enhanced the function of tumor-infiltrating T cells and tumor growth inhibition in a preclinical model [135]. In murine colon, prostate, and breast cancer and fibrosarcoma models, anti-CD73 mAb significantly enhanced the antitumor activity of both anti-CTLA-4 and anti-PD-1 mAbs, although the effects were more prominent with anti-PD-1 mAb [136]. This was attributed to the observation that A2a receptor activation upregulates PD-1 but not CTLA4 on T cells, an important consideration for combinations in clinical trials.

8.4.2 Clinical Trials of Adenosine Signaling Inhibition

Clinical trials of strategies targeting the adenosine generation pathways have been limited thus far. Although antibodies against CD39 have been developed [137], they have not reached human clinical trials; however, an antibody against CD73 (MEDI9447) has entered phase I testing. This antibody noncompetitively inhibits the enzymatic function of soluble and cell-bound CD73 by cross-linking CD73 dimers or otherwise limiting conformational changes necessary for enzymatic function [138]. Preclinical studies have demonstrated amelioration of AMP-mediated immunosuppression and tumor growth inhibition in murine models [139]. In the tumor microenvironment, increased CD8(+) effector cells and activated macrophages were observed following MEDI9447. When combined with anti-PD-1 antibodies, greater antitumor activity was observed for MEDI9447. In the phase I study, solid tumor patients who have progressed, are refractory, or are intolerant to standard therapy are being enrolled to received single agent MEDI9447 or MEDI9447 plus MEDI4736 (an anti-PD-L1 antibody) (NCT02503774). Other companies are developing anti-CD73-based strategies including Bristol-Myers Squibb which also demonstrated enhanced antitumor activity when combined with anti-PD-1 antibody [140]. Innate Pharma, Corvus Pharmaceuticals, and Arcus Biosciences have also recently disclosed CD73 inhibitor programs. No clinical trial data is available yet. Regarding A2a antagonists, PBF-509 is in phase I study development to be combined with an anti-PD-1 antibody in a trial of PBF-509 and PDR001 in patients with advanced non-small cell lung cancer (NCT02403193). The A2a antagonist CPI-444 is also in clinical trials combined with an anti-PD-L1 antibody in phase I/Ib study to evaluate CPI-444 alone and in combination with atezolizumab in advanced cancers (NCT02655822).

8.5 Conclusions

The targeted inhibition of inflammatory mediators to augment immunosuppressive factors within the tumor microenvironment is a rational strategy to improve efficacy of immune checkpoint agents. Disruption of inflammatory signaling pathways particularly involving IDO, TGFβ, and adenosine has compelling evidence demonstrating effects such as inhibition of Tregs and MDSCs while promoting effector T cell function and tumor immunity. Multiple early-phase clinical trials investigating combinational strategies leveraging inflammatory modulators with immune checkpoint therapies are ongoing in numerous malignancies. Importantly, as a substantial portion of patients do not derive clinical benefit from standard immune checkpoint therapies, there is also a critical need for biomarker development to guide therapeutic application and optimize clinical outcomes. Additionally, particular tumor histologies are intrinsically resistant to immune therapies, for example, as seen with pancreatic and colorectal cancers. The mechanisms responsible for mediating these resistant phenotypes are multifactorial; however, inflammatory cytokine dysregulation influences co-localization of tumor-infiltrating lymphocytes (TILs) and PD-L1 expression [141]. Tumors with both TILs present and PD-L1 expressed are believed to have a more favorable response to immune checkpoint therapy compared to tumors with only one or neither present [6]. Targeting immunosuppressive cytokines within the tumor microenvironment may enable induction of response by T cell infiltration in seemingly non-inflamed tumors or overcome acquired resistance mechanisms limiting T cell function. Predictive biomarkers, beyond PD-L1, are needed to guide the clinical use of novel therapeutic combinations to determine patients most likely to derive benefit.

References

1. Larkin J, Chiarion-Sileni V, Gonzalez R et al (2015) Combined nivolumab and Ipilimumab or monotherapy in untreated melanoma. N Engl J Med 373(1):23–34
2. Reck M, Rodriguez-Abreu D, Robinson AG et al (2016) Pembrolizumab versus chemotherapy for PD-L1-positive non-small-cell lung cancer. N Engl J Med 375(19):1823–1833
3. Motzer RJ, Escudier B, McDermott DF et al (2015) Nivolumab versus everolimus in advanced renal-cell carcinoma. N Engl J Med 373(19):1803–1813
4. Wang Q, Wu X (2017) Primary and acquired resistance to PD-1/PD-L1 blockade in cancer treatment. Int Immunopharmacol 46:210–219

5. Hugo W, Zaretsky JM, Sun L et al (2016) Genomic and transcriptomic features of response to anti-PD-1 therapy in metastatic melanoma. Cell 165(1):35–44
6. Teng MW, Ngiow SF, Ribas A, Smyth MJ (2015) Classifying cancers based on T-cell infiltration and PD-L1. Cancer Res 75(11):2139–2145
7. Liu C, Workman CJ, Vignali DA (2016) Targeting regulatory T cells in tumors. FEBS J 283(14):2731–2748
8. Gabrilovich DI (2017) Myeloid-derived suppressor cells. Cancer Immunol Res 5(1):3–8
9. Manegold C, Dingemans AC, Gray JE et al (2017) The potential of combined immunotherapy and antiangiogenesis for the synergistic treatment of advanced NSCLC. J Thorac Oncol 12(2):194–207
10. Mellor AL, Munn DH (2004) IDO expression by dendritic cells: tolerance and tryptophan catabolism. Nat Rev Immunol 4(10):762–774
11. Grohmann U, Bronte V (2010) Control of immune response by amino acid metabolism. Immunol Rev 236:243–264
12. Higuchi K, Hayaishi O (1967) Enzymic formation of D-kynurenine from D-tryptophan. Arch Biochem Biophys 120(2):397–403
13. Shimizu T, Nomiyama S, Hirata F, Hayaishi O (1978) Indoleamine 2,3-dioxygenase. Purification and some properties. J Biol Chem 253(13):4700–4706
14. Munn DH, Zhou M, Attwood JT et al (1998) Prevention of allogeneic fetal rejection by tryptophan catabolism. Science 281(5380):1191–1193
15. Munn DH, Shafizadeh E, Attwood JT, Bondarev I, Pashine A, Mellor AL (1999) Inhibition of T cell proliferation by macrophage tryptophan catabolism. J Exp Med 189(9):1363–1372
16. Metz R, Rust S, Duhadaway JB et al (2012) IDO inhibits a tryptophan sufficiency signal that stimulates mTOR: a novel IDO effector pathway targeted by D-1-methyl-tryptophan. Oncoimmunology. 1(9):1460–1468
17. Mezrich JD, Fechner JH, Zhang X, Johnson BP, Burlingham WJ, Bradfield CA (2010) An interaction between kynurenine and the aryl hydrocarbon receptor can generate regulatory T cells. J Immunol 185(6):3190–3198
18. Fallarino F, Grohmann U, You S et al (2006) The combined effects of tryptophan starvation and tryptophan catabolites down-regulate T cell receptor {zeta}-chain and induce a regulatory phenotype in naive T cells. J Immunol 176:6752–6761
19. Baban B, Chandler P, McCool D, Marshall B, Munn DH, Mellor AL (2004) Indoleamine 2,3-dioxygenase expression is restricted to fetal trophoblast giant cells during murine gestation and is maternal genome specific. J Reprod Immunol 61(2):67–77
20. Munn DH, Mellor AL (2016) IDO in the tumor microenvironment: inflammation, counter-regulation, and tolerance. Trends Immunol 37(3):193–207
21. Munn DH, Mellor AL (2007) Indoleamine 2,3-dioxygenase and tumor-induced tolerance. J Clin Invest 117(5):1147–1154
22. Uyttenhove C, Pilotte L, Theate I et al (2003) Evidence of a tumoral immune resistance mechanism based on tryptophan degradation by indoleamine 2,3-dioxygenase. Nat Med 9(10):1269–1274
23. Boyland E, Williams DC (1955) The estimation of tryptophan metabolites in the urine of patients with cancer of the bladder. Biochem J 60(Annual General Meeting):v
24. Rose DP (1967) Tryptophan metabolism in carcinoma of the breast. Lancet 1(7484):239–241
25. Godin-Ethier J, Hanafi LA, Piccirillo CA, Lapointe R (2011) Indoleamine 2,3-dioxygenase expression in human cancers: clinical and immunologic perspectives. Clin Cancer Res 17(22):6985–6991
26. Katz JB, Muller AJ, Prendergast GC (2008) Indoleamine 2,3-dioxygenase in T-cell tolerance and tumoral immune escape. Immunol Rev 222:206–221
27. Munn DH, Sharma MD, Lee JR et al (2002) Potential regulatory function of human dendritic cells expressing indoleamine 2,3-dioxygenase. Science 297(5588):1867–1870
28. Grohmann U, Fallarino F, Bianchi R et al (2001) IL-6 inhibits the tolerogenic function of CD8 alpha+ dendritic cells expressing indoleamine 2,3-dioxygenase. J Immunol 167(2):708–714

29. Orabona C, Pallotta MT, Volpi C et al (2008) SOCS3 drives proteasomal degradation of indoleamine 2,3-dioxygenase (IDO) and antagonizes IDO-dependent tolerogenesis. Proc Natl Acad Sci U S A 105(52):20828–20833
30. Sharma MD, Baban B, Chandler PR et al (2007) Plasmacytoid dendritic cells from mouse tumor-draining lymph nodes directly activate mature Tregs via indoleamine-2,3-dioxygenase. J Clin Invest 117(9):2570–2582
31. Munn DH, Sharma MD, Hou D et al (2004) Expression of indoleamine 2,3-dioxygenase by plasmacytoid dendritic cells in tumor-draining lymph nodes. J Clin Invest 114(2):280–290
32. Hwu P, Du MX, Lapointe R, Do M, Taylor MW, Young HA (2000) Indoleamine 2,3-dioxygenase production by human dendritic cells results in the inhibition of T cell proliferation. J Immunol 164(7):3596–3599
33. Takikawa O, Kuroiwa T, Yamazaki F, Kido R (1988) Mechanism of interferon-gamma action. Characterization of indoleamine 2,3-dioxygenase in cultured human cells induced by interferon-gamma and evaluation of the enzyme-mediated tryptophan degradation in its anticellular activity. J Biol Chem 263(4):2041–2048
34. Belladonna M, Volpi C, Bianchi R et al (2008) Cutting edge: autocrine TGFbeta sustains default tolerogenesis by IDO-competent dendritic cells. J Immunol 181(8):5194–5198
35. Pallotta MT, Orabona C, Volpi C et al (2011) Indoleamine 2,3-dioxygenase is a signaling protein in long-term tolerance by dendritic cells. Nat Immunol 12(9):870–878
36. Mondanelli G, Bianchi R, Pallotta MT et al (2017) A relay pathway between arginine and tryptophan metabolism confers immunosuppressive properties on dendritic cells. Immunity 46(2):233–244
37. Thomas SR, Terentis AC, Cai H et al (2007) Post-translational regulation of human indoleamine 2,3-dioxygenase activity by nitric oxide. J Biol Chem 282(33):23778–23787
38. Holmgaard RB, Zamarin D, Munn DH, Wolchok JD, Allison JP (2013) Indoleamine 2,3-dioxygenase is a critical resistance mechanism in antitumor T cell immunotherapy targeting CTLA-4. J Exp Med 210(7):1389–1402
39. Hou D, Muller AJ, Sharma MD et al (2007) Inhibition of indoleamine 2,3-dioxygenase in dendritic cells by stereoisomers of 1-methyl-tryptophan correlates with antitumor responses. Cancer Res 67(2):792–801
40. Yue EW, Douty B, Wayland B et al (2009) Discovery of potent competitive inhibitors of indoleamine 2,3-dioxygenase with in vivo pharmacodynamic activity and efficacy in a mouse melanoma model. J Med Chem 52(23):7364–7367
41. Koblish HK, Hansbury MJ, Bowman KJ et al (2010) Hydroxyamidine inhibitors of indoleamine-2,3-dioxygenase potently suppress systemic tryptophan catabolism and the growth of IDO-expressing tumors. Mol Cancer Ther 9(2):489–498
42. Liu X, Shin N, Koblish HK et al (2010) Selective inhibition of IDO1 effectively regulates mediators of antitumor immunity. Blood 115(17):3520–3530
43. Soliman HH, Jackson E, Neuger T et al (2014) A first in man phase I trial of the oral immunomodulator, indoximod, combined with docetaxel in patients with metastatic solid tumors. Oncotarget 5(18):8136–8146
44. Soliman SA HH, Sullivan D, Vanahanian N, Link C (2009) Overcoming tumor antigen anergy in human malignancies using the novel indeolamine 2,3-dioxygenase (IDO) enzyme inhibitor, 1-methyl-D-tryptophan (1MT). J Clin Oncol 27(15s)
45. Beatty GL, O'Dwyer PJ, Clark J et al (2017) First-in-human phase I study of the oral inhibitor of Indoleamine 2,3-Dioxygenase-1 Epacadostat (INCB024360) in patients with advanced solid malignancies. Clin Cancer Res
46. Gibney GT, Hamid O, Gangadhar TC, Lutzky J, Olszanski AJ, Gajewski T, Chmielowski B, Boasberg PD, Zhao Y, Newton RC, Scherle PA, Bowman J, Maleski J, Leopold L, Weber JS (2014) Preliminary results from a phase 1/2 study of INCB024360 combined with ipilimumab (ipi) in patients (pts) with melanoma. J Clin Oncol 32(5s)
47. Gangadhar TC, Hamid O, Smith DC, Bauer TM, Wasser JS, Olszanski AJ, Luke JJ, Balmanoukian AS, Kaufman DR, Zhao Y, Maleski J, Jones MJ, Leopold L, Gajewski TF

(2016) Epacadostat plus pembrolizumab in patients with advanced melanoma and select solid tumors: updated phase 1 results from ECHO-202/KEYNOTE-037. Ann Oncol 27(6):379–400
48. Nathan Bahary IG-L, Cinar P, O'Rourke MA, Somer BG, Nyak-Kapoor A, Lee JS, Munn D, Kennedy EP, Vahanian NN, Link CJ, Wang-Gillam A (2016) Phase 2 trial of the indoleamine 2,3-dioxygenase pathway (IDO) inhibitor indoximod plus gemcitabine/nab-paclitaxel for the treatment of metastatic pancreas cancer: interim analysis. J Clin Oncol 34:Abstract 3020
49. Zakharia Y, McWilliams R, Shaheen M et al (2017) Interim analysis of the Phase 2 clinical trial of the IDO pathway inhibitor indoximod in combination with pembrolizumab for patients with advanced melanoma. *2017 AACR Annual Meeting*
50. Iversen TZ, Engell-Noerregaard L, Ellebaek E et al (2014) Long-lasting disease stabilization in the absence of toxicity in metastatic lung cancer patients vaccinated with an epitope derived from indoleamine 2,3 dioxygenase. Clin Cancer Res 20(1):221–232
51. Bjoern J, Iversen TZ, Nitschke NJ, Andersen MH, Svane IM (2016) Safety, immune and clinical responses in metastatic melanoma patients vaccinated with a long peptide derived from indoleamine 2,3-dioxygenase in combination with ipilimumab. Cytotherapy 18(8):1043–1055
52. Enk A, Jonuleit H, Saloga J, Knop J (1997) Dendritic cells as mediators of tumor-induced tolerance in metastatic melanoma. Int J Cancer 73:309–316
53. Holtzhausen A, Zhao F, Evans K et al (2015) Melanoma-derived Wnt5a promotes local dendritic-cell expression of IDO and Immunotolerance: opportunities for pharmacologic enhancement of immunotherapy. Cancer Immunol Res 3(9):1082–1095
54. Holtzhausen A, Zhao F, Evans K, Hanks BA (2014) Early carcinogenesis involves the establishment of immune privilege via intrinsic and extrinsic regulation of indoleamine 2,3-dioxygenase-1: translational implications in cancer immunotherapy. Front Immunol 5:1–9
55. Muller A, DuHadaway J, Donover P, Sutanto-Ward E, Prendergast G (2005) Inhibition of indoleamine 2,3-dioxygenase, an immunoregulatory target of the cancer suppression gene Bin1, potentiates cancer chemotherapy. Nat Med. 11(3):312–319
56. Hanks BA, Holtzhausen A, Jamieson R et al (2013) Type III TGF-β receptor downregulation generates an immunotolerant tumor microenvironment. J Clin Invest 123(9):3925–3940
57. Lemos H, Mohamed E, Huang L et al (2016) STING promotes the growth of tumors characterized by low antigenicity via IDO activation. Cancer Res 76(8):2076–2081
58. Huang L, Li L, Lemos H et al (2013) Cutting edge: DNA sensing via the STING adaptor in myeloid dendritic cells induces potent tolerogenic responses. J Immunol 191(7):3509–3513
59. Zhao F, Xiao C, Evans K et al (2016) The Wnt5a-Beta-catenin signaling pathway triggers a metabolic switch that drives dendritic cell tolerization in the melanoma microenvironment. *In preparation*
60. Balachandran VP, Cavnar MJ, Zeng S et al (2011) Imatinib potentiates antitumor T cell responses in gastrointestinal stromal tumor through the inhibition of Ido. Nat Med 17(9):1094–1100
61. Basu GD, Tinder TL, Bradley JM et al (2006) Cyclooxygenase-2 inhibitor enhances the efficacy of a breast cancer vaccine: role of IDO. J Immunol 177(4):2391–2402
62. Zhai L, Spranger S, Binder DC et al (2015) Molecular pathways: targeting IDO1 and other tryptophan dioxygenases for cancer immunotherapy. Clin Cancer Res 21(24):5427–5433
63. Zhao F, Evans K, Holtzhausen A, Tsutsui M, Tyler DS, Hanks BA (2015) Targeting the Wnt5a-beta-catenin pathway in the melanoma microenvironment to augment checkpoint inhibitor immunotherapy. J Clin Oncol 33(Suppl):abstr 3054
64. Levy L, Hill CS (2006) Alterations in components of the TGF-beta superfamily signaling pathways in human cancer. Cytokine Growth Factor Rev 17(1-2):41–58
65. Pickup M, Novitskiy S, Moses HL (2013) The roles of TGFbeta in the tumour microenvironment. Nat Rev Cancer 13(11):788–799
66. Oh SA, Li MO (2013) TGF-beta: guardian of T cell function. J Immunol 191(8):3973–3979
67. Massague J (2008) TGFbeta in cancer. Cell 134(2):215–230
68. Ikushima H, Miyazono K (2010) TGFbeta signalling: a complex web in cancer progression. Nat Rev Cancer 10(6):415–424

69. Massague J (2012) TGFbeta signalling in context. Nat Rev Mol Cell Biol 13(10):616–630
70. Yang L, Pang Y, Moses HL (2010) TGF-beta and immune cells: an important regulatory axis in the tumor microenvironment and progression. Trends Immunol 31(6):220–227
71. Li MO, Sanjabi S, Flavell RA (2006) Transforming growth factor-beta controls development, homeostasis, and tolerance of T cells by regulatory T cell-dependent and -independent mechanisms. Immunity 25(3):455–471
72. Liu Y, Zhang P, Li J, Kulkarni AB, Perruche S, Chen W (2008) A critical function for TGF-beta signaling in the development of natural CD4+CD25+Foxp3+ regulatory T cells. Nat Immunol 9(6):632–640
73. Wrzesinski SH, Wan YY, Flavell RA (2007) Transforming growth factor-beta and the immune response: implications for anticancer therapy. Clin Cancer Res 13(18 Pt 1):5262–5270
74. Thomas DA, Massague J (2005) TGF-beta directly targets cytotoxic T cell functions during tumor evasion of immune surveillance. Cancer Cell 8(5):369–380
75. Ghiringhelli F, Puig PE, Roux S et al (2005) Tumor cells convert immature myeloid dendritic cells into TGF-beta-secreting cells inducing CD4+CD25+ regulatory T cell proliferation. J Exp Med 202(7):919–929
76. Tu E, Chia PZ, Chen W (2014) TGFbeta in T cell biology and tumor immunity: angel or devil? Cytokine Growth Factor Rev 25(4):423–435
77. Hargadon KM (2016) Dysregulation of TGFbeta1 activity in cancer and its influence on the quality of anti-tumor immunity. J Clin Med 5(9):76
78. Weber F, Byrne SN, Le S et al (2005) Transforming growth factor-beta1 immobilises dendritic cells within skin tumours and facilitates tumour escape from the immune system. Cancer Immunol Immunother 54(9):898–906
79. Geissmann F, Revy P, Regnault A et al (1999) TGF-beta 1 prevents the noncognate maturation of human dendritic Langerhans cells. J Immunol 162(8):4567–4575
80. Flavell RA, Sanjabi S, Wrzesinski SH, Licona-Limon P (2010) The polarization of immune cells in the tumour environment by TGFbeta. Nat Rev Immunol 10(8):554–567
81. Papaspyridonos M, Matei I, Huang Y et al (2015) Id1 suppresses anti-tumour immune responses and promotes tumour progression by impairing myeloid cell maturation. Nat Commun 6:6840
82. Park BV, Freeman ZT, Ghasemzadeh A et al (2016) TGF-beta1-mediated Smad3 enhances PD-1 expression on antigen-specific T cells in cancer. Cancer Discov 6(12):1366–1381
83. Ngiow SF, Young A, Jacquelot N et al (2015) A threshold level of Intratumor CD8+ T-cell PD1 expression dictates therapeutic response to anti-PD1. Cancer Res 75(18):3800–3811
84. Herbertz S, Sawyer JS, Stauber AJ et al (2015) Clinical development of galunisertib (LY2157299 monohydrate), a small molecule inhibitor of transforming growth factor-beta signaling pathway. Drug Des Devel Ther 9:4479–4499
85. de Gramont A, Faivre S, Raymond E (2017) Novel TGF-beta inhibitors ready for prime time in onco-immunology. Oncoimmunology. 6(1):e1257453
86. Kim S, Buchlis G, Fridlender ZG et al (2008) Systemic blockade of transforming growth factor-beta signaling augments the efficacy of immunogene therapy. Cancer Res 68(24):10247–10256
87. Triplett TA, Tucker CG, Triplett KC et al (2015) STAT3 signaling is required for optimal regression of large established tumors in mice treated with anti-OX40 and TGFbeta receptor blockade. Cancer Immunol Res 3(5):526–535
88. Terabe M, Ambrosino E, Takaku S et al (2009) Synergistic enhancement of CD8+ T cell-mediated tumor vaccine efficacy by an anti-transforming growth factor-beta monoclonal antibody. Clin Cancer Res 15(21):6560–6569
89. Takaku S, Terabe M, Ambrosino E et al (2010) Blockade of TGF-beta enhances tumor vaccine efficacy mediated by CD8(+) T cells. Int J Cancer 126(7):1666–1674
90. Conroy H, Galvin KC, Higgins SC, Mills KH (2012) Gene silencing of TGF-beta1 enhances antitumor immunity induced with a dendritic cell vaccine by reducing tumor-associated regulatory T cells. Cancer Immunol Immunother 61(3):425–431

91. Zhong Z, Carroll KD, Policarpio D et al (2010) Anti-transforming growth factor beta receptor II antibody has therapeutic efficacy against primary tumor growth and metastasis through multieffects on cancer, stroma, and immune cells. Clin Cancer Res 16(4):1191–1205
92. Bueno L, de Alwis DP, Pitou C et al (2008) Semi-mechanistic modelling of the tumour growth inhibitory effects of LY2157299, a new type I receptor TGF-beta kinase antagonist, in mice. Eur J Cancer 44(1):142–150
93. Dituri F, Mazzocca A, Peidro FJ et al (2013) Differential inhibition of the TGF-beta signaling pathway in HCC cells using the small molecule inhibitor LY2157299 and the D10 monoclonal antibody against TGF-beta receptor type II. PLoS One 8(6):e67109
94. Hanks BA, Holtzhausen A, Evans K, Heid M, Blobe GC (2014) Combinatorial TGF-{beta} signaling blockade and anti-CTLA-4 antibody immunotherapy in a murine BRAFV600E-PTEN–/– transgenic model of melanoma. ASCO Meeting Abstracts 32(15 Suppl):3011
95. David Schaer YL, Castaneda S, Inigo I, Surguladze D, Xu X, Nugent D, Murphy M, Hall G, Benhadji K, Guba S, Li T, Kalos M, Driscoll K (2015) Targeting the TGFb pathway with galunisertib, a TGFbRI SMI, promotes anti-tumor immunity leading to durable, complete responses, as monotherapy and in combination with checkpoint inhibition. Paper presented at: 30th Annual Meeting and Associated Programs of the Society for Immunotherapy of Cancer (SITC 2015); November 2015, National Harbor
96. Rodon J, Carducci MA, Sepulveda-Sanchez JM et al (2015) First-in-human dose study of the novel transforming growth factor-beta receptor I kinase inhibitor LY2157299 monohydrate in patients with advanced cancer and glioma. Clin Cancer Res 21(3):553–560
97. Jin CH, Krishnaiah M, Sreenu D et al (2014) Discovery of N-((4-([1,2,4]triazolo[1,5-a]pyridin-6-yl)-5-(6-methylpyridin-2-yl)-1H-imidazol-2 -yl)methyl)-2-fluoroaniline (EW-7197): a highly potent, selective, and orally bioavailable inhibitor of TGF-beta type I receptor kinase as cancer immunotherapeutic/antifibrotic agent. J Med Chem 57(10):4213–4238
98. Son JY, Park SY, Kim SJ et al (2014) EW-7197, a novel ALK-5 kinase inhibitor, potently inhibits breast to lung metastasis. Mol Cancer Ther 13(7):1704–1716
99. Yoon JH, Jung SM, Park SH et al (2013) Activin receptor-like kinase5 inhibition suppresses mouse melanoma by ubiquitin degradation of Smad4, thereby derepressing eomesodermin in cytotoxic T lymphocytes. EMBO Mol Med 5(11):1720–1739
100. Morris JC, Tan AR, Olencki TE et al (2014) Phase I study of GC1008 (fresolimumab): a human anti-transforming growth factor-beta (TGFbeta) monoclonal antibody in patients with advanced malignant melanoma or renal cell carcinoma. PLoS One 9(3):e90353
101. Stevenson JP, Kindler HL, Papasavvas E et al (2013) Immunological effects of the TGFbeta-blocking antibody GC1008 in malignant pleural mesothelioma patients. Oncoimmunology 2(8):e26218
102. Lan Y, Zhang D, Xu C, Marelli B, Qi J, Yu H, Qin G, Xu X, Wang H, Sircar A, Brunkhorst B, Austin E, Radvanyi L, Lo K-M (2017) Preclinical evaluation of M7824 (MSB0011359C), a novel bifunctional fusion protein targeting the PD-L1 and TGFβ pathways. Presented at Keystone Symposia: TGFβ in Immunity, Inflammation and Cancer, Taos, 9–13 January, 2017
103. Lan Y, Zhang D, Xu C, Marelli B, Qi J, Yu H, Qin G, Xu X, Wang H, Sircar A, Brunkhorst B, Austin E, Radvanyi L, Lo K-M. Preclinical evaluation and mechanistic characterization of M7824 (MSB0011359C), a novel bifunctional fusion protein targeting the PD-L1 and TGF-β pathways. Presented at the American Association for Cancer Research (AACR) Annual Meeting 2017; Washington, DC
104. Senzer N, Barve M, Kuhn J et al (2012) Phase I trial of "bi-shRNAifurin/GMCSF DNA/autologous tumor cell" vaccine (FANG) in advanced cancer. Mol Ther 20(3):679–686
105. Di Virgilio F, Adinolfi E (2017) Extracellular purines, purinergic receptors and tumor growth. Oncogene 36(3):293–303
106. Kroemer G, Galluzzi L, Kepp O, Zitvogel L (2013) Immunogenic cell death in cancer therapy. Annu Rev Immunol 31:51–72
107. Trautmann A (2009) Extracellular ATP in the immune system: more than just a "danger signal". Sci Signal 2(56):pe6

108. Allard B, Longhi MS, Robson SC, Stagg J (2017) The ectonucleotidases CD39 and CD73: novel checkpoint inhibitor targets. Immunol Rev 276(1):121–144
109. Stagg J, Smyth MJ (2010) Extracellular adenosine triphosphate and adenosine in cancer. Oncogene 29(39):5346–5358
110. Vaupel P, Mayer A (2016) Hypoxia-driven adenosine accumulation: a crucial microenvironmental factor promoting tumor progression. Adv Exp Med Biol 876:177–183
111. Stagg J, Divisekera U, Duret H et al (2011) CD73-deficient mice have increased antitumor immunity and are resistant to experimental metastasis. Cancer Res 71(8):2892–2900
112. Ohta A, Sitkovsky M (2014) Extracellular adenosine-mediated modulation of regulatory T cells. Front Immunol 5:304
113. Ryzhov S, Novitskiy SV, Goldstein AE et al (2011) Adenosinergic regulation of the expansion and immunosuppressive activity of CD11b+Gr1+ cells. J Immunol 187(11):6120–6129
114. Challier J, Bruniquel D, Sewell AK, Laugel B (2013) Adenosine and cAMP signalling skew human dendritic cell differentiation towards a tolerogenic phenotype with defective CD8(+) T-cell priming capacity. Immunology 138(4):402–410
115. Barbera-Cremades M, Baroja-Mazo A, Pelegrin P (2016) Purinergic signaling during macrophage differentiation results in M2 alternative activated macrophages. J Leukoc Biol 99(2):289–299
116. Hoskin DW, Mader JS, Furlong SJ, Conrad DM, Blay J (2008) Inhibition of T cell and natural killer cell function by adenosine and its contribution to immune evasion by tumor cells (Review). Int J Oncol 32(3):527–535
117. Allard D, Turcotte M, Stagg J (2017) Targeting A2 adenosine receptors in cancer. Immunol Cell Biol 95(4):333–339
118. Kunzli BM, Bernlochner MI, Rath S et al (2011) Impact of CD39 and purinergic signalling on the growth and metastasis of colorectal cancer. Purinergic Signal 7(2):231–241
119. Zhang B, Cheng B, Li FS et al (2015) High expression of CD39/ENTPD1 in malignant epithelial cells of human rectal adenocarcinoma. Tumour Biol: J Int Soc Oncodev Biol Med 36(12):9411–9419
120. Montalban Del Barrio I, Penski C, Schlahsa L et al (2016) Adenosine-generating ovarian cancer cells attract myeloid cells which differentiate into adenosine-generating tumor associated macrophages – a self-amplifying, CD39- and CD73-dependent mechanism for tumor immune escape. J Immunother Cancer 4:49
121. Pulte D, Furman RR, Broekman MJ et al (2011) CD39 expression on T lymphocytes correlates with severity of disease in patients with chronic lymphocytic leukemia. Clin Lymphoma Myeloma Leuk 11(4):367–372
122. Perry C, Hazan-Halevy I, Kay S et al (2012) Increased CD39 expression on CD4(+) T lymphocytes has clinical and prognostic significance in chronic lymphocytic leukemia. Ann Hematol 91(8):1271–1279
123. Cai XY, Ni XC, Yi Y et al (2016) Overexpression of CD39 in hepatocellular carcinoma is an independent indicator of poor outcome after radical resection. Medicine (Baltimore) 95(40):e4989
124. Sun X, Wu Y, Gao W et al (2010) CD39/ENTPD1 expression by CD4+Foxp3+ regulatory T cells promotes hepatic metastatic tumor growth in mice. Gastroenterology 139(3):1030–1040
125. Sitkovsky MV, Hatfield S, Abbott R, Belikoff B, Lukashev D, Ohta A (2014) Hostile, hypoxia-A2-adenosinergic tumor biology as the next barrier to overcome for tumor immunologists. Cancer Immunol Res 2(7):598–605
126. Spychala J, Kitajewski J (2004) Wnt and beta-catenin signaling target the expression of ecto-5′-nucleotidase and increase extracellular adenosine generation. Exp Cell Res 296(2):99–108
127. Xiong L, Wen Y, Miao X, Yang Z (2014) NT5E and FcGBP as key regulators of TGF-1-induced epithelial-mesenchymal transition (EMT) are associated with tumor progression and survival of patients with gallbladder cancer. Cell Tissue Res 355(2):365–374
128. Antonioli L, Yegutkin GG, Pacher P, Blandizzi C, Hasko G (2016) Anti-CD73 in cancer immunotherapy: awakening new opportunities. Trends Cancer 2(2):95–109

129. Yegutkin GG, Marttila-Ichihara F, Karikoski M et al (2011) Altered purinergic signaling in CD73-deficient mice inhibits tumor progression. Eur J Immunol 41(5):1231–1241
130. Ren ZH, Lin CZ, Cao W et al (2016) CD73 is associated with poor prognosis in HNSCC. Oncotarget 7(38):61690–61702
131. Ohta A, Gorelik E, Prasad SJ et al (2006) A2A adenosine receptor protects tumors from antitumor T cells. Proc Natl Acad Sci U S A 103(35):13132–13137
132. Beavis PA, Divisekera U, Paget C et al (2013) Blockade of A2A receptors potently suppresses the metastasis of CD73+ tumors. Proc Natl Acad Sci U S A 110(36):14711–14716
133. Jin D, Fan J, Wang L et al (2010) CD73 on tumor cells impairs antitumor T-cell responses: a novel mechanism of tumor-induced immune suppression. Cancer Res 70(6):2245–2255
134. Loi S, Pommey S, Haibe-Kains B et al (2013) CD73 promotes anthracycline resistance and poor prognosis in triple negative breast cancer. Proc Natl Acad Sci U S A 110(27):11091–11096
135. Beavis PA, Milenkovski N, Henderson MA et al (2015) Adenosine receptor 2A blockade increases the efficacy of anti-PD-1 through enhanced antitumor T-cell responses. Cancer Immunol Res 3(5):506–517
136. Allard B, Pommey S, Smyth MJ, Stagg J (2013) Targeting CD73 enhances the antitumor activity of anti-PD-1 and anti-CTLA-4 mAbs. Clin Cancer Res 19(20):5626–5635
137. Bastid J, Cottalorda-Regairaz A, Alberici G, Bonnefoy N, Eliaou JF, Bensussan A (2013) ENTPD1/CD39 is a promising therapeutic target in oncology. Oncogene 32(14):1743–1751
138. Geoghegan JC, Diedrich G, Lu X et al (2016) Inhibition of CD73 AMP hydrolysis by a therapeutic antibody with a dual, non-competitive mechanism of action. MAbs 8(3):454–467
139. Hay CM, Sult E, Huang Q et al (2016) Targeting CD73 in the tumor microenvironment with MEDI9447. Oncoimmunology. 5(8):e1208875
140. Barnhart BC, Sega E, Yamniuk A et al (2016) Abstract 1476: a therapeutic antibody that inhibits CD73 activity by dual mechanisms. Cancer Res 76(14 Supplement):1476–1476
141. Taube JM, Anders RA, Young GD et al (2012) Colocalization of inflammatory response with B7-h1 expression in human melanocytic lesions supports an adaptive resistance mechanism of immune escape. Sci Transl Med 4(127):127ra137

Chapter 9
Combinations of Genomically and Immune-Targeted Therapies in Early-Phase Clinical Trials

Maulik Patel, Sandip Pravin Patel, and Razelle Kurzrock

Abstract Advances in cancer treatment have evolved from relatively nonspecific application of cytotoxic agents to mechanism-based therapies targeting oncogenic signaling pathways and, more recently, to the development of immune-based therapies that seek to activate patients' own immune system in order to reinitiate the antitumor immune response. Some genomically targeted therapies, in addition to inhibiting molecular pathways driving tumor growth and maintenance, also possess immune-modulatory effects such as increasing tumor immunogenicity, in part by increasing T-cell trafficking into the tumor stroma and enhancing expression of tumor antigens. These observations raise the intriguing possibility that some genomically targeted therapies may be effectively combined with immunotherapies to improve overall clinical outcomes. Here, we discuss the preclinical data that serve as the foundation for testing genomically targeted therapies with immune checkpoint inhibitors, such as monoclonal antibodies targeting cytotoxic T-lymphocyte associated antigen 4, programmed cell death protein 1, and PD-1 ligand 1, as well as the clinical status of key combination trials.

Funding: Funded in part by National Cancer Institute grant P30 CA016672 and the Joan and Irwin Jacobs Fund philanthropic fund.

Author's Disclosures

Dr. Razelle Kurzrock receives research funds from Sequenom, Guardant, Foundation Medicine, Genentech, Pfizer, and Merck Serono, consultant fees from XBiotech and Actuate Therapeutics, and has an ownership interest in Curematch, Inc. Dr. Sandip Patel receives research funding from: Bristol-Myers Squibb, Eli Lilly, Incyte, MedImmune, Pfizer, Roche/Genentech, Xcovery.

M. Patel (✉)
UCSD-Pfizer Clinical Pharmacology-Oncology Fellow – Skaggs School of Pharmacy and Pharmaceutical Sciences, University of California, San Diego, La Jolla, CA, USA
e-mail: Maulikp03@gmail.com

S.P. Patel • R. Kurzrock
Division of Hematology/Oncology, Department of Medicine, University of California, San Diego, Moores Cancer Center, La Jolla, CA, USA
e-mail: spatel@ucsd.edu; rkurzrock@ucsd.edu

S.P. Patel, R. Kurzrock (eds.), *Early Phase Cancer Immunotherapy*, Current Cancer Research, DOI 10.1007/978-3-319-63757-0_9

Keywords Immunotherapy • Targeted therapy • Early-phase clinical trial • Combination therapy • Tumor microenvironment • Immune-checkpoint inhibitors • PD-1 • PD-L1 • CTLA-4 • Anaplastic lymphoma kinase • Epidermal growth factor receptor • Histone deacetylase inhibitor • MAPK pathway • Non-small cell lung cancer • Melanoma

9.1 Introduction

Significant scientific insights over the past two decades have led to the development/approval of targeted therapies that inhibit oncogenic drivers of cancer cell growth, along with therapies that enhances host antitumor immunity. Genomically targeted therapies provide objective clinical responses in an important subset of treated patients. However, these responses are short lived for most patients, with tumor progression occurring within months after initial response [1]. This may be due to the application of these therapies as single agents in late-stage, heavily pretreated patients who have multiple genomic alterations, many of which can mediate resistance. In contrast, the objective response rates (ORRs) with immunotherapy are observed at a much lower frequency, although many of the patients who do respond achieve long-lasting durable remission, including patients with advanced, refractory cancer [2]. Thus, a key question is how can the proportion of patients who respond to immunotherapy be increased to give more patients a chance to achieve a durable clinical remission?

To address this question, many clinical trials (Table 9.1) are underway testing combinations of targeted therapies with immune checkpoint inhibitors. The rationale for combining the two treatment modalities extends beyond the non-overlapping antitumor effects of these therapies on tumor biology and immune biology. It is increasingly being accepted that oncogenic pathways operant in cancer cells disrupt the "cancer-immunity cycle" as proposed by Chen and Mellman [3, 4] (Fig. 9.1), by contributing to the development of immunosuppressive networks within the tumor microenvironment mediated by production of immune-inhibitory soluble factors, upregulation of immune checkpoint receptors, decreasing expression of antigen processing machinery (APM) with resultant loss of expression of tumor-associated antigens (TAAs)/tumor neoantigens, and promoting recruitment and development of immunosuppressive cell populations that collectively contribute to tumor-immune escape [5]. Here, we examine the preclinical and emerging clinical evidence in support of utilizing these two treatment modalities together, the clinical trials that are planned/underway to address key questions, and the feasibility of the combination treatment from safety perspective.

Table 9.1 Key targeted therapy and immunotherapy combination trials in solid malignancies

Clinical trial ID	Status	Indication	Targeted therapy	Immunotherapy	Phase	Scheduling
NCT02224781	Recruiting	Melanoma $(BRAF^{mut})^a$	Dabrafenib + Trametinib	Ipilimumab + Nivolumab	3	Sequential
NCT01940809	Recruiting	Melanoma $(BRAF^{mut})^a$	Dabrafenib or Trametinib or Dabrafenib + Trametinib	Ipilimumab or Ipilimumab + Nivolumab	1	Sequential
NCT02723006	Recruiting	Melanoma $(BRAF^{mut})^a$ or $NRAS^{mut}$	TAK-580	Nivolumab	1	Concurrent
NCT02631447	Recruiting	Melanoma $(BRAF^{mut})^a$	LGX818 + MEK162	Ipilimumab + Nivolumab	2	Sequential
NCT01656642	Recruiting	Melanoma $(BRAF^{mut})^a$	Vemurafenib or Vemurafenib + Cobimetinib	Atezolizumab	1	Concurrent with run-in
NCT02788279	Recruiting	CRC	Cobimetinib	Atezolizumab	3	Concurrent
NCT01988896	Active-Not recruiting	CRC, NSCLC, Melanoma	Cobimetinib	Atezolizumab	1	Concurrent
NCT02625337	Recruiting	Melanoma $(BRAF^{mut})^a$	Dabrafenib + Trametinib	Pembrolizumab	2	Concurrent with run-in
NCT02818023	Recruiting	Melanoma $(BRAF^{mut})^a$	Vemurafenib	Pembrolizumab	1	Concurrent
NCT02130466	Recruiting	Melanoma $(BRAF^{mut})^a$	Dabrafenib or Trametinib or Dabrafenib + Trametinib	Pembrolizumab	1/2	Concurrent
NCT01673854	Completed	Melanoma $(BRAF^{mut})^a$	Vemurafenib	Ipilimumab	2	Sequential
NCT01767454	Completed	Melanoma $(BRAF^{mut})^a$	Dabrafenib or Dabrafenib + Trametinib	Ipilimumab	1	Concurrent with run-in

(continued)

Table 9.1 (continued)

Clinical trial ID	Status	Indication	Targeted therapy	Immunotherapy	Phase	Scheduling
NCT02200562	Active-Not recruiting	Melanoma ($BRAF^{mut}$)[a]	Dabrafenib	Ipilimumab	1/2	Concurrent
NCT02027961	Active-Not recruiting	Melanoma ($BRAF^{mut}$)[a]	Trametinib or dabrafenib + trametinib	Durvalumab	1/2	Concurrent
NCT02323126	Active-Not recruiting	NSCLC (EGFRmut)[b]	EGF816	Nivolumab	2	Concurrent
NCT01998126	Active-Not recruiting	NSCLC ($EGFR^{mut}$)[c] / NSCLC (ALK+)[d]	Erlotinib or Crizotinib	Ipilimumab or Nivolumab	1	Concurrent
NCT02393625	Recruiting	NSCLC (ALK+)[d]	Ceritinib	Nivolumab	1	Concurrent
NCT02013219	Recruiting	NSCLC ($EGFR^{mut}$)[c] / NSCLC (ALK+)[d]	Erlotinib or Alectinib	Atezolizumab	1	Concurrent
NCT02584634	Recruiting	NSCLC (ALK+)[d]	Crizotinib or Lorlatinib	Avelumab	1/2	Concurrent
NCT02574078	Recruiting	NSCLC ($EGFR^{mut}$)[c] / NSCLC (ALK+)[d]	Erlotinib or Crizotinib	Nivolumab	1/2	Concurrent
NCT02364609	Recruiting	NSCLC ($EGFR^{mut}$)[e]	Afatinib	Pembrolizumab	1	Concurrent
NCT02511184	Recruiting	NSCLC (ALK+)[d]	Crizotinib	Pembrolizumab	1	Concurrent
NCT02143466	Recruiting	NSCLC ($EGFR^{mut}$)[f]	Osimertinib	Durvalumab	1	Concurrent
NCT02453620	Recruiting	Breast cancer[g]	Entinostat	Ipilimumab + Nivolumab	1	Concurrent
NCT02635061	Not yet recruiting	NSCLC	ACY-241	Nivolumab	1	Concurrent
NCT01928576	Recruiting	NSCLC	Entinostat + Azacitidine[g]	Nivolumab	2	Concurrent

Clinical trial ID	Status	Indication	Targeted therapy	Immunotherapy	Phase	Scheduling
NCT02935790	Recruiting	Melanoma	ACY-241	Ipilimumab + Nivolumab	1	Concurrent
NCT02954991	Recruiting	NSCLC	Mocetinostat	Nivolumab	2	Concurrent
NCT02708680	Recruiting	Breast cancer[h]	Entinostat	Atezolizumab	1/2	Concurrent
NCT02437136	Recruiting	NSCLC	Entinostat	Pembrolizumab	1/2	Concurrent
NCT02538510	Recruiting	HNSCC	Vorinostat	Pembrolizumab	1/2	Concurrent
NCT02638090	Recruiting	NSCLC	Vorinostat	Pembrolizumab	1/2	Concurrent
NCT02619253	Recruiting	Renal or urothelial cell carcinoma	Vorinostat	Pembrolizumab	1	Concurrent
NCT02697630	Not yet recruiting	Uveal Melanoma	Entinostat	Pembrolizumab	2	Concurrent
NCT02395627	Recruiting	Breast cancer[i]	Vorinostat + Tamoxifen	Pembrolizumab	2	Concurrent and Sequential
NCT02032810	Recruiting	Melanoma	Panobinostat	Ipilimumab	1	Concurrent

[a]$BRAF^{V600E/K}$ mutation
[b]$EGFR^{T790M}$ mutation
[c]$EGFR^{mut}$ erlotinib sensitive
[d]ALK rearranged NSCLC
[e]$EGFR^{mut}$ erlotinib resistant
[f]EGFR mutation positive NSCLC and for T790 M directed TKI patients only- Documented T790 M positive status when the patient started on the previous T790 M directed EGFR TKI
[g]Her2-negative breast cancer
[h]Triple negative breast cancer
[i]Hormone therapy-resistant ER (+) breast cancer

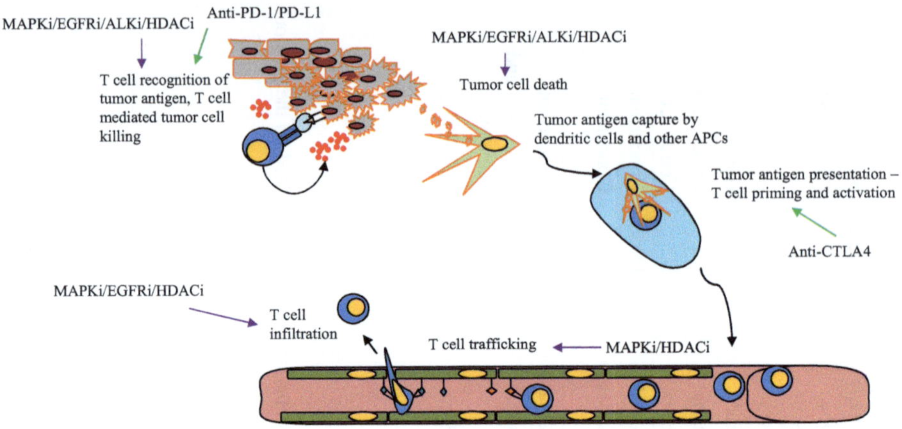

Fig. 9.1 The cancer-immunity cycle as proposed by Chen and Mellman. The development of an antitumor immune response proceeds in a stepwise manner and is initiated by shedding and the capture of tumor antigens by dendritic cells in the tumor microenvironment. These activated dendritic cells enter the tumor draining lymph node and present the tumor antigens to naïve T cells and prime them to become tumor-specific effector T cells. These activated effector T cells enter the circulation, and when appropriate chemotactic signals are present, are effectively trafficked into the tumor stroma where they recognize and carry out target cell lysis of the antigen-presenting tumor cells leading to release of additional antigen to induce subsequent rounds of antitumor immunity. Currently available immune checkpoint inhibitors function at two distinct locales, anti-CTLA4 is thought to promote T-cell priming in the lymph node, and anti-PD-1/PD-L1 are thought to promote T-cell activation and effector T-cell responses at the tumor bed. MAPKi may complement immune checkpoint inhibitors in-part by promoting ICD, enhancing tumor antigen expression, and enhancing T-cell infiltration into the tumor in-part by shutting down expression of immunosuppressive cytokines (e.g., VEGF). EGFRi and ALKi may compliment immune checkpoint inhibitors in-part by promoting ICD, enhancing tumor antigen expression, and enhancing T-cell infiltration. HDACi may compliment immune checkpoint inhibitors in part by promoting ICD, enhancing tumor antigen expression, enhancing expression of ligands recognized by Natural Killer (NK) cells leading to NK cell mediated cytotoxicity, and promoting T-cell infiltration into the tumor bed. Not depicted here are the immune suppressive cells types located in the tumor stroma and their negative impact on the cancer-immunity cycle (see text for details). Abbreviations: *ALKi* Anaplastic lymphoma kinase inhibitor, *APCs* antigen-presenting cells, *EGFRi* epidermal growth factor receptor inhibitor, *HDACi* histone deacetylase inhibitor, *ICD* immunologic cell death, *MAPKi* mitogen-activated protein kinase pathway inhibitors

9.1.1 MAPK Signaling Pathway

The mitogen-activated protein kinase (MAPK) pathway is a well-characterized oncogenic signaling pathway that has a central role in the regulation of cancer cell proliferation, survival, differentiation, and invasion. Diverse array of cytokines and growth factors signaling via G-protein coupled receptors or receptor tyrosine kinases (RTKs) transduce their growth promoting signals through the initial activation of small G-protein Ras. The small G-protein Ras has three family members (H-,

K-, and N-Ras) that function as bimolecular switches. Activated RAS (RAS bound to GTP) interacts with its downstream effectors, of which the best characterized is the RAF family of serine–threonine kinases, consisting of ARAF, BRAF, and CRAF. RAF in-turn activates dual-specificity mitogen-activated protein kinase (MEK1/MEK2). MEK1/MEK2 phosphorylates and activates two closely related extracellular signal-regulated kinases (ERK1 and ERK2). Activated ERK1/ERK2 phosphorylates and regulates the activity of a large roster of effector proteins, which can be localized in cytoplasm and nucleus. Some of the most well-described effectors of ERK1/ERK2 are transcription factors, such as ETS family of transcription factors, which regulate cell proliferation and survival [6, 7].

9.1.1.1 Mutational Activation of MAPK Signaling Pathway in Cancer

The activation of Ras-RAF-MEK-ERK signaling cascade regulates cell proliferation, survival, invasiveness, and migration [6]. It is of no surprise then that many malignancies have mutational oncogenic activation of this pathway (Fig. 9.2). Activating point mutations in *KRAS*, *NRAS*, and *HRAS* are reported to occur in up to 30% of all human malignancies [8, 9], most commonly in *KRAS* codon 12 and 13 resulting in change of glycine to aspartic acid, arginine, or valine. *KRAS* is

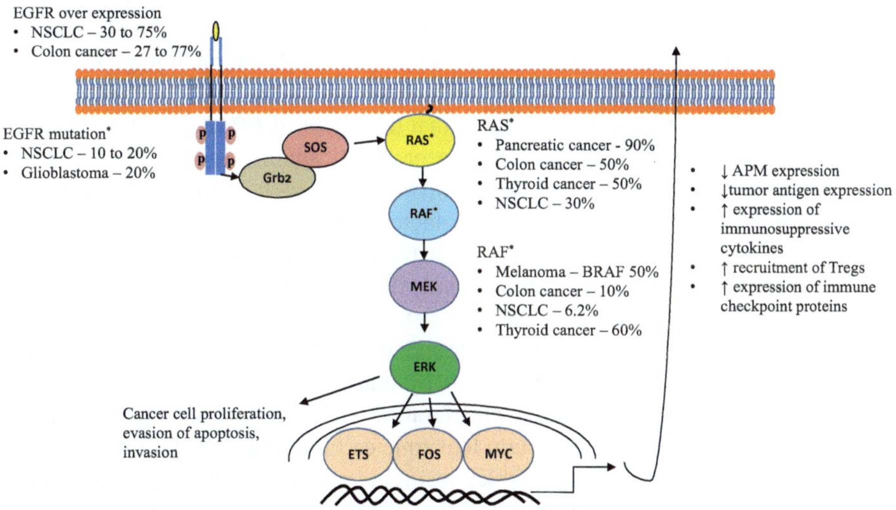

Fig. 9.2 Oncogenic activation of the MAPK signaling pathway. The incidence of mutational activation of the core components of the oncogenic MAPK signaling pathway in select solid malignancies. MAPK pathway activation is well documented to contribute to tumor growth and in promotion of tumor metastasis. In addition to classical oncogenic effects on tumor biology, it is becoming increasingly clear that MAPK pathway activation in tumors (e.g., melanoma, pancreatic cancer) also promotes cancer progression through impairment of antitumor immunity (see text for details). *Mutated in the identified solid malignancies. Abbreviations: *Grb2* growth factor receptor bound-protein 2, *SOS* son of sevenless

mutationally activated in >90% of pancreatic ductal adenocarcinoma [10]. *KRAS* and *NRAS* mutations are found in up to 50% of sporadic colorectal cancers (CRCs), with 40%–45% of tumors harboring *KRAS* mutations [11]. Oncogenic mutations of *BRAF*, of which $BRAF^{V600E}$-activating mutation is by far the most common, are found in approximately 50% of advanced melanomas, up to 60% of thyroid cancer, 10% of colon cancer, and 6.2% of lung cancer [12]. In comparison to activating mutations in *RAS* and *RAF*, similar gain-of-function mutations in MEK1/2 and ERK1/2 are rare in cancer as a whole [7]. In addition to activating mutations in the Ras-RAF-MEK-ERK signaling axis, other operant mechanisms in cancer that contribute to constitutive MAPK activation include, but are not limited to, mutational activation of RTKs, amplification of RTKs, and amplification of individual components of the MAPK signaling cascade, and decreased expression of negative regulators of the MAPK pathway (e.g., sprouty and dual-specificity phosphatases (DUSP5 and DUSP6) [12]. Evidence indicates that one or more of these combinations are often implicated as mechanisms of resistance to targeted therapies [9, 12].

9.1.1.2 MAPK Activation in Tumors Leads to a Protumor Microenvironment Through Production of Immune-Suppressive Factors

Current evidence indicates that constitutive MAPK pathway activation promotes cancer progression through impairment of antitumor immunity. Preclinical and translational studies demonstrate that immune escape by solid malignancies is supported by constitutive MAPK pathway activation in both the tumors and the stroma. One of the earliest studies demonstrated that treatment of *BRAF*-mutant melanoma cell lines with a MEK inhibitor (MEKi) or RNAi against $BRAF^{V600E}$ resulted in decreased expression of immunosuppressive factors, such as interleukin-6 (IL-6), IL-10, and vascular endothelial growth factor (VEGF) [13]. These observations were corroborated in patient samples with metastatic melanoma treated with BRAFi, where decreases in intratumoral IL-6 and IL-8 were observed [14]. Increased IL-1 expression has also been detected from $BRAF^{V600E}$ melanoma cell lines. Increased IL-1 expression was found to partly mediate cyclooxygenase-2 (COX-2) expression and PD-1 expression by tumor-associated fibroblasts found in the stroma, resulting in decreased proliferation and function of tumor-specific T cells [15]. *KRAS* alterations in certain leukemic cell lines have also been implicated in regulating signaling pathways, which result in an autocrine IL-1β production and signaling [16]. Liu et al. demonstrated that $BRAF^{V600E}$ melanoma tumors in mice treated with BRAFi had decreased VEGF production, which was directly correlated to increased T-cell infiltration. These preclinical observations were corroborated with biopsies from patients on treatment with BRAFi. Patient biopsies revealed decreased tumoral VEGF production and increased T-cell infiltration post-BRAFi treatment in comparison to baseline samples [17]. C–C motif chemokine 2 (CCL2) is another soluble factor that promotes immunosuppressive microenvironment and whose expression is thought to be regulated by BRAF/MAPK pathway activation in melanoma. Studies demonstrate that *BRAF*^{V600E} melanoma cells and *BRAF*^{V600E} mouse tumors treated with BRAFi exhibited decreased CCL2 expression. It is postulated that decreased expression of this tumor chemokine results in decreased recruitment of CD4$^+$ regulatory T cells (Tregs) into the stroma, thus promoting CD8$^+$ T-cell function [18]. Constitutive activation of the BRAF/MAPK pathway in melanoma is also implicated to have deleterious effects on the function of dendritic cells found in the tumor microenvironment mediated by immunosuppressive cytokines [19].

Increased production of IL-6 has also been observed in oncogenic *KRAS*-driven colon and pancreatic tumors, as well as from other cellular sources within the tumor microenvironment [20–22]. IL-6 contributes to cancer cell proliferation and metastasis. IL-6 also promotes development of myeloid-derived suppressor cells (MDSCs) that downregulate antitumor immunity [22, 23]. KRAS/MAPK signaling also contributes to expression of COX-2 leading to increased production of prostaglandin E_2 (PGE_2) by the tumor. PGE_2 acting in an autocrine and paracrine manner has a multiplicity of protumorigenic effects [24–26]. In pancreatic cancer, activation of the MAPK pathway by oncogenic KRAS has a significant impact on tumor microenvironment and is recognized to promote pancreatic cancer progression. Oncogenic *KRAS* has been implicated in promoting and maintaining protumorigenic stroma, in part by production of IL-6, PGE_2, and sonic hedgehog [21, 27–29]. Furthermore, these tumors also express granulocyte macrophage-colony stimulating factor (GM-CSF), which recruits MDSCs into the stroma, which negatively regulate antitumor immune responses [30, 31].

9.1.1.3 MAPK Activation in Tumors Prevents Expression of Tumor-Associated Antigens and Tumor Neoantigens

The immunogenicity of a tumor is, in part, regulated by expression and presentation of TAAs and tumor neoantigens. The expression of these antigens by tumor cells is often repressed or completely lost and is a proposed mechanism of immune escape. The mechanism by which antigen expression, processing, and presentation are regulated in tumor cells is not yet completely understood. However, the idea that classical oncogenic pathways, such as the MAPK pathway, may regulate this complex process is being investigated.

Current evidence supports the notion that constitutive MAPK signaling in solid malignancies, such as melanoma, colon, esophageal, and gastric cancers, may negatively regulate MHC Class-I (MHC-I) expression [14, 32–35]. The most abundant evidence comes from preclinical and translational studies conducted with human melanoma cell lines and patient biopsies. Boni and colleagues have demonstrated that BRAFi in *BRAF*^{V600E} -mutant cell lines and MEKi in wild-type melanoma cell lines resulted in increased expression of melanocyte differentiation antigens MART-1, gp100, Tyrp-1, and Tyrp-2. Increased expression of MART-1 and gp100 on these cell lines enhanced their recognition by antigen-specific T cells [36]. Others have similarly reported increased MHC-I expression, melanoma antigen presentation, and enhanced tumor recognition by antigen-specific T cells when the BRAF/MAPK pathway is inhibited [14, 32, 37]. In addition to increased antigen expression, BRAF/MAPK inhibition also has a positive effect on T-cell recruitment and effector function, partly by modulating the tumor microenvironment as discussed previously. Evidence from patients receiving BRAFi treatment that underwent sequential biopsies taken prior to, during, and at progression of melanoma clearly demonstrates increased infiltration of $CD4^+$, $CD8^+$, and PD-1^+ lymphocytes into the tumor stroma over the course of BRAFi treatment [38]. Others have also reported that BRAFi monotherapy in melanoma for 10–14 days increased in totality not only the number of $CD8^+$ tumor-infiltrating lymphocytes (TILs) but also increased clonality [15, 39]. Interestingly, the expression of programmed cell death-ligand 1 (PD-L1) increased over the course of BRAFi treatment when comparing the baseline biopsy to the samples taken at the time of progression, thus potentially implicating an immune-mediated mechanism of resistance to BRAFi monotherapy [38].

In colon cancer, KRAS/MAPK signaling has also been implicated in downregulation of MHC-I expression via negative regulation of the antigen processing machinery [33]. It was demonstrated that MEKi in *KRAS*^{G13D}-mutant cells increased expression of MHC-I, which was attributed to decreased DNA methyltransferase 1 (DNMT1) activity, suggesting that MHC-I expression in these cells may be epigenetically regulated. The increased expression of MHC-I was correlated with enhanced recognition and lysis by HLA-A2 specific $CD8^+$ cytotoxic T cells (CTLs) [40]. In another study, *KRAS*^{G13D}-positive tumors also had increased frequency of MHC-I loss with decreased $CD8^+$ T-cell infiltration in comparison to wild-type *KRAS* tumors [41]. Ebert et al. demonstrated that MEKi in *KRAS*^{G13D} -mutant tumors resulted not only in increased MHC-I expression but also promoted $CD8^+$ antigen-specific T-cell infiltration. Furthermore, combinations of MEKi with anti-PD-L1 yielded durable tumor regression in this colon cancer model [42]. Similar results have also been observed in a preclinical melanoma model with triple combination therapy consisting of BRAFi/MEKi/anti-PD1 treatment [43].

9.1.1.4 MAPK Inhibition with Checkpoint Inhibitors—Clinical Experience

Preclinical and translational evidence supports the testing of MAPK pathway inhibition in combination with immunotherapies in solid malignancies such as metastatic melanoma and colon cancer. However, testing these novel combinations should be conducted with initial decreased doses as combinations with ipilimumab are especially prone to toxicity. In a study reported by Ribas and colleagues that tested the BRAFi vemurafenib in combination with the CTLA-4 blocking antibody, ipilimumab, in patients with *BRAF*^{V600E}-metastatic melanoma, significant liver toxicity was observed. The dose was reduced to vemurafenib 720 mg BID (75% of the full dose), but liver toxicity persisted [44]. This study was subsequently terminated. It is unclear if further dose reduction would have abrogated toxicity.

A second study was a Phase 1/2 trial evaluating the safe use of doublet therapy—BRAFi-dabrafenib + ipilimumab—and triplet therapy—dabrafenib + MEKi-trametinib + ipilimumab—in metastatic *BRAF*$^{V600E/K}$ melanoma, which also had an early termination of the triplet arm due to two of seven patients experiencing colitis followed by intestinal perforation. It was proposed that there may be added toxicity when utilizing these two targeted agents in addition to ipilimumab because the dabrafenib at 150 mg BID + ipilimumab cohort did not experience significant adverse events (AEs) and the study continued enrollment. The added toxicity was proposed to be a result of pharmacodynamic interaction, whereby MAPK pathway inhibition increased immune cell function [45]. Most importantly, initial dose reduction may not have been adequate and may be important when drug combinations are utilized [46, 47].

Despite these earlier challenges, other Phase I studies evaluating safety and efficacy of PD-L1 blocking antibodies in combination with BRAFi and/or MEKi have shown promise. Treatment of patients in a Phase 1 study (NCT02027961) with Stage IIIc/IV melanoma with PD-L1 blocking antibody-MEDI4736 (durvalumab) + trametinib + dabrafenib (Cohort-A), without dabrafenib (Cohort-B), or sequential therapy with trametinib followed by durvalumab (Cohort-C) in patients with BRAF^{V600E} and BRAF^{WT} melanoma, demonstrated safety of the combined durvalumab with trametinib ± dabrafenib at clinically approved doses (for the targeted agents) with manageable safety profiles. Furthermore, an initial efficacy signal was also observed in all cohorts, with 16/24 patient (67%) treated with triplet therapy achieving complete response (CR) or partial response (PR). Of note, these are very early results with duration of response currently unknown. One patient in cohort A experienced dose-limiting toxicity (DLT) of grade 3 thrombocytopenia and one patient in cohort B had reversible grade 3 choroidal effusion. No other serious additive side effects were observed [48]. A similar Phase 1 study testing anti-PD-1 antibody, pembrolizumab + dabrafenib + trametinib reported three patients experiencing DLTs, which were grade 4 neutropenia, grade 4 ALT increase, and grade 3 Aspartate transaminase (AST)/Alanine transaminase (ALT) and gamma-glutamyltransferase increase. The study enrolled 15 patients with 10/15 (67%) experiencing grade 3 or 4 treatment-related AEs with five (33%) discontinuing treatment. A substantial efficacy signal was observed in 9/15 (60%) patients achieving PR [49].

These initial data further support the idea that the constitutive activation of oncogenic pathways, which contributes to development of an immunosuppressive stromal environment and/or evolution of the tumor that allows for immune escape, can be reversed with the addition of inhibitors of the oncogenic pathways in operation. In addition, these results corroborate preclinical in vivo findings that MEK inhibition does not have a detrimental impact on T-cell function [43].

Initial data from Phase 1b study (NCT01988896) in 23 patients with metastatic microsatellite stable (MSS) colorectal cancer, of which 22 harbored *KRAS* mutation, are also encouraging. In this study, the MEKi cobimetinib was given at escalating doses of 20 mg, 40 mg, and 60 mg once-daily, 21 days on, and 7 days off, along with a fixed dose of anti-PD-L1 antibody atezolizumab at 800 mg IV q2weeks. Dose expansion utilized cobimetinib 60 mg and fixed atezolizumab 800 mg. Data indicate that the combination is safe in this patient population, with 8/23 (35%) patients experiencing grade 3 AEs of which the most common were fatigue, rash, and diarrhea. Initial efficacy signal was also observed with 4/23 (17%) patients achieving PR [50]. This is an important initial finding as the vast majority (~95%) of sporadic metastatic CRC are microsatellite stable [51]. A Phase 3 study has been launched to compare the combination therapy with standard treatment in patients with refractory metastatic CRC.

9.1.1.5 Future Directions—Combination Targeted Therapies for MAPK Pathway Inhibitors with Checkpoint Inhibitors

There is clear interest in combining targeted agents inhibiting MAPK pathway and immune checkpoint inhibitors. Clinical trials listed in Table 9.1 will provide a rich mechanistic understanding of how MAPK pathway inhibition impacts intratumoral immunity (NCT01813214) and a deeper understanding of immunotherapy resistance mechanisms and how combination of targeted therapy with immunotherapy may overcome that resistant state (NCT01656642).

The Phase 2 trial NCT01813214 aims to provide prospective clinical data regarding the kinetics of pharmacodynamic effects of vemurafenib ± cobimetinib on intratumoral and host immunity in patients with metastatic $BRAF^{V600E}$ melanoma. The primary outcome is to assess the time course of $CD8^+$ T-cell infiltration into the tumor stroma with vemurafenib ± cobimetinib treatment. Other pharmacodynamic endpoints assessed over time include activation state of the TILs, changes in expression of immunoinhibitory proteins, changes in the tumor and stromal gene expression patterns from "nonimmune" to "proimmune," and determination of tumor cell lysis. Serial biopsies will be collected over 4 weeks to provide rich data, which have clear implications on combination of these targeted therapies with immunotherapies such as check-point inhibitors and adoptive cell transfer therapy.

Several other clinical trials listed in Table 9.1 conducted in melanoma, colon cancer, and NSCLC aim to answer the most pressing clinical questions. Phase 1 (NCT01940809), Phase 1/2 (NCT02130466), Phase 2 (NCT02625337), and Phase 3 (NCT02788279) trials aim to address the question of added benefit of combination therapy over either therapy administered alone, in light of potential toxicity. Phase 2 (NCT02631447), Phase 3 (NCT02224781) trials aim to address the question of ideal sequencing of these agents. There is evidence that intermittent dosing of BRAFi/MEKi in patients with BRAF-mutant melanoma may provide superior tumor control compared to continuous dosing and this is being assessed in a Phase 2 trial (NCT02196181) [52, 53]. In the setting of combination therapies, Phase 1b (NCT01656642) and Phase 2 (NCT02631447) trials aim to address the question of which regimen provides additional safety benefit and tumor control—a regimen consisting of intermittent dosing for targeted therapies in combination with immunotherapy or having a run-in period for targeted therapies followed by immunotherapy alone? The results of these studies may have a significant impact on clinical management for these tumor types.

9.1.1.6 Treatment of NSCLC Molecular Subtypes—EGFR-Mutant (mt) and ALK-Rearranged NSCLC

Over the past decade, our understanding of NSCLC has evolved from defining it as a single disease entity and treating it with one-size-fits all approach to categorizing it as a disease with multiple genomic subgroups. Approximately 85–90% of lung cancer cases are characterized as NSCLC [54]. Two of the most well-defined molecular subtypes of NSCLC are tumors harboring epidermal growth factor receptor (EGFR) mutations and anaplastic lymphoma kinase (ALK) translocations [55, 56]. Targeted treatment with EGFR or ALK tyrosine kinase inhibitors (TKIs) has high-response rates (60–70%) and very high disease control rates (85–95%) [57]. Furthermore, these targeted agents are associated with better median progression-free survival (PFS; 9–14 months) in comparison to platinum-based chemotherapy (5–7 months) [57]. Despite high response rates, most patients treated with these targeted therapies will have disease progression on treatment. Resistance mechanisms that have been identified include acquisition of secondary mutations in targeted genes, gene amplification, and activation of alternate oncogenic pathways. The latter mechanism of resistance has been demonstrated in both molecular subtypes with activation of similar alternate oncogenic pathways contributing to resistance to two different targeted therapies. As an example, resistance to ALKi treatment has been attributed to acquisition of EGFR-activating mutations [58, 59]. For these and other reasons, treatment of these molecular subtypes of NSCLC with combinations of targeted and immunotherapy will be discussed together.

9.1.1.7 EGFR Signaling in NSCLC

EGFR is one of four ErbB family members and often is presented as the prototypic RTK. These receptors contain an extracellular ligand binding domain, a short transmembrane domain, and a cytoplasmic tyrosine kinase domain. Wild-type EGFR signaling is regulated by its ligands EGF, transforming growth factor-α (TGF-α), and amphiregulin [60]. A large body of evidence has demonstrated the oncogenic potential of EGFR signaling in head and neck squamous cell carcinoma, colon, and lung cancer. Overexpression of EGFR and its ligands via gene amplification along with oncogenic activating mutations within the cytoplasmic tyrosine kinase domain establishes signaling networks that regulate cancer cell proliferation, invasion, cell survival, and evasion of immune response [60].

EGFR signaling is initiated as its cognate ligands bind to the extracellular domains inducing homo- or hetero dimerization with other ErbB family members. This interaction promotes the activation of the tyrosine kinase activity and autophosphorylation of various cytoplasmic tyrosine residues and activating the core constituent signaling networks such as the MAPK pathway, phosphatidylinositol 3-kinase (PI3K)—AKT, mammalian target of rapamycin (mTOR) pathway, and signal transducer and activator of transcription (STAT) pathway (Fig. 9.3a). Transcriptional networks regulated by EGFR signaling have also been implicated in regulating tumor microenvironment and the antigen processing machinery, contributing to tumor immune evasion [60].

9.1.1.8 *EGFR* Aberrations in NSCLC

Wild-type EGFR is overexpressed in 30–75% of NSCLC tumors, and *EGFR* gene amplification is observed in ~30–45% NSCLC tumors. However, studies addressing the impact of EGFR overexpression or gene amplification as a predictor of survival after treatment with EGFR TKIs have reported conflicting results [61]. In contrast, clinical data clearly demonstrate improved PFS in patients with somatic mutations in EGFR. Approximately 10–20% of all patients with advanced NSCLC harbor activating mutations within the cytoplasmic kinase domain of EGFR [55]. This number increases to 50% in certain subpopulations such as patients with East Asian ancestry, never smokers, and women, with adenocarcinoma histology [55, 60, 62].

The majority of EGFR mutations occur within exons 18–21 in the tyrosine kinase domain. Up to 45% of the mutations are due to a single nonsynonymous mutation in exon 21, with substitution of arginine for leucine at codon 858--$EGFR^{L858R}$. The other most prevalent mutations, accounting for another 45% of alterations, are in-frame deletions of exon 19, with deletion of E746-A750 ($\mathrm{EGFR}^{\Delta E746-750}$) being the most common [60]. These two alterations have demonstrated to be sensitive to EGFR inhibition with gefitinib, erlotinib, and afatinib [55, 62–64]. As previously discussed, mutation in the tyrosine kinase domain is one mechanism of resistance observed in patients that progress on EGFR TKIs. In fact, the most common EGFR mutation that is associated with first-generation EGFR TKI resistance, as observed in 50% of treated patients, occurs within exon 20 at codon 790--EGFR^{T790M} [61, 65]. Tumors with this mutation are sensitive to osimertinib. Recently, EGFR mutation (EGFR^{C797S}) associated with resistance to second-generation EGFR TKI, osimertinib, was reported [66].

9.1.1.9 *ALK* Translocation in NSCLC

Approximately 3–7% of all NSCLC cases harbor expression of a highly oncogenic chimeric tyrosine kinase fusion protein—echinoderm microtubule-associated protein-like 4-*ALK* (*EML4-ALK*). *EML4-ALK* is a product of chromosome 2p inversion [67]. Patients with ALK-rearranged NSCLC are often younger men, with adenocarcinoma histology, and never or former light smokers [68]. The most common variant identified in NSCLC cases is the *EML4-ALK* fusion variant 1. Other fusion variants of *EML4-ALK* are a product of different fusion breakpoints occurring at exons 2, 6, 13, 14, 15, 18, or 20 of the *EML4* gene [69]. The breakpoint within the *ALK* gene is conserved and contains the entire ALK tyrosine kinase domain [68]. The transcription of the *ALK* fusion oncogene is under the control of the regulatory elements in the promoter region of the fusion partner. The kinase activity is independent of ligand but dependent upon the N-terminal fusion partners' ability to undergo

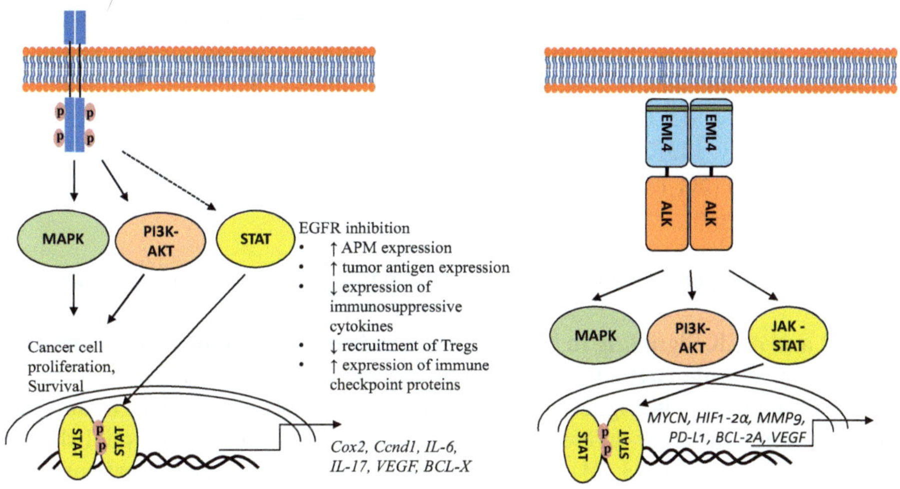

Fig. 9.3 (**a**) EGFR signaling in NSCLC. The major downstream pathways activated by EGFR mutations are MAPK, PI3K-AKT-mTOR, and STAT signaling pathways. Of these, the activation of STAT3 in EGFR mutant NSCLC is thought to be an indirect effect of EGFR signaling (as indicated by *dashed lines*). The increased expression of IL-6, as a result of EGFR signaling, acting in autocrine/paracrine manner contributes to constitutive STAT3 signaling in NSCLC. Transcriptional networks regulated by EGFR signaling in NSCLC (e.g., STAT3) can increase the expression of immunosuppressive cytokines which promotes accumulation and expansion of immune suppressive cell types (e.g., Tregs), and decreases the trafficking of effector T cells. In addition, EGFR signaling in NSCLC increases PD-L1 expression, and decreases NKG2DL expression contributing to tumor-immune escape (see text for details). Abbreviation: *BCL-X* B-cell lymphoma-extra large, *Cyclin D1* Ccnd1. (**b**) *ALK signaling in NSCLC.* EML4 is the most common fusion partner found in ALK translocated NSCLC. EML4-ALK activity is regulated independent of ligand and is dependent on the ability of the fusion partner to undergo dimerization (*green band* representing a coiled-coil domain). The major signaling pathways activated downstream of ALK in NSCLC are MAPK, PI3K-AKT-mTOR, and JAK-STAT pathways which in turn regulate transcription of the indicated genes (e.g., MYCN, VEGF, PD-L1). Currently, the cancer secretome produced by transcriptional networks regulated specifically by ALK signaling is unknown. Additionally, how these soluble factors help establish a protumor microenvironment and promote tumor-immune escape is also not known (see text for details)

dimerization or oligomerization. *EML4* contains a coiled-coil domain that mediates *EML4-ALK* dimerization and constitutive ALK fusion protein activity [67, 68].

9.1.1.10 ALK Signaling in NSCLC

A complete picture of molecular signaling pathways activated by the ALK fusion protein in NSCLC is complex. The N-terminal fusion partner not only regulates kinase activity but also determines its subcellular distribution [56]. This can have a direct impact on the pathways activated by the oncogene. In addition to *EML4-ALK* fusion oncogene, other fusion partners have also been identified, although they are less frequent [70, 71]. The *EML4-ALK* fusion oncogene activates many of the same signaling pathways as those observed in cell lines and clinical samples harboring *EGFR* mutations. Preclinical and translational studies have demonstrated that *EML4-ALK* in NSCLC cell lines and patient derived tumors activate the RAS-MAPK pathway, PI3K-AKT-mTOR pathway, and Janus kinase (JAK)-STAT pathway (Fig. 9.3b) [56, 72].

9.1.1.11 Oncogene-Driven NSCLC—Impact on Tumor Immunogenicity

EGFR and ALK Signaling in NSCLC Tumors Promote Production of Immune-Inhibitory Soluble Factors Activation of oncogenic signaling pathways in tumors has been implicated in triggering immunosuppressive networks, in part by increasing expression of tumor-derived soluble factors that contribute to the establishment of a protumor stroma [73, 74]. A number of cytokines are elevated in patients with lung cancer and their possible role in promoting tumor progression is currently under investigation [75]. However, studies addressing the cytokine profiles associated with *EGFR*- or ALK-aberrant molecular subtypes of NSCLC are lacking. Furthermore, how the cytokine profiles change over the course of treatment with targeted agents is still unclear.

Studies have demonstrated that *EGFR*-mutant NSCLC cell lines and patient-derived tumors express IL-6, and this expression can partially be abrogated by EGFR inhibition [76, 77]. At the same time, *EGFR*-mutant cancer cell lines resistant to erlotinib have also demonstrated increase in IL-6 production when exposed to erlotinib; the latter is proposed as a mechanism of resistance to erlotinib treatment [78, 79]. The increase in IL-6 levels, functioning in an autocrine and paracrine manner, has a direct impact on the tumor itself and on the stroma. Increased IL-6 signaling via IL-6/gp-130/JAK/STAT3 pathway is implicated as a mechanism of resistance for EGFR treatment. IL-6 signaling has a direct effect on tumor cells by increasing phosphorylated STAT3 (pSTAT3) levels [77]. Persistent activation of STAT3 has been noted in 50% of lung adenocarcinomas, and evidence indicates that it contributes to cell cycle progression, prevention of apoptosis, tumor invasion/metastasis, and cell survival [74, 77, 80]. This is in part accomplished through STAT3-mediated transcriptional upregulation of diverse soluble factors, such as VEGF, which can inhibit dendritic cell maturation and promote stromal accumulation of immunosuppressive cells such as MDSCs [81, 82].

VEGF is a validated target in NSCLC and a well-characterized immune suppressive factor in many solid malignancies [83, 84]. Expression of VEGF in NSCLC has been documented in vitro in lung cancer cell lines and in patient tumor biopsies [82]. VEGF expression in *EGFR*-mutant tumors has multiple layers of regulation. In addition to EGFR directly regulating VEGF expression [85], autocrine signaling of IL-6, as observed in *EGFR*-mutant tumors, can also increase VEGF expression [77, 82]. The tumor stroma can also serve as a source of VEGF production, which can also contribute to resistance to EGFR TKIs [86].

IL-8 is another soluble factor that is a positive regulator of tumor cell proliferation, angiogenesis, and metastasis. In NSCLC cell lines, tumor xenografts, and clinical samples, IL-8 production has been correlated with EGFR activity [87, 88]. A clinical biomarker study evaluating small cohort of patients with *EGFR*-mutant NSCLC reported a decrease in IL-8 expression 30 days posttreatment initiation with gefitinib or erlotinib, when compared to baseline [88]. In a more comprehensive immune profiling study, Akbay and colleagues demonstrated in a murine *EGFR*-driven lung cancer model an increase in multiple protumor cytokines such as VEGF, IL-6, TGF-β1, CCL2, and GM-CSF in bronchoalveolar lavage (BAL) samples in comparison to the BAL samples from nontumor-bearing mice [89].

In comparison to *EGFR*-mutant NSCLC subtype, very little is known concerning the way in which ALK signaling in NSCLC may promote the establishment of a protumor microenvironment, perhaps in part through the production of immune-inhibitory soluble factors. One may speculate based on the knowledge that because *EGFR*-mutant and *ALK*- aberrant NSCLC tumors share similar tissue type, share similar core signaling networks leading to regulation of shared transcriptional networks, some of the immune-inhibitory soluble factors known to be produced by *EGFR*-mutant NSCLC tumors may also be generated by *ALK*-aberrant NSCLC tumors. As an example, STAT3 signaling is observed in both molecular subtypes. In NSCLC cell lines and tumor tissues harboring *EML4-ALK*, increased phospho-STAT3 levels are noted, which can be abrogated through pharmacological inhibition of ALK with crizotinib or PF-06463922 [72, 90–92]. STAT3 signaling not only contributes to "traditional oncogenesis" by activating prosurvival signaling pathways within tumor cells but also propagates cross-talk between the tumor microenvironment and the tumor itself through transcriptional regulation of wide range of soluble factors (e.g., VEGF, IL-6, IL-10). These factors signaling in a paracrine manner through their cognate receptors activate STAT3 signaling in stromal MDSCs, dendritic cells, and Tregs in order to further propagate the immunosuppressive tumor microenvironment [74, 81]. The extrapolation of the understanding gained from *EGFR*-mutant tumor biology needs to be confirmed in *ALK*-aberrant NSCLC tumors. A comprehensive understanding of the secretome produced as a result of constitutive oncogenic signaling and the impact these soluble factors may have on establishment of the protumor microenvironment may provide important targets for cancer immunotherapy.

9.1.1.12 Regulation of the Antigen Processing Machinery and Immune-Checkpoint Ligands in *EGFR*-Mutant and *ALK*-Translocated NSCLC

EGFR signaling in NSCLC regulates expression of molecules, which in part determines tumor immunogenicity. In vitro studies utilizing *EGFR*-mutant and wild-type NSCLC cell lines demonstrated that EGFR signaling inhibits expression of natural killer group 2, member D ligands (NKG2DLs—e.g., ULBP1, ULBP2, MICA), which are utilized by natural killer (NK) cells and $CD8^+$ T cells. Inhibition of EGFR signaling with EGFR TKIs in these cancer cell lines increased membrane expression of NKG2D ligand ULBP1 and promoted NK-cell-mediated cytotoxicity [93, 94]. Studies conducted in normal and malignant keratinocytes indicate that EGFR inhibition promotes MHC-I expression. This finding was corroborated in skin biopsies from a limited number of patients who were being treated with erlotinib or cetuximab (monoclonal antibody targeting EGFR) [95]. These findings have also been observed in NSCLC cell lines harboring EGFR mutations. Brea and colleagues demonstrated that treatment of the *EGFR*-mutant NSCLC cell line with afatinib increased MHC-I expression. This was in part due to increases in expression of individual components that make up the antigen-presenting machinery (e.g., TAP1, TAP2, and β_2M) [96]. Furthermore, EGFR signaling in NSCLC has also been implicated in regulating PD-L1 expression and may represent a pathway of immune escape [89, 96–99]. However, a consensus for the signaling pathway downstream of EGFR regulating PD-L1 expression has not been reached, though MAPK pathway and PI3K-AKT-mTOR signaling pathways have been implicated [96, 97]. Nonetheless, preclinical data demonstrated that pharmacological blockage of PD-L1 in a murine EGFR-driven lung cancer model resulted in tumor reduction and greater overall survival [89]. However, the prognostic value of PD-L1 expression in *EGFR*-mutant NSCLC is currently debated [98, 99].

PD-L1 expression is also increased in *ALK*-aberrant NSCLC cell lines and in tumor specimens [97, 98, 100, 101]. Both in vitro and in vivo studies have implicated MEK-ERK and PI3K-AKT-mTOR signaling pathways in regulating PD-L1 expression in *ALK*-aberrant NSCLC [97, 100]. It is interesting to note that two distinct oncogenes, EGFR and ALK, occurring in the same tissue type share common signaling pathways for regulation of PD-L1 expression. However, there is conflicting data concerning which molecular subtype more strongly and frequently expresses PD-L1, which may indicate accessory, as yet unidentified pathways operating in these tumors contributing to PD-L1 expression. It should be noted that other reports have concluded that *EGFR* mutations and PD-L1 expression are not correlated in NSCLC [102]. The high variability in the reported frequency of PD-L1 positivity in these molecular subtypes can in part be explained by the current lack of standardization of PD-L1 testing. Currently, several factors add variability that contributes to the inconsistencies in the reports with regards to PD-L1 positivity: a number of different PD-L1 antibodies and PD-L1 scoring protocols and use of different platforms and different cut-off ranges [103, 104].

9.1.1.13 EGFR and ALK Inhibition in Combination with Immunotherapy—Current Clinical Experience

EGFR- and ALK-driven NSCLC have operating signaling pathways that upregulate PD-L1 expression. Current analysis indicates that increased PD-L1 expression is associated with higher ORR to PD-1/PD-L1 inhibitors in NSCLC [105]. Based on these observations, single-agent PD-1/PD-L1 inhibitors were tested in the clinic in these two molecular subtypes. The results are discouraging as only ~10% of the patients with EGFR mutations had clinical response without any observed survival benefit over chemotherapy [106, 107]. Currently, not much is known regarding response rates in *ALK*-aberrant NSCLC. Retrospective analysis of EGFR- and ALK-driven NSCLC conducted by Gainor and colleagues [101] further support these results. In this analysis, objective responses to PD-1/PD-L1 inhibitors were observed in only 1/28 (3.6%) of *EGFR*-mutant or *ALK*-aberrant NSCLC patient versus confirmed objective response in 7/30 patients (23.3%) with normal *EGFR* and *ALK* genes. Furthermore, in an independent cohort, the tumor immune microenvironment in *EGFR*-mutant ($n = 68$) and *ALK*-rearranged ($n = 27$) NSCLC tumors was assessed. The findings indicate that majority of *EGFR*-mutant tumors lacked concurrent PD-L1 expression and high $CD8^+$ TILs. Similar results were seen in *ALK*-rearranged lung cancers. Furthermore, analysis of paired, pre- and post-TKI resistant biopsies revealed an increase in PD-L1 expression in 12/57 (21%) of EGFRi-resistant biopsies without an observed change in the presence of $CD8^+$ TILs. Analysis of ALKi-resistant biopsies did not significantly differ from pretreatment in regards to PD-L1 expression and presence of $CD8^+$ TILs [101]. The lack of response reported may be due to the innate immune resistance conferred by the constitutive oncogenic signaling (EGFR and ALK) upregulating PD-L1, whereas in adaptive immune resistance, the stimuli for tumoral upregulation of PD-L1 are the inflammatory signals (e.g., IFN-γ) produced during an active antitumor immune response [108]. The former mechanism of upregulating PD-L1 may confer resistance to single-agent checkpoint inhibitors [108]. Additionally, the lack of response may also be related to the low tumor nonsynonymous somatic mutational burden associated with these molecular subtypes as these patients are often never smokers. The study by Rizvi and colleagues clearly demonstrated that the response to anti-PD-1 treatment in NSCLC was associated with high nonsynonymous mutational burden resulting in higher tumor neoantigen load [109–111]. Beyond resistance, a recent study suggests that some patients with *EGFR* mutations may experience accelerated tumor growth—hyperprogression—on anti-PD1/PD-L1 checkpoint inhibitors. Early studies suggest that patients with *MDM2* amplification or *EGFR* alterations may be more vulnerable to this problem. The etiology of hyperprogression is still under investigation. However, it is plausible that combining checkpoint inhibitors with *MDM2* or *EGFR* inhibitors could ameliorate the accelerated progression [112, 113].

From these data and other studies, the strategy of using combinations of PD-1/PD-L1 inhibitors and targeted agents has emerged. Additional rationale for this approach is based on the observation that the highly active targeted therapies, such as EGFR and ALK TKIs, increase tumor cell apoptosis with resultant increase in tumor antigen shedding, which may promote immune cell influx into the stroma, with resultant increase in proinflammatory cytokine production. This may lead to synergistic activity with PD-1/PD-L1 inhibitors as the targeted treatment may help establish an antitumor microenvironment in part by shutting down oncogene -driven expression of immunosuppressive factors and the use of PD-1/PD-L1 inhibitors would overcome the adaptive immune resistance brought on by the production of inflammatory cytokines in the stromal compartment [114]. Furthermore, it is suggested that inhibition of ALK in the tumor-infiltrating T cells located in the tumor stromal compartment may promote an increase of antitumor T-cell proliferation [115]. Preliminary results from studies combining targeted therapies and immunotherapy in these two molecular subtypes of NSCLC are discussed below.

Interim analysis from an ongoing Phase 1 study (NCT01454102) assessing the safety and response of nivolumab 3 mg/kg IV q2weeks plus erlotinib 150 mg QD in EGFR (mt) NSCLC revealed that the combination treatment may provide durable clinical benefit with an acceptable safety profile. The study has enrolled 21 patients, with only one patient that was TKI naïve at enrollment. Grade 3 or 4 treatment-related AEs were observed in 4/21 patients (19%): increase in AST ($n = 2$) or ALT ($n = 1$) and weight loss and diarrhea (one patient each). Two patients discontinued the treatment due to Grade 3 AST increase and Grade 2 nephritis. No pneumonitis of any grade was observed. In this study ORR was reported in 4/21 (19%) of the patients and 24 week PFS was 47%. The TKI-naïve patient had achieved a PR with duration of response (DOR) of 24.3 weeks and was ongoing at the time of data cut-off. The interim results suggest that combination therapy may provide durable clinical benefit with acceptable safety profile in TKI refractory advanced *EGFR*-mutant NSCLC [116].

Another Phase 1 study (NCT02088112) assessed the safety and efficacy of the anti-PD-L1 antibody durvalumab 10 mg/kg IV q2weeks in combination with gefitinib 250 mg QD in TKI-naïve NSCLC patients with confirmed *EGFRi*-sensitizing mutations. The study had two arms: in Arm 1, patients ($n = 10$) are treated with a combination of durvalumab and gefitinib; in Arm 2, patients ($n = 10$) are first treated with gefitinib for 4 weeks prior to starting the combination treatment. At the time of data cut-off, follow up was ≥3 months for all patients. The combination treatment was considered to be tolerable. Grade 3 or 4 treatment-related AEs that led to discontinuation occurred in 4/20 (20%) patients, all in Arm 2, with three patients experiencing increased AST and/or ALT, and one patient experiencing pneumonitis. At ≥ 8 weeks, out of 19 evaluable patients, 7/9 (77.8%) patients in Arm 1 and 8/10 (80%) patients in Arm 2 had documented responses. These initial findings of activity further support evaluation of combination treatment in TKI-naïve, *EGFR*-mutant NSCLC patients [117].

In contrast to the previous findings, two other clinical trials (NCT02143466 and NCT02454933) both testing a next generation EGFR TKI osimertinib, targeting the *EGFR* T790 M mutation, used in combination with durvalumab in patients with *EGFR*-mutant NSCLC in both treatment- naïve and EGFR TKI resistance due to T790 M mutation, reported mixed results. Preliminary data from NCT02143466 indicate that the combination of osimertinib 80 mg QD, and durvalumab at 3 mg/kg or 10 mg/kg IV q2weeks is active, as 20/31 (65%) of patients had achieved PR. However, the safety profile was not optimal. In this study, 13/34 (38%) of treated patients had experienced pneumonitis with five of the patients experiencing Grade 3 or 4 pneumonitis. The frequency of pneumonitis occurring with combination treatment was significantly greater than that reported for osimertinib (2.9%) and durvalumab (2%) when used as single agents suggesting that there is synergistic toxicity when these two specific agents are used together because current experience with erlotinib or gefitinib with PD-1/PD-L1 inhibitors seem not to result in this

AE at this high rate. Based on these findings NCT02454933 trial was prematurely halted with no future plans of pursing this combination [118]. It is, therefore, unclear if dose reduction would have salvaged this study.

9.1.1.14 Future Directions—EGFR and ALK TKI with Immunotherapy

Although the data are premature, there are positive efficacy signals from limited number of Phase 1 studies testing combinations of EGFR TKIs with checkpoint inhibitors. Additionally, results from several of these studies also highlight the need for careful monitoring for immune and other toxicities and also suggest that dose reduction is in order, at least initially, when administering combinations. The potential safety concern with coadministration of EGFR TKIs and immunotherapy agents is the occurrence of overlapping toxicities involving various organ systems such as skin, gastrointestinal tract, liver, and lung. The safety data from some studies with EGFR TKIs combined with anti-PD1/PD-L1 antibody demonstrate that these combinations can be safely administered together. Ultimately larger trials will be needed to address if combination treatment in EGFR TKI-naïve or -experienced patients provides substantial benefits over the use of EGFR TKIs as monotherapy.

Similarly, combination treatment with crizotinib (or next generation ALK TKIs) and immune check point inhibitors are currently being tested in multiple Phase 1 studies (Table 9.1). The potential safety concerns of interest for testing ALK TKIs with immunotherapy are the overlapping toxicities effecting the gastrointestinal tract, liver, and lung. All currently approved ALK TKIs (crizotinib, ceritinib, and alectinib) have the potential to cause pneumonitis, hepatotoxicity, and gastrointestinal-related AEs. Currently, we do not have adequate preliminary data regarding the safety and tolerability of these two combinations for treatment of *ALK*-aberrant NSCLC. These ongoing studies will provide the initial data to help determine if patients with this molecular subtype can have their initial tumor responses consolidated into long-lived durable responses.

9.1.1.15 Histone Deacetylase Inhibitors (HDACis) and Immunotherapy

Immunotherapy confers a durable response predominantly to "immunogenic" tumors characterized as tumors with high somatic nonsynonymous mutational burden, high pretreatment expression of PD-1/PD-L1 on tumor cells and infiltrating immune cells, and high pretreatment levels of TILs [109, 119–122]. However, many tumors are not characterized as "immunogenic," hence the modest percentages of patients treated with immunotherapy achieving durable clinical response. Thus, far, we have discussed how oncogene regulated signaling pathways within tumors can promote a protumor microenvironment. Additional mechanism by which tumor immunogenicity may be regulated is by reversible epigenetic modifications. Accumulating evidence suggests that pharmacological agents targeting one class of epigenetic modifiers—histone deacetylases (HDACs)—can promote antitumor immune responses by increased expression of a variety of mediators and effectors involved in immune system activation.

9.1.1.16 Epigenetic Modification Overview—HDAC in Cancer Development and Progression

Cancer is a disease initiated and fueled by germline/somatic aberrations within the genome. These aberrations often directly impact the epigenetic regulatory proteins leading to the acquisition of a cancer epigenome that contributes to the induction and maintenance of the cancer. Conrad Waddington in 1961 coined the term epigenetics to describe reversible, heritable genetic changes that impact cellular phenotype without incurring any changes in DNA sequences [123, 124]. Currently, the term epigenetics is used to describe the dynamic processes that regulate chromatin structure and how it impacts DNA-based processes of transcription, DNA replication, and repair [123].

Chromatin is a macromolecular complex consisting of DNA and histone proteins. The basic functional subunit of chromatin is a nucleosome, which consists of an octamer of four core histone proteins (H2A, H2B, H3, and H4), which serves as the scaffold for the negatively charged DNA that is wrapped around the histone octamer core. Covalent modifications made directly on the DNA and histones by epigenetic regulators alter chromatin structure through noncovalent interactions within and between nucleosomes; this process has a direct effect on gene transcription [123, 125]. The best-studied epigenetic modification is DNA methylation. However, the most diverse epigenetic modifications occur on the N-terminal tails of histones and include methylation, acetylation, phosphorylation, ubiquitination, sumoylation, proline isomerization, and ADP ribosylation [123, 125].

Epigenetic modifications are dynamically controlled by epigenetic regulators that can be divided into three distinct functional groups: (i) epigenetic writers, such as DNA methyltransferases or histone acetyltransferases that lay down specific epigenetic marks on DNA or N-terminal tail of histones, respectively; (ii) epigenetic readers, such as bromodomain containing BET (bromodomain and extraterminal) family of proteins, which recognize specific epigenetic marks and help recruit other chromatin modifiers or remodeling complexes to alter chromatin structure and function; and (iii) epigenetic erasers—such as HDACs—which are a family of enzymes that reverse the covalent modification such as acetylation on N-terminal tails of histones [125]. Pharmacological inhibitors for DNA methyltransferases and HDACs are currently approved for treatment of range of malignancies, along with great interest and progress made toward developing pharmacological inhibitors of BET family of proteins [124]. Here, we focus primarily on HDACis.

There are three classical classes of HDACs (Class I, II (a and b), IV) that require Zn^{2+} for catalytic activity. Class III HDACs, also referred to as sirtuins, which differ in structure and function from other deacetylases, require NAD^{+} for activity. Class I HDACs (HDAC 1–3 and 8) are primarily localized in the nucleus and are the major mediators of histone deacetylation. Class IIa HDACs (HDAC 4, 5, 7, and 9), Class

IIb HDACs (HDAC 6 and 10) are able to shuttle between nucleus and cytoplasm or are restricted to the cytoplasm [125, 126]. With the ability to change subcellular localization, the main protein substrates for Class II HDACs can be histone and nonhistone proteins. HDAC 11 is the only identified HDAC in Class IV, which also is able to shuttle between nucleus and cytoplasm [125, 127].

HDACs are one example of epigenetic enzymes that are often deregulated in human tumors, primarily through altered expression or inappropriate recruitment to certain gene loci via binding to oncogenic fusion proteins [125]. In fact, aberrant recruitment of HDACs by oncogenic fusion proteins to certain gene loci leads to HDAC-mediated gene silencing and contributes to leukemogenesis [125, 127]. As an example, the oncogenic fusion protein acute myeloid leukemia 1-eight-twenty-one (AML1-ETO) found in patients with t(8;21) AML recruits class I HDAC-containing complexes to repress AML1 target genes, thus preventing myeloid differentiation and resulting in cellular transformation [128]. As a consequence, HDACis are potent inducers of terminal differentiation and apoptosis in AML1-ETO expressing leukemia [125, 127, 129].

Somatic mutations in HDACs are not prominent in cancer [123, 130]. However, overexpression of individual HDACs in several solid malignancies such as breast, lung, colon, liver, and gastric cancers is correlated with a decrease in both disease-free and overall survival [127, 131–135]. The overexpression of HDACs in these cancers is correlated to key events in tumorigenesis such as cell cycle progression, cell proliferation, and resistance to apoptosis [125, 127]. HDACs can contribute to these key events through their actions on histone and nonhistone targets. As a principle mechanism, overexpression of Class I HDACs has been linked to epigenetic silencing of tumor suppressor genes such as cyclin-dependent kinase inhibitor (*CDKN1A*), DNA repair genes—ataxia telangiectasia and Rad3 (*ATR*) and breast cancer 1, early onset (*BRCA1*) [127, 136, 137]. In addition, HDACs, either directly or indirectly, regulate the activity of an ever-growing list of nonhistone proteins, which include transcription factors (e.g., p53, STATS, Bcl6, FoxP3), DNA repair proteins (e.g., Ku70), chaperones (e.g., heat-shock protein 90 HSP90), and cytoskeletal proteins (e.g., α-tubulin). Post-translational regulation of these nonhistone proteins by HDACs can lead to altered transcription factor activity and changes in gene transcription, dysregulation of cellular signaling pathways, and inhibition of protein degradation contributing to key biological processes of apoptosis, cell cycle regulation, and differentiation [127, 136, 138, 139].

9.1.1.17 HDACs—Epigenetic Regulators of Tumor Immunogenicity

The protumorigenic effects of HDACs via regulation of cell cycle progression, resistance to apoptosis, and cell proliferation are well studied. In addition to these effects, accumulating evidence implicates HDACs in promoting tumor immune escape through various mechanisms resulting in tumor progression. These mechanisms include regulating expression of immunosuppressive soluble factors by tumor cells, increased resistance to immune cell-mediated apoptosis, and reduced immune recognition of tumor cells. Here, we will discuss the growing preclinical and clinical evidence that supports the use of HDACis in combination with immune checkpoint inhibitors, as a way to overcome tumor immune escape.

Cancer cells can promote immune escape through development of an immunosuppressive tumor microenvironment via production of cytokines and growth factors (e.g., VEGF, TGF-β, IL-6). Indeed, HDACs have been implicated in regulation of VEGF production in cancer cells by both epigenetic and nonepigenetic-mediated mechanisms [140]. In HepG2, a hepatocellular carcinoma cell line and Lewis lung carcinoma tumor model, HDAC activity was demonstrated to be increased under hypoxic conditions leading to upregulation of VEGF expression [141]. Overexpression of HDAC1 in HepG2 cells also increased VEGF expression [141]. Mazumdar and colleagues demonstrated that VEGF production in basal-type breast cancer cell lines is regulated by corepressor for element-1-silencing transcription factor (CoREST1). HDAC1/2 dimer along with lysine-specific demethylase-1 (LSD1) make up the catalytic core of this large multiprotein transcriptional corepressor complex, CoREST1 [142]. Downregulation of CoREST1 expression decreased VEGF production in vitro and in vivo [143]. The increase in VEGF production by these tumor cells promotes angiogenesis to fuel tumor growth. In addition to promoting angiogenesis, VEGF along with other angiogenic growth factors produced by tumors have a direct impact on tumor vasculature by downregulating endothelial adhesion molecules such as intercellular adhesion molecule-1 (ICAM-1) and vascular cell adhesion molecule-1 (VCAM-1), which are critical for efficient chemotaxis of leukocytes [144–146]. VEGF-mediated downregulation of ICAM-1 decreases leukocyte and tumor vessel interactions, ultimately limiting leukocyte endothelial transmigration into the tumor stroma [144, 147]. In addition, immune escape can also occur through inhibiting expression of chemokines responsible for recruitment of effector T cells to the tumor site. Zheng and colleagues, clearly demonstrated in lung cancer cell lines and multiple lung tumor models that expression of CCL5, C-X-C motif chemokine 9 (CXCL9), and CXCL10 is negatively regulated by HDACs [148]. The use of pan-HDACis, romidepsin and vorinostat, increased expression of these T-cell chemokines by the tumor and resulted in recruitment of $CD4^+$ and $CD8^+$ T cells into the tumor stroma [148]. Romidepsin treatment alone in syngeneic immune-competent tumor-bearing mice stabilized the disease, which was dependent on the production of T-cell chemokines, and the subsequent recruitment of the effector T cells into the tumor compartment [148]. Furthermore, romidepsin increased PD-L1 expression on tumor cells and that combined treatment of anti-PD-1 antibody and romidepsin led to significant reduction in tumor growth and, in the majority of the mice, complete rejection of the tumor, which was not observed in mice treated with either single agent therapies [148]. These reports demonstrate the role of HDACs in regulating expression of soluble factors, which prevents accumulation of effector T cells in the tumor compartment as a mechanism of immune escape. Ongoing comprehensive studies addressing the role of HDACs in regulating the cancer secretome, and how it impacts the communication networks between tumor, tumor stroma, and stromal resident immune cells will be critical in understanding the part played by HDACs in promoting tumor immune escape and potentially providing new therapeutic targets.

9.1.1.18 HDACi Mediated Regulation of Tumor-Immunogenicity—Regulation of Antigen-Presenting Machinery and Immune-Stimulatory and Immune-Inhibitory Molecule Expression

HDACis may regulate tumor immunogenicity through various mechanisms. HDACis, such as vorinostat, induce immunogenic cell death. Immunogenic cell death is a process by which cell death promotes an immune response, as the dying cells present signals such as calreticulin translocation, ATP release, and high mobility group box-1 (HMGB1) protein release from the dying cells, which are sensed by antigen-presenting cells (APCs) leading to APC infiltration, engulfment of dying cell antigens, and ultimately MHC-dependent activation of T cells, thus promoting activation, proliferation, and infiltration of cytotoxic T-lymphocytes and other immune cells into the tumor stroma to mediate tumor destruction [149, 150]. Christiansen and colleagues demonstrated that vorinostat-induced apoptosis of a colon cancer cell line increased surface expression of calreticulin and release of HMGB1. It was suggested that HDACi-mediated apoptosis was found to be critical for tumor eradication [151]. Indeed, the follow-up report confirmed that vorinostat promoted calreticulin surface expression, ATP and HMGB1 release in vivo in a colon cancer mouse model [152]. Furthermore, even though vorinostat-induced apoptosis in both immune-competent and immune-compromised tumor-bearing mice, only the immune-competent mice treated with vorinostat had long-term anti-cancer effects, indicating that an intact immune system is required for therapeutic effects of vorinostat [152].

HDACis also improve tumor immunogenicity by transcriptional regulation of NKG2DL [153]. Multiple reports now have clearly demonstrated that HDACis such as, trichostatin A (TSA), sodium valproate, and vorinostat, increases the expression of MICA, MICB, and ULBP1–ULBP3 in various epithelial tumor cell lines and in Ewing sarcoma cell lines [154–157]. Importantly, valproate-induced increase in MICA and MICB was not observed in primary nonmalignant human hepatocytes [154]. Furthermore, the expression of these NKG2DLs enhanced NK cell-mediated cytotoxicity [154, 156–159].

In addition to increasing expression of NKG2DLs, HDACis also increases tumor cell recognition by immune cells by increasing expression of APM, MHC-I, and MHC-II (Fig. 9.4) [160]. This is best exemplified in melanoma where several studies support the role of HDACs in epigenetic regulation of APM expression. LAQ824, a Class I and II HDACi, demonstrated an increase in MHC-I and TAA expression, and promoted survival of gp100 melanoma antigen-specific T cells thus contributing to tumor eradication in melanoma mouse model [161]. In another study, TSA-induced expression of TAP-1 was also observed in murine prostate, lung, and melanoma cancer cell lines. The increase in TAP-1 along with other APM components,

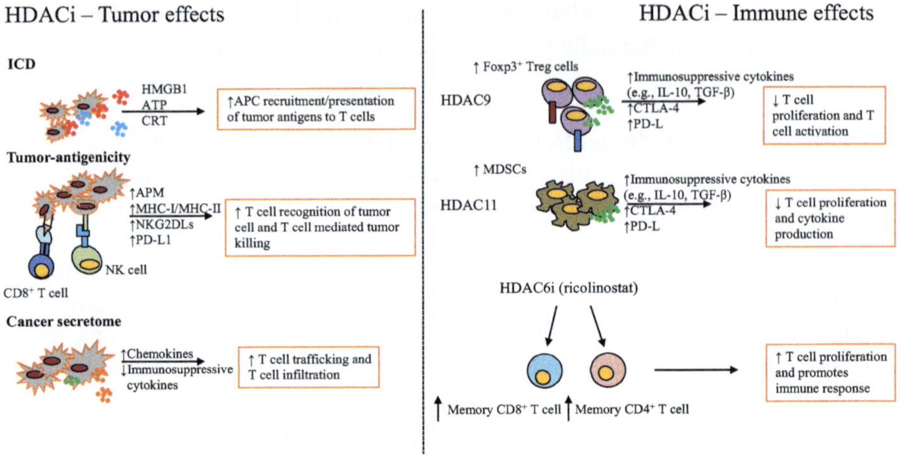

Fig. 9.4 Role of HDACis in regulating antitumor immunity. HDACis can promote antitumor immune response through direct effects on cancer cells through histone and nonhistone mediated actions. HDACis can promote ICD, increase expression of tumor-associated antigens/neoantigens, NKG2DLs, and chemokines thus enhancing various aspects of the cancer-immunity cycle and promoting an effective antitumor immune response. In addition, HDACis decrease tumor expression of immunosuppressive cytokines which further promotes T cell/NK cell recruitment into the tumor stroma and T cell/NK cell function. HDACis may also prevent an effective antitumor immune response by increasing proliferation and function of immune regulatory cells (e.g., Tregs, MDSCs). It should be noted that these effects are seen with use of pan-HDACis, and the effect of class or isoform specific HDACis on the immune system is not completely understood (see text for details). As an example, pharmacological inhibition or genetic abrogation of HDAC9 and HDAC11 has been implicated in positively regulating Treg and MDSCs functions, respectively

increased surface expression of MHC-I and enhanced CTL-mediated tumor cell killing [162]. Khan and colleagues reported that TSA and VPA not only increased the expression of MHC-I, TAP1, TAP2, and Tapsin, along with other components of APM in melanoma cell line but also increased the expression of costimulatory molecules CD40 and B7-2 [163]. The role of HDAC6 in regulating the expression of MHC-I and TAAs in human and murine melanoma cell lines has also been investigated. Pharmacological inhibition with specific HDAC6i or by genetic abrogation of HDAC6 expression increased MHC-I expression along with melanoma-specific antigens (e.g., gp100 and MART-1). Furthermore, it was demonstrated that inhibition of HDAC6 delayed tumor progression, which was dependent on an intact immune system [164]. In addition to these findings in melanoma, pharmacological inhibition of Class I HDACs with entinostat, along with genetic inhibition of HDAC1 in human prostate and breast cancer cell lines, resulted in increased MHC-I and TAA expression (e.g., CEA, brachyury, MUC1, and prostate specific antigen), which contributed to efficient antigen-specific CTL-mediated tumor cell lysis [165]. In addition to the increase in expression of TAA, APM, MHC-I, and MHC-II in melanoma, HDACs have also been implicated in regulating the expression of PD-L1/L2. Pan-HDACi (belinostat) or Class I HDACis (LBH589, MS275, and MGCD0103) all increased PD-L1 expression on melanoma cell lines and human tumor samples in vitro in a dose-dependent manner, with LBH589 promoting the greatest increase in PD-L1 expression. Mechanistically, it was demonstrated that LBH589 increased histone acetylation at the *PD-L1* promoter. The combination of PD-L1 blockade with LBH589 resulted in significant delay in tumor progression and increase in OS in this murine model, which was not observed when either agents were administered alone [166]. Collectively, the current preclinical and translational evidence supports the rationale for combining HDACis with immunotherapy.

9.1.1.19 HDACis Impact on Immune Cells

HDACs have pleotropic effects with large body of evidence suggesting that HDACis produce anti-inflammatory effects in immune cells by playing a role in regulation of both innate and adaptive immunity [125, 153, 167]. The data suggest that HDACis can promote or inhibit effector lymphocyte function. This is dependent on cell type, activation status of the effector cells, and the use of pan-HDACi or Class-specific HDACis [139, 153]. Furthermore, HDACs also have positive and negative effects on development of regulatory immune cells (e.g., Tregs, MDSCs) [125, 153, 160]. As an example, HDAC9 knockout (KO) mice have elevated numbers of Tregs potentially through its regulation of Foxp3 [168]. Indeed, TSA increased *Foxp3* gene expression and regulated Foxp3 activity, leading to enhanced production and function of Tregs in vivo, which was primarily attributed to HDAC9. In addition to increase in Foxp3 expression, TSA also increased expression of IL-10, CTLA-4, and PD-1, while repressing expression of IL-2 by Tregs [169]. HDAC11 also negatively regulates IL-10 expression in APCs and MDSCs [170, 171]. MDSCs isolated from HDAC11 KO tumor-bearing mice were more immune suppressive in comparison to the MDSCs isolated from wild-type tumor-bearing mice. This was translated into higher tumor growth kinetics in HDAC11 KO mice in comparison to WT mice [171]. Interestingly, the addition of entinostat (Class I HDACi) to anti-PD-1 and anti-CTLA-4 antibody treatment for four T1 tumor-bearing mice led to a dramatic reduction in circulating and tumor-infiltrating granulocytic-MDSCs (G-MDSCs), which correlated with sustained tumor regression. Co-culture experiments with G-MDSCs and $CD8^+$ T cells, revealed that entinostat directly suppresses G-MDSCs inhibitory function on $CD8^+$ T cells [172]. Thus, based on the current evidence it is clear that the effects of HDACis on the immune system are diverse and context specific (Fig. 9.4). More studies are required to further understand the role of specific HDACs, along with the macromolecular chromatin remodeling complexes that they are part of, in regulating effector T-cell function, development of immune suppressive cell types, and the impact of these immune suppressive cell populations on immunotherapy outcomes.

9.1.1.20 HDACi with Checkpoint Inhibitors—Current Clinical Experience

Several HDACis have been approved by US FDA for treatment of hematological malignancies either as single agent or as combination with other anticancer agents [139]. However, the efficacy of HDACis as single agents in solid malignancies is modest. As an example, pan-HDACi, panobinostat, is not active as a single agent in treatment of patients with metastatic melanoma, even though posttreatment biopsies from these patients did indicate increase in MHC-I expression and increased $CD8^+$ T-cell infiltration [173]. As discussed above, a large body of evidence supports the use of combination therapy of HDACi with anti-PD-1/PD-L1, anti-CTLA-4, and adoptive cell transfer therapies. Adding to the evidence is a recent study, utilizing HDAC6-specific inhibitor (ricolinostat). Combination of ricolinostat with anti-CTLA-4 or anti-PD-1 treatments inhibited melanoma tumor growth in vivo [174]. Treatment of murine T cells with ricolinostat in vitro promoted enhanced central memory T-cell formation and strong anti-melanoma activity in vivo [174]. This observation was corroborated in a translational study, which demonstrated enhanced proliferation and function of patient-derived $CD8^+$ T cells from patient TILs during ex vivo expansion. In addition, ricolinostat promoted central memory $CD4^+$ and $CD8^+$ T-cell formation during ex vivo expansion [175]. Based on the current evidence multiple clinical trials testing the combination of HDACi with anti-PD-1/PD-L1 and anti-CTLA-4 are underway to test if the observations made in the lab can be translated into achieving higher rate of durable clinical responses (Table 9.1).

The three HDACis with most safety information currently being tested in the clinic with checkpoint inhibitors include vorinostat, panobinostat, and entinostat. The safety profile of these agents when utilized as single agent is known. The most frequent toxicities with these HDACi are fatigue, nausea, and diarrhea [176]. Panobinostat product label carries two black-box warnings, (1) up to 25% of patients have experienced severe diarrhea and (2) severe arrhythmias and fatal cardiac events have occurred with panobinostat [177]. In addition, these agents also cause myelosuppression with thrombocytopenia, neutropenia, and anemia being the most common [176–178]. Vorinostat-specific toxicities include pulmonary embolism 4/86 (5%) and hyperglycemia [178]. Hyperglycemia of grade 2 or higher has also been reported in a Phase 1 trial of entinostat [179].

Preliminary results from ENCORE 601, a Phase 1b/2 trial, of entinostat in combination with pembrolizumab were reported with positive safety and tolerability data. At the time of reporting, $n = 9$ patients with advanced NSCLC were enrolled ($n = 6$ at the entinostat 3 mg qweekly and $n = 3$ at 5 mg qweekly) with pembrolizumab 200 mg IV q3weeks in 21-day cycles [180]. Only one of nine patients experienced a DLT, a grade 3 elevation of alkaline phosphatase and bilirubin, at entinostat 3 mg dose level. This was considered a manifestation of immune-related hepatitis and was successfully managed by withholding study medications and administration of corticosteroids [180]. At the time of reporting, stable disease was observed in 3/6 patients evaluated thus far, with longest ongoing patient in cycle 8. Circulating MDSCs were decreased from baseline in two of three patients. Based on this preliminary data, additional subjects will be recruited for the dose confirmation phase [180]. It will be important to observe the early safety and tolerability data and have a clinical management plan available for some of the potential overlapping toxicities between the two treatment modalities.

9.1.1.21 Future Directions—HDACis with Immune Checkpoint Inhibitors

We currently have very limited safety information regarding the use of HDACis with immune checkpoint inhibitors for treatment of solid malignancies. The preliminary safety data from the ongoing Phase 1/2 studies will be very important in understanding the feasibility of utilizing these two pharmacotherapeutic modalities together. The potential overlapping toxicities on the hematopoietic, gastrointestinal, and hepatic organ systems should be monitored closely. Most of the studies listed in Table 9.1 are designed to identify the optimal safe and tolerable dose of the HDACi when given concomitantly with standardized dose of checkpoint inhibitors. The question of whether sequencing the HDACis with checkpoint inhibitors may provide superior safety and potential therapeutic benefit will be addressed in the study NCT02437136 (entinostat + pembrolizumab), as it contains an additional cohort of patients that will be pretreated with entinostat for 2 weeks prior to coadministration of pembrolizumab with entinostat. An interesting feature of NCT02437136 and NCT02638090 (vorinostat + pembrolizumab) is the inclusion of patients who previously failed checkpoint inhibitors. The rationale being that the failure of immunotherapy is perhaps in part due to lack of tumor immunogenicity, which may be epigenetically silenced. Identification of biomarkers of response/resistance to combination therapy will be important. Assessment of histone acetylation status and changes in expression of immune-related genes as assessed in peripheral blood mononuclear cells and in the tumor compartment in response to combination therapy may provide valuable insight into predictors of response (NCT02635061).

Pan-HDACis and class-specific HDACis are being tested in multiple solid malignancies without enriching for specific molecular subtypes. As an example, clinical trials NCT02635061 (ACY-241 + nivolumab + ipilimumab), NCT02437136, and NCT02638090 are enrolling patients irrespective of NSCLC molecular subtype (e.g., EGFR (mt) or ALK translocation (+)) as currently there is no information regarding the role of oncogenic drivers in regulating the HDACi mediated tumor immune-modulatory effects. If these initial studies prove positive and can be confirmed within larger clinical trials, the potential for making an impact in treatment of NSCLC and other solid malignancies, irrespective of mutational status is tremendous. In other words, many more patients potentially can benefit from positive outcomes of these studies in comparison to other targeted and immune checkpoint inhibitor modalities currently being tested.

9.1.1.22 Conclusion

Here, we have reviewed the current preclinical and translational evidence, which strongly supports that targeted therapies may synergize with checkpoint inhibitors by enhancing various aspects of cancer-immunity cycle to promote immune-mediated tumor control/elimination. Currently available clinical data, although preliminary, yield positive efficacy signals with mixed safety signals as previously discussed [44, 45, 118]. Thus, one of the key questions to be addressed by ongoing clinical trial is the possibility of synergistic toxicities. Furthermore, these studies will also help identify the appropriate dose, timing, and sequencing of the therapies that would not only maximize the antitumor immune response, but also would identify the safe and tolerable regimen for the combination therapy which will hopefully be tested in larger confirmatory trials. In addition, these studies will also help identify biomarkers of response/resistance, which may better enable patient selection for combination therapies.

Beyond the combination therapies discussed here, several other combinations of targeted therapies with immune checkpoint inhibitors are also being assessed in the clinic. Combination of VEGF inhibitors with immune checkpoint inhibitors are also being tested as large body of evidence indicates potential synergies with these two combinations [4, 181, 182]. In addition, combination of checkpoint inhibitors with other traditional therapeutic modalities, such as radiation therapy and chemotherapy, are also being tested as these modalities too have demonstrated to enhance various aspects of cancer immunity [160, 183–185]. Finally, novel molecular pathways operating in immunologically "cold" tumors have been identified and preliminary data indicates that targeting these pathways (e.g., WNT/β-catenin, PTEN/PI3K) may promote conversion into immunologically "hot" tumors [186, 187]. Ultimately, the hope is that these combination strategies will not only increase the response rates, but also promote the consolidation of the responses into long-term durable remission.

References

1. Eroglu Z, Ribas A (2016) Combination therapy with BRAF and MEK inhibitors for melanoma: latest evidence and place in therapy. Ther Adv Med Oncol 8(1):48–56
2. Robert C et al (2015) Pembrolizumab versus Ipilimumab in advanced melanoma. N Engl J Med 372(26):2521–2532
3. Chen Daniel S, Mellman I (2013) Oncology meets immunology: the cancer-immunity cycle. Immunity 39(1):1–10
4. Hughes PE, Caenepeel S, Wu LC (2016) Targeted therapy and checkpoint immunotherapy combinations for the treatment of cancer. Trends Immunol 37:462–476
5. Mittal D, Gubin MM, Schreiber RD, Smyth MJ (2014) New insights into cancer immunoediting and its three component phases — elimination, equilibrium and escape. Curr Opin Immunol 27:16–25
6. Roberts PJ, Der CJ (2007) Targeting the Raf-MEK-ERK mitogen-activated protein kinase cascade for the treatment of cancer. Oncogene 26(22):3291–3310

7. Caunt CJ, Sale MJ, Smith PD, Cook SJ (2015) MEK1 and MEK2 inhibitors and cancer therapy: the long and winding road. Nat Rev Cancer 15(10):577–592
8. Forbes SA et al (2015) COSMIC: exploring the world's knowledge of somatic mutations in human cancer. Nucleic Acids Res 43(D1):D805–D811
9. Santarpia L, Lippman SL, El-Naggar AK (2012) Targeting the mitogen-activated protein kinase RAS-RAF signaling pathway in cancer therapy. Expert Opin Ther Targets 16(1):103–119
10. Eser S, Schnieke A, Schneider G, Saur D (2014) Oncogenic KRAS signalling in pancreatic cancer. Br J Cancer 111(5):817–822
11. Fernández-Medarde A, Santos E (2011) Ras in cancer and developmental diseases. Genes Cancer 2(3):344–358
12. Holderfield M, Deuker MM, McCormick F, McMahon M (2014) Targeting RAF kinases for cancer therapy: BRAF-mutated melanoma and beyond. Nat Rev Cancer 14(7):455–467
13. Sumimoto H, Imabayashi F, Iwata T, Kawakami Y (2006) The BRAF–MAPK signaling pathway is essential for cancer-immune evasion in human melanoma cells. J Exp Med 203(7):1651–1656
14. Frederick DT et al (2013) BRAF inhibition is associated with enhanced melanoma antigen expression and a more favorable tumor microenvironment in patients with metastatic melanoma. Clin Cancer Res 19(5):1225–1231
15. Khalili JS et al (2012) Oncogenic BRAF(V600E) promotes stromal cell-mediated immunosuppression via induction of interleukin-1 in melanoma. Clin Cancer Res 18(19):5329
16. Beaupre DM et al (1999) Autocrine interleukin-1β production in leukemia. Cancer Res 59(12):2971
17. Liu C et al (2013) BRAF inhibition increases tumor infiltration by T cells and enhances the antitumor activity of adoptive immunotherapy in mice. Clin Cancer Res 19(2):393
18. Knight DA et al (2013) Host immunity contributes to the anti-melanoma activity of BRAF inhibitors. J Clin Invest 123(3):1371–1381
19. Ott P, Bhardwaj N (2013) Impact of MAPK pathway activation in BRAFV600 melanoma on T cell and dendritic cell function. Front Immunol 4:346
20. Catanzaro JM et al (2014) Oncogenic Ras induces inflammatory cytokine production by upregulating the squamous cell carcinoma antigens SerpinB3/B4. Nat Commun 5:3729
21. Lesina M et al (2011) Stat3/Socs3 activation by IL-6 transsignaling promotes progression of pancreatic intraepithelial neoplasia and development of pancreatic cancer. Cancer Cell 19(4):456–469
22. West NR, McCuaig S, Franchini F, Powrie F (2015) Emerging cytokine networks in colorectal cancer. Nat Rev Immunol 15(10):615–629
23. Bunt SK et al (2007) Reduced inflammation in the tumor microenvironment delays the accumulation of myeloid-derived suppressor cells and limits tumor progression. Cancer Res 67(20):10019
24. Bissonnette M et al (2000) Mutational and nonmutational activation of p21ras in rat colonic azoxymethane-induced tumors: effects on mitogen-activated protein kinase, cyclooxygenase-2, and cyclin D1. Cancer Res 60(16):4602–4609
25. Fujishita T, Kajino-Sakamoto R, Kojima Y, Taketo MM, Aoki M (2015) Antitumor activity of the MEK inhibitor trametinib on intestinal polyp formation in ApcΔ716 mice involves stromal COX-2. Cancer Sci 106(6):692–699
26. Wang D, DuBois RN (2009) The role of COX-2 in intestinal inflammation and colorectal cancer. Oncogene 29(6):781–788
27. Charo C et al (2013) PGE(2) regulates pancreatic stellate cell activity via the EP4 receptor. Pancreas 42(3):467–474
28. Collins MA et al (2012) Oncogenic Kras is required for both the initiation and maintenance of pancreatic cancer in mice. J Clin Invest 122(2):639–653
29. Thayer SP et al (2003) Hedgehog is an early and late mediator of pancreatic cancer tumorigenesis. Nature 425(6960):851–856

30. Pylayeva-Gupta Y, Lee Kyoung E, Hajdu Cristina H, Miller G, Bar-Sagi D (2012) Oncogenic kras-induced GM-CSF production promotes the development of pancreatic neoplasia. Cancer Cell 21(6):836–847
31. Bayne Lauren J et al (2012) Tumor-derived granulocyte-macrophage colony-stimulating factor regulates myeloid inflammation and T cell immunity in pancreatic cancer. Cancer Cell 21(6):822–835
32. Kono M et al (2006) Role of the mitogen-activated protein kinase signaling pathway in the regulation of human melanocytic antigen expression. Mol Cancer Res 4(10):779
33. Atkins D et al (2004) MHC class I antigen processing pathway defects, ras mutations and disease stage in colorectal carcinoma. Int J Cancer 109(2):265–273
34. Mimura K et al (2013) The MAPK pathway is a predominant regulator of HLA-A expression in esophageal and gastric cancer. J Immunol 191(12):6261–6272
35. El-Jawhari JJ et al (2014) Blocking oncogenic RAS enhances tumour cell surface MHC class I expression but does not alter susceptibility to cytotoxic lymphocytes. Mol Immunol 58(2):160–168
36. Boni A et al (2010) Selective BRAFV600E inhibition enhances T-cell recognition of melanoma without affecting lymphocyte function. Cancer Res 70(13):5213
37. Sapkota B, Hill CE, Pollack BP (2013) Vemurafenib enhances MHC induction in BRAFV600E homozygous melanoma cells. OncoImmunology 2(1):e22890
38. Kakavand H et al (2015) PD-L1 expression and tumor-infiltrating lymphocytes define different subsets of MAPK inhibitor–treated melanoma patients. Clin Cancer Res 21(14):3140
39. Cooper ZA et al (2013) BRAF inhibition is associated with increased clonality in tumor-infiltrating lymphocytes. OncoImmunology 2(10):e26615
40. Sers C et al (2009) Down-regulation of HLA Class I and NKG2D ligands through a concerted action of MAPK and DNA methyltransferases in colorectal cancer cells. Int J Cancer 125(7):1626–1639
41. Koelzer VH et al (2015) Active immunosurveillance in the tumor microenvironment of colorectal cancer is associated with low frequency tumor budding and improved outcome. Transl Res 166(2):207–217
42. Ebert Peter JR et al (2016) MAP kinase inhibition promotes T cell and anti-tumor activity in combination with PD-L1 checkpoint blockade. Immunity 44(3):609–621
43. Hu-Lieskovan S et al (2015) Improved antitumor activity of immunotherapy with BRAF and MEK inhibitors in BRAF(V600E) melanoma. Sci Transl Med 7(279):279ra241–279ra241
44. Ribas A, Hodi FS, Callahan M, Konto C, Wolchok J (2013) Hepatotoxicity with combination of vemurafenib and ipilimumab. N Engl J Med 368(14):1365–1366
45. Minor DR, Puzanov I, Callahan MK, Hug BA, Hoos A (2015) Severe gastrointestinal toxicity with administration of trametinib in combination with dabrafenib and ipilimumab. Pigment Cell Melanoma Res 28(5):611–612
46. Nikanjam M, Liu S, Kurzrock R (2016) Dosing targeted and cytotoxic two-drug combinations: lessons learned from analysis of 24,326 patients reported 2010 through 2013. Int J Cancer 139(9):2135–2141
47. Liu S, Nikanjam M, Kurzrock R (2016) Dosing de novo combinations of two targeted drugs: towards a customized precision medicine approach to advanced cancers. Oncotarget 7(10):11310–11320
48. Ribas ABM, Lutzky J, Lawrence PD, Robert C et al (2015) Phase I study combining anti-PD-L1 (MEDI4736) with BRAF (dabrafenib) and/or MEK (trametinib) inhibitors in advanced melanoma. ASCO Annual Meeting, J Clin Oncol 33, 2015 (suppl; abstr 3003)
49. Ribas A HS, Lawrence DP, Atkinson V et al (2016) Pembrolizumab (pembro) in combination with dabrafenib (D) and trametinib (T) for BRAF-mutant advanced melanoma: phase 1 KEYNOTE-022 study. ASCO Annual Meeting 2016, J Clin Oncol 34, 2016 (suppl; abstr 3014)
50. Bendell JKW, Chee EC et al (2016) Safety and efficacy of cobimetinib (cobi) and atezolizumab (atezo) in a Phase 1b study of metastatic colorectal cancer (mCRC). ESMO 18th World Congress of Gastrointestinal Cancer, (abstr LBA-01)

51. ASCO-POST (2016) Anti–PD-L1 immunotherapy shows response in microsatellite-stable metastatic colorectal cancer in combination with MEK inhibition
52. Thakur MD, Stuart DD (2013) The evolution of melanoma resistance reveals therapeutic opportunities. Cancer Res 73(20):6106
53. Moriceau G et al (2015) Tunable-combinatorial mechanisms of acquired resistance limit the efficacy of BRAF/MEK cotargeting but result in melanoma drug addiction. Cancer Cell 27(2):240–256
54. Molina JR, Yang P, Cassivi SD, Schild SE, Adjei AA (2008) Non–small cell lung cancer: epidemiology, risk factors, treatment, and survivorship. Mayo Clin Proc Mayo Clin 83(5):584–594
55. Rosell R et al (2009) Screening for epidermal growth factor receptor mutations in lung cancer. N Engl J Med 361(10):958–967
56. Hallberg B, Palmer RH (2013) Mechanistic insight into ALK receptor tyrosine kinase in human cancer biology. Nat Rev Cancer 13(10):685–700
57. Thomas A, Liu SV, Subramaniam DS, Giaccone G (2015) Refining the treatment of NSCLC according to histological and molecular subtypes. Nat Rev Clin Oncol 12(9):511–526
58. Katayama R et al (2012) Mechanisms of acquired crizotinib resistance in ALK-rearranged lung cancers. Sci Transl Med 4(120):120ra117–120ra117
59. Gainor JF et al (2016) Molecular mechanisms of resistance to first- and second-generation ALK inhibitors in ALK-rearranged lung cancer. Cancer Discov 6(10):1118
60. Sharma SV, Bell DW, Settleman J, Haber DA (2007) Epidermal growth factor receptor mutations in lung cancer. Nat Rev Cancer 7(3):169–181
61. Soria J-C, Mok TS, Cappuzzo F, Jänne PA (2012) EGFR-mutated oncogene-addicted non-small cell lung cancer: current trends and future prospects. Cancer Treat Rev 38(5):416–430
62. Pao W et al (2004) EGF receptor gene mutations are common in lung cancers from "never smokers" and are associated with sensitivity of tumors to gefitinib and erlotinib. Proc Natl Acad Sci U S A 101:13306–13311
63. Kancha RK, von Bubnoff N, Peschel C, Duyster J (2009) Functional analysis of epidermal growth factor receptor (EGFR) mutations and potential implications for EGFR targeted therapy. Clin Cancer Res 15(2):460
64. Yang JC-H et al (2015) Afatinib versus cisplatin-based chemotherapy for EGFR mutation-positive lung adenocarcinoma (LUX-Lung 3 and LUX-Lung 6): analysis of overall survival data from two randomised, phase 3 trials. Lancet Oncol 16(2):141–151
65. Pao W et al (2005) Acquired resistance of lung adenocarcinomas to gefitinib or erlotinib is associated with a second mutation in the EGFR kinase domain. PLoS Med 2(3):e73
66. Thress KS et al (2015) Acquired EGFR C797S mutation mediates resistance to AZD9291 in non-small cell lung cancer harboring EGFR T790M. Nat Med 21(6):560–562
67. Soda M et al (2007) Identification of the transforming EML4-ALK fusion gene in non-small-cell lung cancer. Nature 448(7153):561–566
68. Katayama R, Lovly CM, Shaw AT (2015) Therapeutic targeting of anaplastic lymphoma kinase in lung cancer: a paradigm for precision cancer medicine. Clin Cancer Res 21(10):2227
69. Choi YL et al (2008) Identification of novel isoforms of the EML4-ALK transforming gene in non–small cell lung cancer. Cancer Res 68(13):4971
70. Takeuchi K et al (2012) RET, ROS1 and ALK fusions in lung cancer. Nat Med 18(3):378–381
71. Rikova K et al (2007) Global survey of phosphotyrosine signaling identifies oncogenic kinases in lung cancer. Cell 131(6):1190–1203
72. Zou HY et al (2015) PF-06463922, an ALK/ROS1 inhibitor, overcomes resistance to 1(st) and 2(nd) generation ALK inhibitors in pre-clinical models. Cancer Cell 28(1):70–81
73. Ott PA (2015) Combined BRAF and MEK inhibition in BRAF V600E mutant melanoma: a synergistic and potentially safe combination partner with immunotherapy. Ann Transl Med; Vol 3, No 20 (November 2015): Ann Transl Med 3:313
74. Yu H, Kortylewski M, Pardoll D (2007) Crosstalk between cancer and immune cells: role of STAT3 in the tumour microenvironment. Nat Rev Immunol 7(1):41–51

75. Marrugal Á, Ojeda L, Paz-Ares L, Molina-Pinelo S, Ferrer I (2016) Proteomic-based approaches for the study of cytokines in lung cancer. Dis Markers 2016:2138627
76. Fukuyama T et al (2007) Cytokine production of lung cancer cell lines: correlation between their production and the inflammatory/immunological responses both in vivo and in vitro. Cancer Sci 98(7):1048–1054
77. Gao SP et al (2007) Mutations in the EGFR kinase domain mediate STAT3 activation via IL-6 production in human lung adenocarcinomas. J Clin Invest 117(12):3846–3856
78. Lee H-J et al (2014) Drug resistance via feedback activation of stat3 in oncogene-addicted cancer cells. Cancer Cell 26(2):207–221
79. Kim SM et al (2012) Activation of IL-6R/JAK1/STAT3 signaling induces de novo resistance to irreversible EGFR inhibitors in non-small cell lung cancer with T790M resistance mutation. Mol Cancer Ther 11:2254–2264
80. Haura EB, Zheng Z, Song L, Cantor A, Bepler G (2005) Activated epidermal growth factor receptor–stat-3 signaling promotes tumor survival <em>In vivo</em> in non–small cell lung cancer. Clin Cancer Res 11(23):8288
81. Wang T et al (2004) Regulation of the innate and adaptive immune responses by Stat-3 signaling in tumor cells. Nat Med 10(1):48–54
82. Yeh HH, Lai WW, Chen HHW, Liu HS, Su WC (2006) Autocrine IL-6-induced Stat3 activation contributes to the pathogenesis of lung adenocarcinoma and malignant pleural effusion. Oncogene 25(31):4300–4309
83. Sandler A et al (2006) Paclitaxel–carboplatin alone or with bevacizumab for non–small-cell lung cancer. N Engl J Med 355(24):2542–2550
84. Hato T, Zhu AX, Duda DG (2016) Rationally combining anti-VEGF therapy with checkpoint inhibitors in hepatocellular carcinoma. Immunotherapy 8(3):299–313
85. Pore N et al (2006) EGFR tyrosine kinase inhibitors decrease VEGF expression by both hypoxia-inducible factor (HIF)-1–independent and HIF-1–dependent mechanisms. Cancer Res 66(6):3197
86. Naumov GN et al (2009) Combined vascular endothelial growth factor receptor and epidermal growth factor receptor (EGFR) blockade inhibits tumor growth in xenograft models of EGFR inhibitor resistance. Clin Cancer Res 15(10):3484
87. Sunaga N et al (2012) Oncogenic KRAS-induced interleukin-8 overexpression promotes cell growth and migration and contributes to aggressive phenotypes of non-small cell lung cancer. Int J Cancer 130(8):1733–1744
88. Umekawa K et al (2013) Plasma RANTES, IL-10, and IL-8 levels in non–small-cell lung cancer patients treated with EGFR-TKIs. BMC Res Notes 6(1):139
89. Akbay EA et al (2013) Activation of the PD-1 pathway contributes to immune escape in EGFR-driven lung tumors. Cancer Discov 3(12):1355
90. Koh J et al (2016) EML4-ALK enhances programmed cell death-ligand 1 expression in pulmonary adenocarcinoma via hypoxia-inducible factor (HIF)-1α and STAT3. Oncoimmunology 5(3):e1108514
91. Hamedani FS et al (2014) Crizotinib (PF-2341066) induces apoptosis due to downregulation of pSTAT3 and BCL-2 family proteins in NPM-ALK+ anaplastic large cell lymphoma. Leuk Res 38(4):503–508
92. Sun Y et al (2013) ALK Inhibitor PF02341066 (Crizotinib) increases sensitivity to radiation in non–small cell lung cancer expressing EML4-ALK. Mol Cancer Ther 12(5):696
93. Kim H et al (2011) EGFR inhibitors enhanced the susceptibility to NK cell-mediated lysis of lung cancer cells. J Immunother 34:372–381
94. He S et al (2013) Enhanced interaction between natural killer cells and lung cancer cells: involvement in gefitinib-mediated immunoregulation. J Transl Med 11(1):186
95. Pollack BP, Sapkota B, Cartee TV (2011) Epidermal growth factor receptor inhibition augments the expression of MHC class I and II genes. Clin Cancer Res 17(13):4400
96. Brea EJ et al (2016) Kinase regulation of human MHC class I molecule expression on cancer cells. Cancer Immunol Res 4(11):936

97. Lastwika KJ et al (2016) Control of PD-L1 expression by oncogenic activation of the AKT–mTOR pathway in non–small cell lung cancer. Cancer Res 76(2):227
98. D'Incecco A et al (2015) PD-1 and PD-L1 expression in molecularly selected non-small-cell lung cancer patients. Br J Cancer 112(1):95–102
99. Azuma K et al (2014) Association of PD-L1 overexpression with activating EGFR mutations in surgically resected nonsmall-cell lung cancer. Ann Oncol 25(10):1935–1940
100. Ota K et al (2015) Induction of PD-L1 expression by the EML4–ALK oncoprotein and downstream signaling pathways in non–small cell lung cancer. Clin Cancer Res 21(17):4014
101. Gainor JF et al (2016) EGFR Mutations and ALK rearrangements are associated with low response rates to PD-1 pathway blockade in non-small cell lung cancer: a retrospective analysis. Clin Cancer Res 22(18):4585
102. Huynh TG et al (2016) Programmed cell death ligand 1 expression in resected lung adenocarcinomas: association with immune microenvironment. J Thorac Oncol 11(11):1869–1878
103. Goodman A, Patel SP, Kurzrock R (2017) PD-1-PD-L1 immune-checkpoint blockade in B-cell lymphomas. Nat Rev Clin Oncol 14(4):203–220
104. Khagi Y, Kurzrock R, Patel SP (2017) Next generation predictive biomarkers for immune checkpoint inhibition. Cancer Metastasis Rev 36(1):179–190
105. Garon EB et al (2015) Pembrolizumab for the treatment of non–small-cell lung cancer. N Engl J Med 372(21):2018–2028
106. Borghaei H et al (2015) Nivolumab versus docetaxel in advanced nonsquamous non–small-cell lung cancer. N Engl J Med 373(17):1627–1639
107. Herbst RS et al (2016) Pembrolizumab versus docetaxel for previously treated, PD-L1-positive, advanced non-small-cell lung cancer (KEYNOTE-010): a randomised controlled trial. Lancet 387(10027):1540–1550
108. Pardoll DM (2012) The blockade of immune checkpoints in cancer immunotherapy. Nat Rev Cancer 12(4):252–264
109. Rizvi NA et al (2015) Mutational landscape determines sensitivity to PD-1 blockade in non–small cell lung cancer. Science (New York, NY) 348(6230):124–128
110. Snyder A et al (2014) Genetic basis for clinical response to CTLA-4 blockade in melanoma. N Engl J Med 371(23):2189–2199
111. Yadav M et al (2014) Predicting immunogenic tumour mutations by combining mass spectrometry and exome sequencing. Nature 515(7528):572–576
112. Champiat S et al (2016) Hyperprogressive disease (HPD) is a new pattern of progression in cancer patients treated by anti-PD-1/PD-L1. Clin Cancer Res 23:1920–1928
113. Kato S et al (2017) Hyper-progressors after immunotherapy: analysis of genomic alterations associated with accelerated growth rate. Clin Cancer Res 23(15):4242–4250
114. Gettinger S, Politi K (2016) PD-1 Axis inhibitors in EGFR- and ALK-driven lung cancer: lost cause? Clin Cancer Res 22(18):4539
115. Zhou P et al (2014) In vivo discovery of immunotherapy targets in the tumor microenvironment. Nature 506(7486):52–57
116. Rizvi AN, Chow LQ, Borghaei H, Shen Y et al (2014) Safety and response with nivolumab (anti-PD-1; BMS-936558, ONO-4538) plus erlotinib in patients (pts) with epidermal growth factor receptor mutant (EGFR MT) advanced NSCLC. J Clin Oncol 32(5s):8022
117. Gibbons LD CQ, Kim D, Kim S, Yeh T et al (2016) Efficacy, safety and tolerability of MEDI4736 (durvalumab [D]), a human IgG1 anti-programmed cell death-ligand-1 (PD-L1) antibody, combined with gefitinib (G): a phase I expansion in TKI-naïve patients (pts) with EGFR mutant NSCLC. ELCC 2016 (abstr 57O)
118. Ahn MYJ, Yu H et al (2016) Osimertinib combined with durvalumab in EGFR-mutant non-small cell lung cancer: results from the TATTON phase Ib trial. ELCC 2016, (abstr136O)
119. Patel SP, Kurzrock R (2015) PD-L1 Expression as a predictive biomarker in cancer immunotherapy. Mol Cancer Ther 14(4):847
120. Herbst RS et al (2014) Predictive correlates of response to the anti-PD-L1 antibody MPDL3280A in cancer patients. Nature 515:563–567

121. Taube JM et al (2014) Association of PD-1, PD-1 ligands, and other features of the tumor immune microenvironment with response to anti-PD-1 therapy. Clin Cancer Res: Off J Am Assoc Cancer Res 20(19):5064–5074
122. Tumeh PC et al (2014) PD-1 blockade induces responses by inhibiting adaptive immune resistance. Nature 515(7528):568–571
123. Dawson Mark A, Kouzarides T (2012) Cancer epigenetics: from mechanism to therapy. Cell 150(1):12–27
124. Dawson MA, Kouzarides T, Huntly BJP (2012) Targeting epigenetic readers in cancer. N Engl J Med 367(7):647–657
125. Falkenberg KJ, Johnstone RW (2014) Histone deacetylases and their inhibitors in cancer, neurological diseases and immune disorders. Nat Rev Drug Discov 13(9):673–691
126. West AC, Smyth MJ, Johnstone RW (2014) The anticancer effects of HDAC inhibitors require the immune system. OncoImmunology 3(1):e27414
127. West AC, Johnstone RW (2014) New and emerging HDAC inhibitors for cancer treatment. J Clin Invest 124(1):30–39
128. Peterson LF, Zhang D-E (2004) The 8;21 translocation in leukemogenesis. Oncogene 23(24):4255–4262
129. Insinga A et al (2005) Inhibitors of histone deacetylases induce tumor-selective apoptosis through activation of the death receptor pathway. Nat Med 11(1):71–76
130. Hornig E, Heppt MV, Graf SA, Ruzicka T, Berking C (2016) Inhibition of histone deacetylases in melanoma—a perspective from bench to bedside. Exp Dermatol 25(11):831–838
131. Weichert W et al (2008) Class I histone deacetylase expression has independent prognostic impact in human colorectal cancer: specific role of class I histone deacetylases in vitro and in vivo. Clin Cancer Res 14(6):1669
132. Krusche CA et al (2005) Histone deacetylase-1 and -3 protein expression in human breast cancer: a tissue microarray analysis. Breast Cancer Res Treat 90(1):15–23
133. Minamiya Y et al (2011) Expression of histone deacetylase 1 correlates with a poor prognosis in patients with adenocarcinoma of the lung. Lung Cancer 74(2):300–304
134. Rikimaru T et al (2007) Clinical significance of histone deacetylase 1 expression in patients with hepatocellular carcinoma. Oncology 72(1–2):69–74
135. Weichert W (2009) HDAC expression and clinical prognosis in human malignancies. Cancer Lett 280(2):168–176
136. Glozak MA, Seto E (2007) Histone deacetylases and cancer. Oncogene 26(37):5420–5432
137. Eot-Houllier G, Fulcrand G, Magnaghi-Jaulin L, Jaulin C (2009) Histone deacetylase inhibitors and genomic instability. Cancer Lett 274(2):169–176
138. Ocker M (2010) Deacetylase inhibitors – focus on non-histone targets and effects. World J Biol Chem 1(5):55–61
139. Terranova-Barberio M, Thomas S, Munster PN (2016) Epigenetic modifiers in immunotherapy: a focus on checkpoint inhibitors. Immunotherapy 8(6):705–719
140. Ellis L, Hammers H, Pili R (2009) Targeting tumor angiogenesis with histone deacetylase inhibitors. Cancer Lett 280(2):145–153
141. Kim MS et al (2001) Histone deacetylases induce angiogenesis by negative regulation of tumor suppressor genes. Nat Med 7(4):437–443
142. Bantscheff M et al (2011) Chemoproteomics profiling of HDAC inhibitors reveals selective targeting of HDAC complexes. Nat Biotech 29(3):255–265
143. Mazumdar S et al (2015) CoREST1 promotes tumor formation and tumor stroma interactions in a mouse model of breast cancer. PLoS One 10(3):e0121281
144. Hellebrekers DMEI et al (2006) Epigenetic regulation of tumor endothelial cell anergy: silencing of intercellular adhesion molecule-1 by histone modifications. Cancer Res 66(22):10770
145. Hellebrekers DMEI et al (2007) Identification of epigenetically silenced genes in tumor endothelial cells. Cancer Res 67(9):4138
146. Griffioen AW, Damen CA, Martinotti S, Blijham GH, Groenewegen G (1996) Endothelial intercellular adhesion molecule-1 expression is suppressed in human malignancies: the role of angiogenic factors. Cancer Res 56(5):1111

147. Dirkx AEM et al (2003) Tumor angiogenesis modulates leukocyte-vessel wall interactions in vivo by reducing endothelial adhesion molecule expression. Cancer Res 63(9):2322
148. Zheng H et al (2016) HDAC inhibitors enhance T-cell chemokine expression and augment response to PD-1 immunotherapy in lung adenocarcinoma. Clin Cancer Res 22(16):4119
149. Kroemer G, Galluzzi L, Kepp O, Zitvogel L (2013) Immunogenic cell death in cancer therapy. Annu Rev Immunol 31(1):51–72
150. Scaffidi P, Misteli T, Bianchi ME (2002) Release of chromatin protein HMGB1 by necrotic cells triggers inflammation. Nature 418(6894):191–195
151. Christiansen AJ et al (2011) Eradication of solid tumors using histone deacetylase inhibitors combined with immune-stimulating antibodies. Proc Natl Acad Sci 108(10):4141–4146
152. West AC et al (2013) An intact immune system is required for the anticancer activities of histone deacetylase inhibitors. Cancer Res 73(24):7265
153. Kroesen M et al (2014) HDAC inhibitors and immunotherapy; a double edged sword? Oncotarget 5(16):6558–6572
154. Armeanu S et al (2005) Natural killer cell-mediated lysis of hepatoma cells via specific induction of NKG2D ligands by the histone deacetylase inhibitor sodium valproate. Cancer Res 65:6321–6329
155. Skov S et al (2005) Cancer cells become susceptible to natural killer cell killing after exposure to histone deacetylase inhibitors due to glycogen synthase kinase-3–dependent expression of MHC class I–related chain A and B. Cancer Res 65(23):11136
156. Lopez-Soto A, Folgueras AR, Seto E, Gonzalez S (2009) HDAC3 represses the expression of NKG2D ligands ULBPs in epithelial tumour cells: potential implications for the immunosurveillance of cancer. Oncogene 28(25):2370–2382
157. Berghuis D et al (2012) Histone deacetylase inhibitors enhance expression of NKG2D ligands in Ewing sarcoma and sensitize for natural killer cell-mediated cytolysis. Clinical Sarcoma Research 2(1):8
158. Skov S et al (2005) Cancer cells become susceptible to natural killer cell killing after exposure to histone deacetylase inhibitors due to glycogen synthase kinase-3-dependent expression of MHC class I-related chain A and B. Cancer Res 65:6321–6329
159. Verhoeven DH et al (2008) NK cells recognize and lyse Ewing sarcoma cells through NKG2D and DNAM-1 receptor dependent pathways. Mol Immunol 45:3917–3925
160. Chacon AJ, Schutsky K, Powell JD (2016) The impact of chemotherapy, radiation and epigenetic modifiers in cancer cell expression of immune inhibitory and stimulatory molecules and anti-tumor efficacy. Vaccine 4(4):43
161. Vo DD et al (2009) Enhanced antitumor activity induced by adoptive T-cell transfer and adjunctive use of the histone deacetylase inhibitor LAQ824. Cancer Res 69(22):8693
162. Setiadi AF et al (2008) Epigenetic enhancement of antigen processing and presentation promotes immune recognition of tumors. Cancer Res 68(23):9601
163. Khan ANH, Gregorie CJ, Tomasi TB (2008) Histone deacetylase inhibitors induce TAP, LMP, Tapasin genes and MHC class I antigen presentation by melanoma cells. Cancer Immunol Immunother 57(5):647–654
164. Woan KV et al (2015) Targeting histone deacetylase 6 mediates a dual anti-melanoma effect: enhanced antitumor immunity and impaired cell proliferation. Mol Oncol 9(7):1447–1457
165. Gameiro SR, Malamas AS, Tsang KY, Ferrone S, Hodge JW (2016) Inhibitors of histone deacetylase 1 reverse the immune evasion phenotype to enhance T-cell mediated lysis of prostate and breast carcinoma cells. Oncotarget 7(7):7390–7402
166. Woods DM et al (2015) HDAC Inhibition upregulates PD-1 ligands in melanoma and augments immunotherapy with PD-1 blockade. Cancer Immunol Res 3:1375–1385
167. Leggatt GR, Gabrielli B (2012) Histone deacetylase inhibitors in the generation of the antitumour immune response. Immunol Cell Biol 90(1):33–38
168. De Zoeten EF, Wang L, Sai H, Dillmann WH, Hancock WW (2010) Inhibition of HDAC9 increases T regulatory cell function and prevents colitis in mice. Gastroenterology 138(2):583–594

169. Tao R et al (2007) Deacetylase inhibition promotes the generation and function of regulatory T cells. Nat Med 13(11):1299–1307
170. Villagra A et al (2009) The histone deacetylase HDAC11 regulates the expression of interleukin 10 and immune tolerance. Nat Immunol 10(1):92–100
171. Sahakian E et al (2015) Histone deacetylase 11: a novel epigenetic regulator of myeloid derived suppressor cell expansion and function. Mol Immunol 63(2):579–585
172. Kim K et al (2014) Eradication of metastatic mouse cancers resistant to immune checkpoint blockade by suppression of myeloid-derived cells. Proc Natl Acad Sci 111(32):11774–11779
173. Ibrahim N et al (2016) A phase I trial of panobinostat (LBH589) in patients with metastatic melanoma. Cancer Med 5(11):3041–3050
174. Cheng FLS, Wang H, Chen J, Villagra A et al (2016) In vitro and in vivo antimelanoma activity of ricolinostat, a selective HDAC6 inhibitor with immunomodulatory properties. ASCO Annual Meeting, J Clin Oncol 34, 2016 (suppl; abstr e21075)
175. Laino AS, Woods DM, Sarnaik A, Quayle S et al (2016) Selective histone deacetylase inhibition augments melanoma immunotherapy. ASCO Annual Meeting 2016, J Clin Oncol 34, 2016 (suppl; abstr e14521)
176. Lane AA, Chabner BA (2009) Histone deacetylase inhibitors in cancer therapy. J Clin Oncol 27(32):5459–5468
177. FDA (FARYDAK® (panobinostat) [package insert] (2015) Novartis Pharmaceuticals Corporation. February 2015. http://www.accessdata.fda.gov/drugsatfda_docs/label/2015/205353s000lbl.pdf
178. FDA (ZOLINZA® (vorinostat) [package insert] (2015) Merck Sharp & Dohme Corp., December 2015. https://www.merck.com/product/usa/pi_circulars/z/zolinza/zolinza_pi.pdf
179. Pili R et al (2012) Phase I study of the histone deacetylase inhibitor entinostat in combination with 13-cis retinoic acid in patients with solid tumours. Br J Cancer 106(1):77–84
180. Johnson MLAA, Ramalingam SS, Janne PA et al (2016) Preliminary results of ENCORE 601, a phase 1b/2, open-label study of entinostat (ENT) in combination with pembrolizumab (PEMBRO) in patients with non-small cell lung cancer (NSCLC). ASCO Annual Meeting 2016, J Clin Oncol 34, 2016 (suppl; abstr e20659)
181. Vanneman M, Dranoff G (2012) Combining immunotherapy and targeted therapies in cancer treatment. Nat Rev Cancer 12(4):237–251
182. Ott PA, Hodi FS, Buchbinder EI (2015) Inhibition of immune checkpoints and vascular endothelial growth factor as combination therapy for metastatic melanoma: an overview of rationale, preclinical evidence, and initial clinical data. Front Oncol 5:202
183. Kalbasi A, June CH, Haas N, Vapiwala N (2013) Radiation and immunotherapy: a synergistic combination. J Clin Invest 123(7):2756–2763
184. Bernstein MB, Krishnan S, Hodge JW, Chang JY (2016) Immunotherapy and stereotactic ablative radiotherapy (ISABR): a curative approach? Nat Rev Clin Oncol 13(8):516–524
185. Galluzzi L, Buqué A, Kepp O, Zitvogel L, Kroemer G (2015) Immunological effects of conventional chemotherapy and targeted anticancer agents. Cancer Cell 28(6):690–714
186. Spranger S, Bao R, Gajewski TF (2015) Melanoma-intrinsic [bgr]-catenin signalling prevents anti-tumour immunity. Nature 523(7559):231–235
187. Peng W et al (2016) Loss of PTEN promotes resistance to T cell–mediated immunotherapy. Cancer Discov 6(2):202

Chapter 10
Thoracic Immunotherapy

Peter Vu and Lyudmila Bazhenova

Abstract Immunotherapies for lung cancer using tumor cell or antigen-based vaccines to generate immune memory have been unsuccessful in all randomized, phase 3 clinical trials. Therapeutics targeting PD-1/L1 interactions have been the most efficacious immunotherapies to date and mark a paradigm shift in the treatment of thoracic malignancies, although the benefits have been limited to a minority of patients. Emerging immunotherapy strategies have involved combining programmed death blockade with agents that target T-cell activation (e.g., platinum-based chemotherapy, radiotherapy, ipilimumab, and tremelimumab), T-cell infiltration into tumors (e.g., erlotinib, ramucirumab, and bevacizumab), and effector T-cell killing (e.g., BMS-986016). Most early studies with these combinations have been promising; however, some treatment regimens (e.g., durvalumab plus osimertinib, nivolumab plus ipilimumab 3 mg/kg) have had unacceptable safety profiles, and particular attention should be paid to the potential for new toxicities with combination immunotherapies.

Keywords Non-small cell lung cancer (NSCLC) • Small cell lung cancer (SCLC) • Malignant pleural mesothelioma (MPM) • Thymic epithelial tumors (TET) • Immune checkpoint inhibitors • Programmed cell death protein 1 (PD-1) • Cytotoxic T-lymphocyte antigen-4 (CTLA-4) • Vascular endothelial growth factor (VEGF) • Lymphocyte-activation gene 3 protein (LAG-3) • Abscopal effect • Pembrolizumab • Nivolumab • Atezolizumab • Durvalumab • Avelumab • Ipilimumab • Tremelimumab • BMS-986016 • Erlotinib • Gefitinib • Osimertinib • Ramucirumab • Bevacizumab

10.1 Introduction

Thoracic malignancies are the leading cause of cancer-related deaths in the world [1] and include non-small cell lung cancer (NSCLC), small cell lung cancer (SCLC), malignant pleural mesothelioma (MPM), and thymic epithelial tumors (TET). Historically, immunotherapies for lung cancer using tumor cell or antigen-based

P. Vu (✉) • L. Bazhenova
UC San Diego, Moores Cancer Center, San Diego, CA, USA
e-mail: p0vu@ucsd.edu; Lbazhenova@ucsd.edu

S.P. Patel, R. Kurzrock (eds.), *Early Phase Cancer Immunotherapy*, Current Cancer Research, DOI 10.1007/978-3-319-63757-0_10

vaccines to generate immune memory have been unsuccessful in all randomized, phase 3 clinical trials [2–4]. Patients who do not benefit from immunotherapies have either immunologic ignorance (inability of the immune system to recognize tumor-specific antigens) or have developed active immune escape mechanisms. Proposed methods for immune escape involve failures in (1) T-cell activation and recruitment (e.g., due to low nonsynonymous mutation burden, upregulation of cytotoxic T-lymphocyte antigen-4 (CTLA-4)), (2) T-cell trafficking and infiltration into tumors (e.g., high expression of vascular endothelial growth factor (VEGF), fibroblast growth factors), and (3) T-cell recognition and killing of tumor cells (e.g., high expression of programmed cell death protein 1 (PD-1), lymphocyte-activation gene 3 protein (LAG-3), T-cell immunoglobulin mucin-3 (TIM-3), TIGIT) [5, 6].

Increased understanding of these cancer immune evasion mechanisms led to the development of monoclonal antibodies (e.g., nivolumab, pembrolizumab) targeting a co-inhibitory receptor, PD-1, on T cells. These agents became known as immune checkpoint inhibitors and became the first FDA-approved immunotherapies in lung cancer based on significant improvements in median overall survival (OS), objective response rate (ORR), and duration of response (DOR) compared to chemotherapy [7–12]. Current and future immunotherapy investigations are utilizing checkpoint inhibitors as a backbone in combination with potentially synergistic agents designed to address one or more immune escape mechanisms, with the aim of increasing efficacy and response rates [13].

10.2 NSCLC

Management of patients with metastatic lung cancer relies on the presence or absence of actionable mutations. Therapy targeting EGFR-sensitizing mutations (10% prevalence among Caucasians and up to 50% prevalence among Asians) [14], translocations in EML4-ALK (2–7% prevalence) [15], or ROS1 (1–2% prevalence) [16] have led to significant improvements in outcomes. For patients without these mutations, the standard of care for the first-line treatment of advanced NSCLC is either a platinum-based chemotherapy doublet [17] or pembrolizumab [11].

10.2.1 FDA-Approved Immunotherapies

10.2.1.1 First Line

Pembrolizumab is a highly selective, humanized IgG4 monoclonal antibody against PD-1 that is recommended as first-line therapy in patients with a high level of tumor-programmed death-ligand 1 (PD-L1) expression whose EGFR, EML4-ALK, or ROS1 status is negative or unknown [18]. This recommendation is based on the results of KEYNOTE-024, a pivotal phase 3, randomized (1:1), multicenter, open-label, active-control trial in previously untreated metastatic NSCLC with a tumor proportion score (TPS) of ≥50%. In this trial, PD-L1 expression was determined before randomization using PD-L1 antibody clone 22C3. A total of 305 patients were randomized to receive either pembrolizumab 200 mg every 3 weeks (until progressive disease (PD), unacceptable toxicity, or a maximum of 35 cycles) or the investigator's choice of platinum-based chemotherapy for four to six cycles. At a median follow-up of 11.2 months (range, 6.3–19.7), pembrolizumab demonstrated significant improvements in OS (hazard ratio for death (HR), 0.60; 95% CI, 0.41–0.89; *P* = 0.005), progression-free survival (PFS) of 10.3 months (95% CI, 6.7–not reached) compared to 6.0 months (95% CI, 4.2–6.2), and ORR of 45% (95% CI, 37–53) compared to 28% (95% CI, 21–36) in the chemotherapy arm. In addition, there were fewer severe (grades 3–5) treatment-related adverse events (TRAEs) in the pembrolizumab arm compared to chemotherapy (26.6% vs. 53.3%) [11].

10.2.1.2 Subsequent Therapy

Pembrolizumab has also demonstrated efficacy in previously treated patients. KEYNOTE-010 was a phase 2/3, multicenter, open-label, active-control trial in which patients who had PD following platinum-based chemotherapy and a PD-L1 TPS of at least 1% were randomized (1:1:1) to receive pembrolizumab at 2 mg/kg every 3 weeks (low dose), 10 mg/kg every 3 weeks (high dose), or docetaxel 75 mg/m^2 every 3 weeks until unacceptable toxicity or PD. A total of 1033 patients were randomized and stratified by PD-L1 expression (TPS ≥ 50% vs. 1–49%), performance status (PS), and geographic region. For all patients, median OS was 10.4 months (HR, 0.71; 95% CI, 0.58–0.88; *P* = 0.0008) for low-dose pembrolizumab, 12.7 months (HR, 0.61; CI, 0.49–0.75; P <0.0001) for high-dose pembrolizumab, and 8.5 months for docetaxel. For the subgroup of patients with TPS ≥ 50%, median OS was significantly longer with low-dose pembrolizumab (14.9 vs. 8.2 months; HR, 0.54; 95% CI, 0.38–0.77; *P* = 0.0002) and high-dose pembrolizumab (17.3 vs. 8.2 months; HR, 0.50; CI, 0.36–0.70; P <0.0001) compared to docetaxel [9].

Similarly, nivolumab is a fully humanized IgG4 antibody against PD-1. It has been studied in the first-line setting in patients with PD-L1 expression ≥5% (CheckMate 026), but failed to demonstrate any difference in PFS, ORR, or median OS when compared to the investigator's choice of platinum-based doublet chemotherapy [19]. On the other hand, positive results were seen when nivolumab was administered after disease progression following one prior platinum-based chemotherapy doublet regimen. Two-phase 3 randomized (1:1), open-label, multicenter, active-control trials in squamous cell (CheckMate 017) and non-squamous (CheckMate 057) were conducted. The results of both studies were favorable for median OS, ORR, and DOR compared to docetaxel. Specifically, CheckMate 017 randomized 272 squamous cell NSCLC patients to either nivolumab 3 mg/kg every 2 weeks or docetaxel 75 mg/m^2 every 3 weeks until unacceptable toxicity or PD. Median OS was 9.2 months (95% CI, 7.3–13.3) with nivolumab compared with 6.0 months (95% CI, 5.1–7.3) for docetaxel (HR, 0.59; 95% CI, 0.44 to 0.79;

Table 10.1 PD-L1 assays utilized in NSCLC clinical trials

Drug	Companion anti-PD-L1 assay	PD-L1-positive expression level cutoff
Pembrolizumab	Dako/Agilent 22C3	≥50% of tumor cells [11]
Nivolumab	Dako/Agilent 28–8	≥1, 5, or 10% of tumor cells [7]
Atezolizumab	Ventana SP142	≥1, 5, or 50% of tumor cells or ≥1, 5, or 10% of immune cells [10]
Avelumab	Dako/Merck 73–10	≥1, 5, or 25% of tumor cells or ≥10% of immune cells [21]
Durvalumab	Ventana SP263	≥25% of tumor cells [22]

Several studies have evaluated the staining characteristics and concordance between PD-L1 assays and have concluded that most assays perform similarly except for Ventana SP142, which stains fewer tumor cells and identifies fewer PD-L1-positive patients. For all assays, immune cell staining for PD-L1 is significantly less reliable than tumor cell staining [23–25]

P <0.001). Squamous cell patients benefited from nivolumab irrespective of PD-L1 expression level [7].

CheckMate 057 utilized the same trial design as CheckMate 017 in a non-squamous NSCLC population. A total of 582 patients were randomized, with an ORR of 19% in the nivolumab arm and 12% in the docetaxel arm. Median OS was 12.2 months (95% CI, 9.7–15.0) with nivolumab compared to 9.4 months (95% CI, 8.1–10.7) with docetaxel (HR, 0.73; 96% CI, 0.59–0.89; *P* = 0.002). In contrast to squamous cell tumors studied in CheckMate 017, PD-L1 expression levels of ≥1%, ≥5%, and ≥10% in this non-squamous population were all associated with significant improvements in median OS (range, 17.7–19.9 months vs. 9.8–10.5 months), PFS (range, 4.2–5 months vs. 2.1 months), and ORR (range, 32–38% vs. 10–16%) when treated with nivolumab [8]. One possible explanation for the discrepancy between PD-L1 expression and benefit noted in squamous versus non-squamous tumors is because PD-L1 expression was evaluated retrospectively using archival tumor tissue, and the PD-L1 protein has been noted to deteriorate after 6 months, leading to unreliable staining [20]. Table 10.1 summarizes the various PD-L1 assays currently being used in clinical trials.

Atezolizumab is a humanized IgG1 monoclonal antibody targeting PD-L1 rather than the PD-1 receptor (e.g., pembrolizumab and nivolumab), allowing inhibition of both PD-1 and B7-1 interactions, which may lead to enhanced immune responses. It is indicated for use in metastatic NSCLC patients with PD during or after platinum-based chemotherapy, irrespective of PD-L1 expression or histologic subtype. It was studied in a phase 3 randomized (1:1), open-label, multicenter, active-control trial with 850 patients assigned to receive atezolizumab 1200 mg every 3 weeks or docetaxel 75 mg/m^2 every 3 weeks until PD or unacceptable toxicity. Median OS was longer for atezolizumab compared to docetaxel (13.8 vs. 9.6 months; HR 0.74; 95% CI, 0.63–0.87, *P* = 0.0004). Notably, survival benefit increased with higher PD-L1 expression but was still observed in PD-L1-negative tumors. Median OS was 20.5 for atezolizumab vs. 8.9 months for docetaxel (HR, 0.41; 95% CI, 0.27–0.64) among tumors with high levels of PD-L1 expression, defined as ≥50%

of tumor cells or ≥10% of tumor-infiltrating immune cells assessed using the Ventana SP142 IHC assay [12]. As a result, atezolizumab monotherapy is currently being evaluated in a randomized (1:1), phase 3 trial (IMpower 110, 111) against standard first-line chemotherapy (cisplatin or carboplatin plus pemetrexed or gemcitabine) in patients selected for high PD-L1 expression [26].

10.2.2 Emerging Immunotherapies

10.2.2.1 Other Checkpoint Inhibitors in Development

Durvalumab is a selective, high-affinity human IgG1 monoclonal antibody that blocks PD-L1. As part of a phase 1/2 dose-escalation and expansion study in advanced solid tumors, the treatment-naive NSCLC cohort consisted of 304 patients (47% non-squamous, 53% squamous). About half (51%) had a high level of PD-L1 expression, defined as ≥25% staining of tumor cells using the Ventana SP263 assay. Durvalumab was administered every 2 weeks at a dose of 10 mg/kg for up to 12 months. Results suggested that PD-L1-positive tumors had higher ORR (25 vs. 6%) and longer median OS (17.8 vs. 8.2 months) compared to PD-L1-negative tumors when administered as second-line therapy. Responses were not associated with histologic subtype. Grade 3–5 TRAEs were seen in 10% of patients, with one treatment-related death due to pneumonia and a TRAE discontinuation rate of 5% [27].

This data led to the phase 2, single-arm ATLANTIC trial, where durvalumab was administered as a single agent to patients who failed two or more prior systemic therapies (at least one must have been platinum based). Patients were divided into three subgroups by PD-L1 expression level (negative/low, was less than 25%; high, was at least 25%; very high, was at least 90%). Preliminary data showed that durvalumab produced durable responses and that ORR and disease control rate (DCR, defined as CR, PR, or SD for at least 24 weeks) correlated with tumor PD-L1 expression level. The ORR was 7.5% (95% CI, 3.1–14.9) for PD-L1 negative/low ($n = 93$), 16.4% (95% CI, 10.8–23.5) for PD-L1 high ($n = 146$) and 30.9% (95% CI, 20.2–43.3) for PD-L1 very high ($n = 68$), and DCR was 20.4%, 28.8%, and 38.2%, respectively [28]. A randomized, phase 3 study comparing durvalumab monotherapy to a platinum-based chemotherapy doublet in the first-line setting recently started enrollment (NCT03003962).

Avelumab is a fully human IgG1 antibody against PD-L1. What makes avelumab unique compared to other checkpoint inhibitors is that it maintains antibody-dependent cell-mediated cytotoxicity (ADCC) function and therefore may be more effective than other checkpoint inhibitors. Conversely, other PD-1/L1 inhibitors have been purposely engineered to eliminate Fc-effector function to reduce the risk of ADCC-mediated depletion of T cells expressing PD-L1 [29]. Currently, not enough data is available to conclude whether avelumab's ability to mediate ADCC is beneficial, harmful, or has no effect compared to other checkpoint inhibitors. Preliminary results of a phase 1b trial that enrolled 145 patients treated with avelumab 10 mg/kg every 2 weeks as monotherapy for first-line NSCLC showed it was clinically active and tolerable. The most common AEs were infusion reactions and fatigue. Grade 3–5 TRAEs occurred in 9% of patients, and immune-related adverse events (irAE) occurred in 2.8%. No deaths were attributed to treatment. The DCR was 64% with an unconfirmed ORR of 18.7% [30]. Based on this data, a randomized (1:1), multicenter, phase 3 trial (JAVELIN Lung 100) comparing avelumab to platinum-based doublet chemotherapy for treatment-naive PD-L1-positive tumors was initiated and enrollment is ongoing [31].

An early trial using avelumab in patients who have progressed after platinum-based chemotherapy has also demonstrated promising results. As part of a dose expansion cohort in NSCLC, an open-label phase 1b study enrolled 184 unselected patients to receive avelumab as subsequent therapy. ORR was 12% (22 of 184); among these patients, 83% had a response lasting at least 24 weeks. The DCR was 50% (92 of 184). Median OS was 8.4 months (95% CI, 7.3–10.6) and median DOR was not reached (95% CI, 48.1–not evaluable) [21]. TRAEs were similar to those discussed above when avelumab was given as initial therapy.

Also, lymphocyte-activation gene-3 (Lag-3) is another immune checkpoint protein that is expressed at high levels in tumors that have progressed after treatment with PD-1/L1 inhibitors [32]. It functions as an immune modulator by inhibiting effector T cells and promoting regulatory T-cell activity [33]. A monoclonal antibody, BMS-986016, has been developed that binds and inhibits the activity of LAG-3 on tumor-infiltrating lymphocytes (TILs). It is currently being tested in combination with nivolumab and/or ipilimumab for patients with advanced lung cancer in a phase 2 clinical trial (FRACTION-Lung, NCT02750514) in hopes of improving ORR, DOR, and PFS.

10.2.2.2 Emerging Checkpoint Inhibitor Chemotherapy Combinations

In preclinical studies, platinum-based chemotherapy has demonstrated the ability to stimulate higher levels of PD-L1 expression within tumor cells in a dose-dependent fashion [34–36]. In addition, chemotherapy may be synergistic with immune checkpoint inhibitors by inducing an immunogenic form of cell death, eliminating immunosuppressive cells, or releasing tumor-specific antigens for T-cell activation [37–40]. Thus, adding chemotherapy to checkpoint inhibition has the potential to increase the antigen pool for T-cell recognition and thus improve response rates.

The first checkpoint inhibitor studied in combination with chemotherapy for NSCLC was ipilimumab, a recombinant anti-CTLA-4 antibody. A randomized (1:1:1), double-blind, multicenter phase 2 trial assigned 204 untreated patients to receive either ipilimumab concurrently with carboplatin and paclitaxel, "phased" ipilimumab to start after two cycles of carboplatin and paclitaxel, or chemotherapy alone. Compared to chemotherapy alone, only the phased ipilimumab arm improved ORR (32 vs. 18%) and PFS by 1.1 months (HR, 0.72; $P = 0.05$) when assessed using the immune-related response criteria (irRC). Survival benefit was not observed on either the concurrent or phased ipilimumab schedule. Of note, improvements in

PFS with phased ipilimumab occurred primarily in lung tumors with squamous cell histology [41]. As a result, a phase 3 trial was conducted comparing ipilimumab given in a phased schedule vs. placebo in addition to paclitaxel and carboplatin for the first-line treatment of squamous cell lung cancer. Enrollment is complete, but results have not been published.

More recently, the combination of pembrolizumab with standard first-line chemotherapy was tested in a randomized (1:1), open-label, multicenter phase 2 trial (KEYNOTE-021). The primary outcome measure was ORR. PD-L1 expression was not required for enrollment. A total of 123 patients were randomized to receive 4 cycles of pembrolizumab 200 mg plus standard carboplatin and pemetrexed followed by up to 24 months of pembrolizumab or chemotherapy with carboplatin and pemetrexed alone. The combination arm demonstrated improved ORR (55% vs. 29%, $p = 0.0016$) and median PFS (13.0 vs. 8.9 months; HR, 0.53, 95% CI, 0.31–0.91, $p = 0.0102$) compared to chemotherapy alone. Severe TRAEs were more frequent in those receiving combination therapy with pembrolizumab and chemotherapy (39% vs. 26%), but there was no difference in treatment discontinuation related to AEs. Most importantly, more than half (12 of 21) of PD-L1-negative patients achieved a response to combination therapy (ORR, 57%; 95% CI, 34–79) [42]. This data further supports the concept that chemotherapy may improve tumor immunogenicity when given with PD-1 inhibitors and may become a first-line treatment option for patients who have low or negative PD-L1 expression. Two phase 3 trials (KEYNOTE-189, KEYNOTE-407) comparing platinum plus pemetrexed chemotherapy with or without pembrolizumab are ongoing.

Nivolumab has also been studied in combination with platinum-based doublet chemotherapy in treatment-naive patients with similarly encouraging results [43, 44]. The FDA-approved monotherapy dosing regimen for nivolumab is 3 mg/kg every 2 weeks; however, this phase 1 trial evaluated the safety and tolerability of nivolumab 10 mg/kg every 3 weeks in combination with gemcitabine-cisplatin for squamous tumors ($n = 12$), pemetrexed-cisplatin for non-squamous tumors ($n = 15$), paclitaxel-carboplatin for all histologies ($n = 15$), or nivolumab 5 mg/kg every 3 weeks with paclitaxel-carboplatin ($n = 14$). No dose-limiting toxicities (DLTs) were observed in the first 6 weeks of treatment. Grade 3–4 TRAEs occurred in 45% of patients; however, treatment discontinuation related to AEs was 21% and mostly occurred during nivolumab monotherapy. Although sample sizes were small, the 2-year OS rate for nivolumab 5 mg/kg plus paclitaxel-carboplatin was 62% compared to 25–33% in the other cohorts. Consistent with results from the pembrolizumab trial (KEYNOTE-021) discussed above, patients with negative or low PD-L1 expression responded to combination treatment with similar ORR (43% vs. 48%, respectively) and DOR (5.8 months vs. 6.3 months) to patients who were PD-L1 positive (defined as ≥1%) [43].

Atezolizumab in combination with chemotherapy for first-line therapy is currently being investigated in four global, phase 3, randomized, open-label trials based on positive responses seen in early trials [45]. IMpower130 plans to enroll 650 patients with non-squamous histology to receive atezolizumab with carboplatin plus nab-paclitaxel. IMpower131 is a three-arm study that plans to enroll 1025 squamous cell patients randomized to receive atezolizumab with carboplatin plus paclitaxel, atezolizumab with carboplatin plus nab-paclitaxel, or chemotherapy alone. IMpower132 plans to enroll 568 non-squamous NSCLC patients to receive atezolizumab with cisplatin or carboplatin plus pemetrexed. Lastly, IMpower150 plans to enroll 1200 patients to evaluate the benefit of adding bevacizumab to atezolizumab with carboplatin plus paclitaxel in lung cancer patients with non-squamous histology [46]. Overall, the addition of chemotherapy to checkpoint inhibition appears to be a promising therapeutic strategy that will likely be of most benefit to patients whose tumors have negative or low PD-L1 expression and were less likely to respond to checkpoint inhibitor monotherapy.

10.2.2.3 Dual Checkpoint Inhibitor Combinations

Combining two immune checkpoint inhibitors (anti-PD-1/L1 and anti-CTLA-4) aimed at different T-cell regulation steps to enhance the immune response has demonstrated increased ORR and improved outcomes in metastatic melanoma and renal cell carcinoma, albeit with increased frequency and severity of TRAEs [47, 48].

As part of a dose-finding cohort within the phase 1/2 KEYNOTE-021 trial, reduced dose pembrolizumab 2 mg/kg every 3 weeks was studied in combination with ipilimumab 1 mg/kg in NSCLC patients after PD on at least one prior regimen. Among 45 patients enrolled, 24% experienced grade 3–5 TRAEs that led to treatment discontinuation in four patients. ORR was 24%, disease control rate was 64%, and median duration of response was 13.8 months. Efficacy was not associated with PD-L1 expression. The investigators determined the combination of reduced dose pembrolizumab with ipilimumab was tolerable and had similar response rates to standard dose pembrolizumab monotherapy [49]. Given the significant response to pembrolizumab monotherapy in lung cancer [11], it is not surprising that the addition of CTLA-4 inhibition did not enhance response rates beyond pembrolizumab.

On the other hand, results from a phase 1 trial (CheckMate 012) in chemotherapy-naive patients combining nivolumab with ipilimumab suggested that dual checkpoint inhibition was synergistic in NSCLC. Six different dosing regimens were tested and the two most tolerable regimens that demonstrated clinical activity were standard dose nivolumab (3 mg/kg every 2 weeks) plus ipilimumab 1 mg/kg every 12 weeks ($n = 38$) or every 6 weeks ($n = 39$). Ipilimumab given more frequently (every 3 weeks) or at higher doses (3 mg/kg) resulted in treatment-related discontinuation AEs in 33% of patients and 6% treatment-related deaths. When ipilimumab was given every 12 weeks, ORR was 47% compared to 38% when given every 6 weeks. Although responses were seen at all levels of PD-L1 expression, there was a trend toward improved responses as expression level increased (ORR was 57% for PD-L1 $\geq$ 1% and 92% for PD-L1 $\geq$ 50%). Serious (grade 3–4) TRAEs (32 vs. 28%) and discontinuation rates (11 vs. 13%) were similar between the 12-week and 6-week cohorts, respectively [50]. As a result, this checkpoint inhibitor combination is being investigated further in CheckMate 227, a randomized, open-label, multicenter phase 3 trial that compares nivolumab alone, nivolumab plus ipilimumab every 6 weeks, nivolumab plus platinum-based doublet chemotherapy, and standard of care chemotherapy. Results are potentially practice changing and expected as early as the end of 2017. Unfortunately, this trial does not include a treatment arm that combines dual checkpoint inhibition (e.g., nivolumab plus ipilimumab) with chemotherapy.

Durvalumab has also been studied in combination with tremelimumab, a selective human IgG2 CTLA-4 inhibitor, in several trials. Results of a phase 1 open-label dose-escalation study ($n = 102$) found that the maximally tolerated dose was durvalumab 20 mg/kg every 4 weeks with tremelimumab 1 mg/kg every 4 weeks. The most common AEs included diarrhea, fatigue, pruritus, colitis, and elevated lipase. Grade 3–4 TRAEs occurred in 42% of patients and resulted in discontinuation in 28% of patients. There were three treatment-related deaths. Toxicities were mostly manageable and responses were seen in both PD-L1 positive (defined as ≥25% using the Ventana SP263 assay) and PD-L1-negative/low patients (defined as <25%) [22, 51, 52]. Several randomized, open-label, multicenter, phase 3 trials are evaluating the combination of durvalumab plus tremelimumab against chemotherapy in the first-line setting (NEPTUNE, MYSTIC) or as subsequent therapy (ARCTIC) [53–55].

In addition, a small cohort of 24 treatment-naive NSCLC patients were enrolled in a phase 1 safety and tolerability study using platinum-based doublet chemotherapy in combination with durvalumab 15 mg/kg every 3 weeks with or without tremelimumab. Four checkpoint inhibitor regimens were assessed: durvalumab without tremelimumab ($n = 5$), durvalumab plus a single dose of tremelimumab 1 mg/kg ($n = 5$), durvalumab plus tremelimumab 1 mg/kg every 6 weeks ($n = 7$), or durvalumab plus tremelimumab 3 mg/kg every 6 weeks ($n = 7$). Preliminary results were encouraging, with an ORR of 52.9% (95% CI, 28–77) and mostly non-severe (grade 2 or less) AEs. Two patients in the tremelimumab 1 mg/kg every 6 weeks cohort experienced DLTs (febrile neutropenia, pneumonitis) [56]. This combination of dual checkpoint inhibition (i.e., durvalumab plus tremelimumab) with or without platinum-based chemotherapy will be further evaluated in a randomized, phase 2 study (NCT03057106) by the Canadian Cancer Trials Group.

10.2.2.4 Checkpoint Inhibitors Combined with Targeted Therapies

The basis for combining immune checkpoint inhibition with targeted therapy is based on the observation that BRAF and MEK inhibition in melanoma led to pro-inflammatory changes in the tumor microenvironment that may improve T lymphocyte function [57]. In lung cancer, a meta-analysis of EGFR-mutated NSCLC patients who received either nivolumab (Checkmate 057), pembrolizumab (KEYNOTE 010), or atezolizumab (POPLAR) as subsequent therapy for NSCLC demonstrated no improvement in OS ($n = 186$, HR = 1.05, 95% CI: 0.70–1.55, $p < 0.81$) [58]. A possible explanation for the observed lack of benefit may be that patients with actionable mutations in EGFR, EML4-ALK, and ROS1 tend to have a significantly lower mutation burden [59]. In addition, patients with actionable mutations in NSCLC rarely have high expression of PD-L1 (defined as TPS ≥ 50% using anti-PD-L1 clone 22C3 pharmDx kit) [60, 61].

A phase 1b study evaluated the combination of erlotinib 150 mg daily with atezolizumab 1200 mg IV every 3 weeks following a 7-day run-in period with erlotinib alone. The study enrolled 28 patients with EGFR-mutant NSCLC, regardless of PD-L1 status. There were no DLT and no cases of pneumonitis; 39% of patients experienced serious (grade 3–4) TRAEs and 5 patients stopped therapy due to AEs. Notably, tumor biopsies obtained after erlotinib run-in showed an increase in intratumoral CD8+ T cells compared to paired pretreatment biopsies in 8 of 13 patients. The combination appeared safe, although ORR and PFS were similar to erlotinib monotherapy [62].

Durvalumab was also studied in combination with gefitinib. Preliminary data from an open-label, multicenter phase 1 trial that enrolled 20 patients with EGFR-mutant NSCLC demonstrated the combination was tolerable and active. Durvalumab 10 mg/kg every 2 weeks was given either concurrently or after 4 weeks of treatment with gefitinib 250 mg daily. The most common TRAEs were diarrhea and transaminase elevation. One patient developed pneumonitis, and four patients discontinued treatment due to AEs [63].

The development of resistance to targeted therapy in most patients with EGFR-mutant lung cancer after 9–13 months of treatment led to the development of osimertinib, an irreversible EGFR-TKI selective for both sensitizing and T790 M resistance mutations. Osimertinib significantly improved PFS and ORR compared to chemotherapy in EGFR secondary-resistant patients [64]. One of the first studies to examine checkpoint inhibition combined with targeted therapy in NSCLC utilized durvalumab at either 3 mg/kg or 10 mg/kg every 2 weeks given concurrently with osimertinib 80 mg daily. The phase 1b trial demonstrated positive response rates (ORR, 43% in Part A and 70% in Part B); however, the study was stopped due to the surprisingly high incidence of interstitial lung disease in 38% (13 of 34) of patients [65]. As a result, several other studies evaluating PD-1/L1 inhibition in combination with targeted therapies in lung cancer have been suspended.

10.2.2.5 Checkpoint Inhibitors Combined with Angiogenesis Inhibitors

In addition to promoting angiogenesis, preclinical studies have demonstrated that VEGF is immunosuppressive. VEGF can inhibit dendritic cell maturation, stimulate expansion of suppressive immune cell subsets (e.g., regulatory T cells, myeloid-derived suppressor cells), and can inhibit T-cell infiltration into the tumor microenvironment by interfering with adhesion molecules required for CD8+ T lymphocyte migration [66–70].

Ramucirumab is a human IgG1 antibody that inhibits VEGF signaling by binding specifically to VEGF receptor-2. When ramucirumab was combined with docetaxel in second-line therapy for NSCLC, there was an improvement in median OS from 9.1 to 10.5 months [71]. Thus, ramucirumab is being investigated in combination with pembrolizumab in a phase 1a/b study in NSCLC, gastric, gastroesophageal junction, urothelial, and biliary tract cancers. Preliminary data with 91 patients enrolled (21 patients with NSCLC) showed the combination was tolerable and active with a DCR of 85%. Grade 3–4 TRAE occurred in 7% of patients [72]. Similarly, ramucirumab is also being combined with durvalumab in a phase 1 study in gastrointestinal and NSCLC (NCT02572687).

Nivolumab has also been studied in combination with bevacizumab, a humanized anti-VEGF monoclonal IgG1 antibody, for maintenance therapy in patients who have not progressed on first-line chemotherapy. The phase 1 study assigned 12 non-squamous patients to nivolumab 5 mg/kg with bevacizumab 15 mg/kg every 3 weeks and 21 patients (8 squamous, 13 non-squamous) to nivolumab 3 mg/kg every 2 weeks. Preliminary results demonstrated longer median PFS of 37.1 weeks in the non-squamous combination cohort compared to 21.4 weeks in the non-squamous nivolumab only cohort. Squamous patients who received nivolumab only had a median PFS of 16 weeks. ORR was similar in the combination and monotherapy arms (8 vs. 10%, respectively). Four patients in each arm had treatment-related discontinuation AEs [73]. Bevacizumab is also being studied in a phase 3 trial in combination with atezolizumab and carboplatin plus pemetrexed (IMpower150) [46].

10.2.2.6 Checkpoint Inhibitors Combined with Radiotherapy

Radiation therapy (RT) has traditionally been used to treat local disease. However, by adjusting the dose and fractionation schedule of ionizing radiation, the effect on tumors can vary from mild inflammation to programmed cell death. This process of tumor cell death can lead to the presentation of tumor-specific antigens on MHC molecules and potentially T-cell recognition and activation of the innate and adaptive immune system. As a result, an abscopal effect (tumor regression outside of the field of irradiation) may be seen [74].

Abscopal effects with RT alone are extremely rare, which has led to the successful trial of combination strategies in preclinical models using anti-CTLA-4 antibodies and a fractionated (6 Gy in 5 fractions on consecutive days) RT regimen [75]. The first case report of an abscopal response in a lung cancer patient treated with ipilimumab while undergoing RT was published in 2013 [76]. This informed the development of a phase 2 trial in metastatic NSCLC patients using ipilimumab 3 mg/kg every 3 weeks for 9 weeks plus RT (6 Gy × 5 daily fractions), with the first dose of ipilimumab given within 24 h of starting RT. Preliminary results showed abscopal responses in 9 of 12 patients [77]. The National Cancer Institute will begin a randomized, phase 2 trial in NSCLC and colorectal cancer evaluating the safety and efficacy of combination immunotherapy using durvalumab plus tremelimumab with or without high- or low-dose RT. RT will start 2 weeks after the first dose of the checkpoint inhibitor combination, with high-dose RT administered daily over 10 days for up to 3 fractions and low-dose RT given twice a day on weeks 2, 6, 10, and 14 (NCT02888743).

10.3 SCLC

Systemic chemotherapy with cisplatin or carboplatin plus etoposide has been the mainstay of treatment in SCLC for decades. Platinum-based chemotherapy results in excellent initial responses in 60 to 70% of patients [78]; however, the majority develops recurrent disease within months. Topotecan has demonstrated ORR 16.9% and is the only FDA-approved treatment in the second-line setting [79]. All other cytotoxic agents have failed to demonstrate a meaningful improvement in outcomes when evaluated in large, randomized trials. Multiple genomic profile studies have shown that SCLC tumors are characterized by inactivating mutations in tumor suppressor genes TP53 and RB1 with very few actionable driver mutations. In addition, SCLC has a very high nonsynonymous mutational burden (approximately 7.4–8.6 per million base pairs) [80, 81], and therefore may be more responsive to immune checkpoint inhibitors [82]. At this time, there are no FDA-approved immunotherapies for the treatment of SCLC.

10.3.1 First Line

Many are hopeful that immunotherapy in SCLC may be at least as successful as it has been in NSCLC. Ipilimumab was first studied in SCLC in combination with carboplatin plus paclitaxel as initial therapy for ES-SCLC in a phase 2 trial. A total of 130 patients were randomized (1:1:1) to ipilimumab 10 mg/kg administered concurrently with carboplatin plus paclitaxel every 3 weeks, to ipilimumab given in a phased schedule to start after two doses of carboplatin plus paclitaxel, or to chemotherapy alone. Following completion of 18 weeks of chemotherapy, ipilimumab or placebo was given every 12 weeks as maintenance therapy until PD. Interestingly, only the phased dosing schedule of ipilimumab demonstrated an improvement in PFS compared to chemotherapy alone (6.4 vs. 5.3 months; HR, 0.64; $P = 0.03$) when assessed using irRC. There was no difference in PFS when evaluated using modified WHO criteria and no difference in OS between groups [83].

Unfortunately, similar results were obtained when the phased dosing schedule for ipilimumab was expanded to a phase 3 trial. A total of 1132 patients were randomized (1:1) to either phased ipilimumab in combination with cisplatin or carboplatin plus etoposide or chemotherapy plus placebo. Among 954 patients who received treatment, the addition of ipilimumab to standard chemotherapy for ES-SCLC did not prolong survival (median OS 11.0 vs. 10.9 months; HR, 0.94; 95% CI, 0.81–1.09) or PFS (median PFS, 4.6 vs. 4.4 months; HR, 0.85; 95% CI, 0.75–0.97) [84]. Thus, anti-CTLA-4 therapy is likely ineffective in SCLC and consistent with results from NSCLC trials with ipilimumab.

The first programmed death pathway inhibitor studied in SCLC with clinical data in the first-line setting was atezolizumab. It was administered as a single agent to 17 patients with ES-SCLC as part of the phase 1a portion of the phase 1/3

IMpower133 trial. In this unselected population, treatment was tolerable and could generate responses in 6% of patients. Two of 17 patients remained on treatment for at least 12 months. These results informed the development of the randomized (1:1), multicenter, double-blinded, placebo-controlled, phase 3 portion of the IMpower133 study examining the safety and efficacy of carboplatin plus etoposide with or without atezolizumab as first-line therapy. Atezolizumab 1200 mg or placebo will be given every 3 weeks with chemotherapy for four cycles and then as maintenance therapy until PD. An enrollment of 400 patients is expected and PD-L1 expression is not required [85].

10.3.2 Maintenance Therapy

Based on responses and tolerable AEs seen in the phase 1/2 CheckMate 032 trial discussed earlier, a randomized phase 3 trial (CheckMate 451) evaluating the role of nivolumab or nivolumab plus ipilimumab compared to placebo as maintenance therapy for ES-SCLC is being conducted. Eligible patients have had stable disease or better responses to first-line platinum-based doublet chemotherapy and are not required to have positive PD-L1 expression [86]. In addition, a phase 2 study with a planned recruitment of 54 patients evaluating pembrolizumab as maintenance therapy following standard first-line chemotherapy for SCLC has recently completed enrollment. The primary outcome measure will be PFS and secondary outcome measure will be OS.

10.3.3 Subsequent Therapy

Pembrolizumab monotherapy was studied within a phase 1b trial that enrolled PD-L1-positive (defined as TPS $\geq$ 1%) ES-SCLC patients who had progressed on platinum-based chemotherapy. Initially, 147 patients were screened and 42 (29%) patients were found to be PD-L1 positive. A total of 24 PD-L1-positive patients received pembrolizumab 10 mg/kg every 2 weeks until PD or unacceptable toxicity. Nine of 24 patients achieved a response (ORR, 37.5%; 95% CI, 18.8–59.4%) with 1 CR. Median PFS was 1.9 months; however, the median OS was 9.7 months and 12-month OS rate was 35.7%. There was one treatment-related death due to colitis and only two grade 3–4 TRAEs [87–89]. This very encouraging data suggests that pembrolizumab is effective in SCLC and can generate durable responses like what has been observed in other tumor types. Furthermore, several new trials plan to utilize pembrolizumab in treatment-naive SCLC, including pembrolizumab in combination with cisplatin/carboplatin plus etoposide (NCT03066778), pembrolizumab plus chemotherapy with or without RT (NCT02934503), and pembrolizumab monotherapy (NCT02580994). These trials have the potential to be practice changing when results become available in the next several years.

Nivolumab is another checkpoint inhibitor studied in SCLC that has reported promising results. CheckMate-032 is an open-label, multicenter, phase 1/2 trial conducted in patients with either LS-SCLC or ES-SCLC with PD after platinum-based chemotherapy. At interim analysis, a total of 216 patients had been assigned to receive nivolumab 3 mg/kg alone (n = 98) or nivolumab plus ipilimumab followed by nivolumab maintenance (n = 118). Nivolumab plus ipilimumab was evaluated at three dose levels: nivolumab 1 mg/kg plus ipilimumab 1 mg/kg (n = 3), nivolumab 1 mg/kg plus ipilimumab 3 mg/kg (n = 61), or nivolumab 3 mg/kg plus ipilimumab 1 mg/kg (n = 54). ORR ranged from 19 to 33% in the combination cohorts and 10% in the monotherapy cohort, with no difference in PFS between groups (range, 1.4–2.6 months) or OS at 1 year (range, 33–43%). Responses did not correlate with PD-L1 expression. Grade 3–4 TRAEs ranged from 13% in patients receiving nivolumab alone up to 30% in patients treated with nivolumab 1 mg/kg plus ipilimumab 3 mg/kg, with two treatment-related deaths in the latter group [90]. Other checkpoint inhibitors being studied in SCLC includes durvalumab plus tremelimumab in relapsed SCLC (NCT02937818) and durvalumab plus tremelimumab in combination with chemotherapy for untreated ES-SCLC (Caspian, NCT03043872).

10.4 Mesothelioma

Malignant pleural mesothelioma (MPM) is an aggressive neoplasm associated with asbestos exposure with a poor prognosis and limited treatment options. It is often diagnosed at a late stage, thus only 10–15% of cases are resectable [91]. The only FDA-approved treatment option for unresectable, advanced MPM is cisplatin plus pemetrexed as initial therapy [92]. In relapsed disease, the median OS is 6 months. Histologically, it is categorized as predominantly epithelioid (associated with a more favorable prognosis), sarcomatoid (more aggressive), or biphasic (a mixture of both). Significant gene mutations in MPM include CDKN2A, NF2, BAP1, TP53, SETD2, DDX3X, ULK2, RYR2, CFAP45, SETDB1, and DDX51; however, the overall frequency of protein-altering somatic mutations in MPM is low compared to other cancers [93].

10.4.1 Checkpoint Inhibitors

Hypothesis generating data from single-arm, open-label trials with tremelimumab monotherapy for MPM patients with PD after first-line treatment demonstrated that anti-CTLA-4 therapy was safe and appeared effective [94, 95]. This led to development of the DETERMINE study, a randomized (2:1), double-blind, phase 2b study (n = 571) comparing tremelimumab (10 mg/kg every 4 weeks for 7 doses, then every 12 weeks until PD) to placebo as second- or third-line therapy for

MPM. Unfortunately, there was no significant difference in survival between tremelimumab and placebo (median OS, 7.7 vs. 7.3 months; HR, 0.92; 95% CI, 0.76–1.12, $p = 0.408$), indicating that single-agent CTLA-4 inhibition in previously treated MPM is likely ineffective [96].

PD-L1 inhibition has recently been explored in MPM. As part of the phase 1 JAVELIN solid tumor trial, a cohort of 53 patients with relapsed MPM were treated with avelumab 10 mg/kg every 2 weeks with promising results. Treatment was tolerable, with the most common minor TRAEs being infusion reactions, fatigue, and chills. Only 4 of 53 patients experienced a grade 3–4 TRAE. Unconfirmed objective responses were seen in 9.4% with a disease control rate of 56.6% for the entire cohort. There was a statistically insignificant trend toward increased ORR (14.3 vs. 8.0%) and PFS (17.1 vs. 7.4 weeks) in the 14 patients with PD-L1 expression of ≥5% compared to PD-L1-negative tumors [97].

Likewise, PD-1 inhibition with pembrolizumab was studied as part of a multicohort trial in patients with solid tumors expressing PD-1 in at least 1% of cells (KEYNOTE-028). The phase 1b cohort consisted of 25 patients with MPM (72% epithelioid, 8% sarcomatoid, 8% biphasic, 12% unknown) who received pembrolizumab 10 mg/kg every 2 weeks as first-, second-, or third-line treatment. Pembrolizumab was tolerable, with grade 3–4 TRAEs reported in 20% of patients and zero treatment-related discontinuations or deaths. An objective response was seen in 20% of patients with a median DOR of 12 months (95% CI, 3.7–not reached). The clinical benefit rate (defined as CR, PR, or SD for at least 6 months) was 40% and median OS was 18.0 months (95% CI, 9.4–not reached). Of note, a total of 83 patients with MPM were initially screened and 45.8% were found to express PD-1 [98]. This study demonstrated that pembrolizumab is clinically active in PD-1-positive MPM and can lead to durable responses. As a result, pembrolizumab will be explored in a randomized, open-label, phase 3 trial (PROMISE-meso) in relapsed MPM and compared to salvage chemotherapy using gemcitabine or vinorelbine using a primary endpoint of PFS.

10.4.2 Combination Strategies

Clinical trial development in MPM has followed a similar trajectory to that of NSCLC and SCLC, albeit at a slower pace likely due to fewer affected patients. Thus, most combination strategies have involved adding immune checkpoint inhibition to chemotherapy or combining CTLA-4 and PD-1/L1 inhibition. These trials are in early stages of development and plan to begin enrolling patients in 2017.

Two clinical trials are evaluating the utility of chemotherapy with cisplatin plus pemetrexed in combination with a PD-1/L1 inhibitor. In the single-arm, phase 2 DREAM study, durvalumab 1125 mg will be given concurrently with cisplatin and pemetrexed for six cycles and then continued as maintenance therapy. The trial will enroll the first six participants as part of a safety run-in and then expand enrollment to a total of 54 patients. The primary endpoint will be PFS at 6 months and ORR; other study outcomes include TRAEs, OS, and correlative biomarkers [99]. In addition, pembrolizumab is being evaluated in the front-line setting in a potentially practice-changing phase 2, randomized, three-arm trial (NCT02784171). The study will compare standard of care chemotherapy with cisplatin plus pemetrexed to pembrolizumab plus chemotherapy or pembrolizumab alone and utilize PFS as the primary outcome measure.

Although ineffective as a single-agent, tremelimumab is being combined with durvalumab in an open-label, phase 2 study (NIBIT-MESO-1) for patients who have failed chemotherapy. A planned 40 patients will be assigned to receive tremelimumab 1 mg/kg every 4 weeks for 4 doses and durvalumab 20 mg/kg every 4 weeks for 12 doses. There is no requirement for PD-L1 expression for enrollment and the primary outcome measure is ORR [100].

10.5 Thymic Epithelial Tumors

Thymic epithelial tumors (TETs) are rare neoplasms (1.3 cases per million) that originate from the thymus and consist of thymomas and thymic carcinomas [101]. Thymomas are classified by morphology (types A, AB, B1-B3) that reflects different maturational stages of the thymic epithelial progenitor cell. Types B2 and B3 tend to be more aggressive, with a 15% incidence of metastatic disease [102]. In thymomas, dysplastic proliferation of thymic epithelial cells frequently results in abnormal T-cell selection and autoimmune paraneoplastic syndromes such as myasthenia gravis [103]. Thymic carcinomas make up about 12% of TETs, have lost thymus-like morphological features, and rarely present with paraneoplastic syndromes. Thymic carcinomas are histologically subclassified into squamous cell (most common), undifferentiated, and others [102]. Overall, thymic carcinomas are more aggressive, more likely to metastasize, and have a poorer prognosis than thymomas with 5-year survival rates of 55% compared to 90% [104].

Optimal management of TETs involves evaluation for complete surgical resection [105]. For unresectable disease or patients who have undergone an incomplete surgical resection, radiation therapy and/or systemic chemotherapy with a platinum-based regimen is often recommended. There is no consensus on the optimal management for recurrence after systemic treatment [104]. Unlike other thoracic malignancies, there are few actionable mutations and limited data available for the treatment of TETs. In a DNA sequencing and immunohistochemical analysis of 112 cases of TETs with various histologies, 4 of 112 (3.8%) tumors harbored c-KIT mutations and all occurred in thymic carcinomas. There were no ALK rearrangements or mutations in EGFR, BRAF, KRAS, HER2, or PDGFR [106].

10.5.1 Checkpoint Inhibitors

Recently, the use of PD-1/L1 inhibitors for the treatment of TETs has been reported in a few small trials based on several clinicopathological studies demonstrating significant PD-1/L1 expression in both thymic carcinomas and thymomas. In a sample of 112 TETs, PD-L1 expression (defined as staining in at least 10% of tumor cells) was seen in 65% (13 of 20) of thymic carcinomas and 18% (16 of 87) of thymomas. There was no relationship between PD-L1 expression and survival [106]. These results are consistent with findings by Katsuya et al. (2015), where PD-L1 expression was seen in 70% (26 of 37) thymic carcinomas and 23% (22 of 102) thymomas [107]. Notably, both studies utilized the same PD-L1 antibody clone (E1L3N). Other estimates for the frequency of PD-L1 expression range from 50–100% in thymic carcinomas [108–112] and 54–92% in thymomas [108–110, 112, 113]. In addition, Naidoo et al. (2015) has also demonstrated that other checkpoints, such as TIM-3, are frequently expressed at a high level in TETs and may be the target of future immunotherapy studies [114].

In a group of eight patients with TETs (seven thymomas, one thymic carcinoma) who failed one or more prior therapies, avelumab was given at either 10 mg/kg or 20 mg/kg every 2 weeks until PD or unacceptable toxicity. Patients with a history of autoimmune disease were ineligible for the study. There were four PR, three SD, and one PD. Treatment was tolerable, although a relatively high number of irAEs occurred that included three patients with myositis and one with enteritis. Interestingly, three patients treated at the higher dose of avelumab had pre- and posttreatment biopsies performed. Posttreatment, one patient had necrotic tissue without viable tumor, and the other two patients had diffuse, membranous PD-L1 staining in epithelial cells along with fewer regulatory immune cells [115]. The clinical significance of these histologic differences remains to be seen.

Recently, a cohort of 30 patients (planned enrollment of 41 patients) with advanced thymic carcinoma who failed one or more prior therapies were treated as part of a phase 2 trial with pembrolizumab 200 mg given every 3 weeks. Patients with thymomas were not included in this study. Results were reported for 24 patients who demonstrated an ORR of 25% (1 CR, 5 PR) and a median PFS of 36 weeks. The most common TRAEs were hepatic enzyme elevations in nearly all patients (n = 24), asthenia (n = 7), enteritis (n = 5). Grade 3–4 TRAEs occurred in four patients who developed severe asthenia, hepatitis, pancreatitis, myositis, and myocarditis requiring pacemaker placement. Other irAEs seen included polymyositis, type 1 diabetes mellitus, and bullous pemphigoid [116]. Although PD-1 inhibition appears efficacious in thymic carcinomas, significant attention should be paid to irAE in future studies.

Notably, medullary thymic epithelial cells normally express tissue-specific antigens to aid in the positive and negative selection of T cells to maintain immune self-tolerance. However, this same selection mechanism may also lead to the deletion of effector T cells capable of recognizing tumor-specific antigens and thus contribute to a tumor's ability to escape immune surveillance [117, 118]. Khan et al. (2014) have shown that inhibiting T-cell tolerance can increase the number of tumor-specific effector T cells, which could potentially lead to enhanced antitumor immune responses [118]. Since the thymus plays a large role in central immune tolerance, it may be difficult to predict the safety and efficacy of cancer immunotherapies on TETs.

10.6 Conclusion

Although therapeutics targeting PD-1/L1 interactions have been the most efficacious immunotherapies to date and mark a paradigm shift in the treatment of thoracic malignancies, the benefits have been limited to a minority of patients. These patients tend to have a higher nonsynonymous mutational burden, higher levels of PD-L1 expression on tumor cells, and preexisting TIL within the tumor microenvironment. Patients who do not benefit from programmed death pathway inhibitors have been theorized to possess one or more immune escape mechanisms. Therefore, emerging immunotherapy strategies have involved combining programmed death blockade with agents that target T-cell activation (e.g., platinum-based chemotherapy, radiotherapy, ipilimumab, and tremelimumab), T-cell infiltration into tumors (e.g., erlotinib, ramucirumab, and bevacizumab), and effector T-cell killing (e.g., BMS-986016). Most early studies with these combinations have been promising; however, some treatment regimens (e.g., durvalumab plus osimertinib, nivolumab plus ipilimumab 3 mg/kg) have had unacceptable safety profiles and attention should be paid to the potential for new toxicities with combination immunotherapies.

References

1. Torre LA, Bray F, Siegel RL, Ferlay J, Lortet-Tieulent J, Jemal A (2015) Global cancer statistics, 2012. CA Cancer J Clin 65:87–108
2. Vansteenkiste JF, Cho BC, Vanakesa T et al (2016) Efficacy of the MAGE-A3 cancer immunotherapeutic as adjuvant therapy in patients with resected MAGE-A3-positive non-small-cell lung cancer (MAGRIT): a randomised, double-blind, placebo-controlled, phase 3 trial. Lancet Oncol 17:822–835
3. Butts C, Socinski MA, Mitchell PL et al (2014) Tecemotide (L-BLP25) versus placebo after chemoradiotherapy for stage III non-small-cell lung cancer (START): a randomised, double-blind, phase 3 trial. Lancet Oncol 15:59–68
4. Giaccone G, Bazhenova LA, Nemunaitis J et al (2015) A phase III study of belagenpumatucel-L, an allogeneic tumour cell vaccine, as maintenance therapy for non-small cell lung cancer. Eur J Cancer 51:2321–2329
5. Kim JM, Chen DS (2016) Immune escape to PD-L1/PD-1 blockade: seven steps to success (or failure). Ann Oncol 27:1492–1504
6. Chen DS, Mellman I (2013) Oncology meets immunology: the cancer-immunity cycle. Immunity 39:1–10

7. Brahmer J, Reckamp KL, Baas P et al (2015) Nivolumab versus docetaxel in advanced squamous-cell non-small-cell lung cancer. N Engl J Med 373:123–135
8. Borghaei H, Paz-Ares L, Horn L et al (2015) Nivolumab versus docetaxel in advanced non-squamous non-small-cell lung cancer. N Engl J Med 373:1627–1639
9. Herbst RS, Baas P, Kim D-W et al (2016) Pembrolizumab versus docetaxel for previously treated, PD-L1-positive, advanced non-small-cell lung cancer (KEYNOTE-010): a randomised controlled trial. Lancet 387:1540–1550
10. Fehrenbacher L, Spira A, Ballinger M et al (2016) Atezolizumab versus docetaxel for patients with previously treated non-small-cell lung cancer (POPLAR): a multicentre, open-label, phase 2 randomised controlled trial. Lancet 387:1837–1846
11. Reck M, Rodríguez-Abreu D, Robinson AG et al (2016) Pembrolizumab versus chemotherapy for PD-L1-positive non-small-cell lung cancer. N Engl J Med 375:1823–1833
12. Rittmeyer A, Barlesi F, Waterkamp D et al (2017) Atezolizumab versus docetaxel in patients with previously treated non-small-cell lung cancer (OAK): a phase 3, open-label, multicentre randomised controlled trial. Lancet 389:255–265
13. Ott PA, Stephen Hodi F, Kaufman HL, Wigginton JM, Wolchok JD (2017) Combination immunotherapy: a road map. J Immunother Cancer. doi:10.1186/s40425-017-0218-5
14. Hirsch FR, Bunn PA Jr (2009) EGFR testing in lung cancer is ready for prime time. Lancet Oncol 10:432–433
15. Kwak EL, Bang Y-J, Camidge DR et al (2010) Anaplastic lymphoma kinase inhibition in non-small-cell lung cancer. N Engl J Med 363:1693–1703
16. Gainor JF, Shaw AT (2013) Novel targets in non-small cell lung cancer: ROS1 and RET fusions. Oncologist 18:865–875
17. Azzoli CG, Giaccone G, Temin S (2010) American Society of Clinical Oncology clinical practice guideline update on chemotherapy for stage IV non–small-cell lung cancer. J Oncol Pract 6:39–43
18. Ettinger DS, Wood DE, Aisner DL et al (2017) NCCN guidelines version 4.2017 non-small cell lung cancer. In: National comprehensive cancer network. https://www.nccn.org/professionals/physician_gls/pdf/nscl.pdf. Accessed 4 Mar 2017
19. Socinski M, Creelan B, Horn L et al (2016) NSCLC, metastaticCheckMate 026: a phase 3 trial of nivolumab vs investigator's choice (IC) of platinum-based doublet chemotherapy (PT-DC) as first-line therapy for stage iv/recurrent programmed death ligand 1 (PD-L1)−positive NSCLC. Ann Oncol. doi:10.1093/annonc/mdw435.39
20. Grigg C, Rizvi NA (2016) PD-L1 biomarker testing for non-small cell lung cancer: truth or fiction? J Immunother Cancer. doi:10.1186/s40425-016-0153-x
21. Gulley JL, Rajan A, Spigel DR et al (2017) Avelumab for patients with previously treated metastatic or recurrent non-small-cell lung cancer (JAVELIN solid tumor): dose-expansion cohort of a multicentre, open-label, phase 1b trial. Lancet Oncol. doi:10.1016/S1470-2045(17)30240-1
22. Antonia S, Goldberg SB, Balmanoukian A et al (2016) Safety and antitumour activity of durvalumab plus tremelimumab in non-small cell lung cancer: a multicentre, phase 1b study. Lancet Oncol 17:299–308
23. Scheel AH, Dietel M, Heukamp LC et al (2016) Harmonized PD-L1 immunohistochemistry for pulmonary squamous-cell and adenocarcinomas. Mod Pathol 29:1165–1172
24. Hirsch FR, McElhinny A, Stanforth D et al (2017) PD-L1 immunohistochemistry assays for lung cancer: results from phase 1 of the blueprint PD-L1 IHC assay comparison project. J Thorac Oncol 12:208–222
25. Rimm DL, Han G, Taube JM et al (2017) A prospective, multi-institutional, pathologist-based assessment of 4 immunohistochemistry assays for PD-L1 expression in non-small cell lung cancer. JAMA Oncol. doi:10.1001/jamaoncol.2017.0013
26. Herbst RS, De Marinis F, Jassem J, Lam S, Mocci S, Sandler A, Lopez-Chavez A, Deng Y, Giaccone G, Spigel DR (2016) PS01.56: IMpower110: phase III trial comparing 1L Atezolizumab with chemotherapy in PD-L1-selected chemotherapy-naive NSCLC patients: topic: medical oncology. J Thorac Oncol 11:S304–S305

27. Antonia SJ, Brahmer JR, Khleif S et al (2016) Phase 1/2 study of the safety and clinical activity of durvalumab in patients with non-small cell lung cancer (NSCLC). Ann Oncol. doi:10.1093/annonc/mdw383.16
28. Garassino M, Vansteenkiste J, Kim J-H, Léna H, Mazières J, Powderly J, Dennis P, Huang Y, Wadsworth C, Rizvi N (2017) PL04a.03: durvalumab in ≥3rd-line locally advanced or metastatic, EGFR/ALK wild-type NSCLC: results from the phase 2 ATLANTIC study. J Thorac Oncol 12:S10–S11
29. Boyerinas B, Jochems C, Fantini M, Heery CR, Gulley JL, Tsang KY, Schlom J (2015) Antibody-dependent cellular cytotoxicity activity of a novel anti-PD-L1 antibody Avelumab (MSB0010718C) on human tumor cells. Cancer Immunol Res 3:1148–1157
30. Jerusalem G, Chen F, Spigel D et al (2017) OA03.03 JAVELIN solid tumor: safety and clinical activity of Avelumab (anti-PD-L1) as first-line treatment in patients with advanced NSCLC. J Thorac Oncol 12:S252
31. Reck M, DeGreen HP, Rose AL et al (2016) Avelumab (MSB0010718C; anti-PD-L1) vs platinum-based doublet as first-line treatment for metastatic or recurrent PD-L1-positive non-small-cell lung cancer: the phase 3 JAVELIN Lung 100 trial. In: 2016 ASCO annual meeting. http://meetinglibrary.asco.org/content/164274-176. Accessed 12 Mar 2017
32. Koyama S, Akbay EA, Li YY et al (2016) Adaptive resistance to therapeutic PD-1 blockade is associated with upregulation of alternative immune checkpoints. Nat Commun 7:10501
33. Anderson AC, Joller N, Kuchroo VK (2016) Lag-3, Tim-3, and TIGIT: co-inhibitory receptors with specialized functions in immune regulation. Immunity 44:989–1004
34. Zhang P, Ma Y, Lv C et al (2016) Upregulation of programmed cell death ligand 1 promotes resistance response in non-small-cell lung cancer patients treated with neo-adjuvant chemotherapy. Cancer Sci 107:1563–1571
35. Grabosch S, Zeng F, Zhang L, Strange M, Brozick J, Edwards RP, Vlad A (2015) PD-L1 biology in response to chemotherapy in vitro and in vivo in ovarian cancer. J Immunother Cancer 3:P302
36. Peng J, Hamanishi J, Matsumura N et al (2015) Chemotherapy induces programmed cell death-ligand 1 overexpression via the nuclear factor- B to foster an immunosuppressive tumor microenvironment in ovarian cancer. Cancer Res 75:5034–5045
37. Apetoh L, Ladoire S, Coukos G, Ghiringhelli F (2015) Combining immunotherapy and anticancer agents: the right path to achieve cancer cure? Ann Oncol 26:1813–1823
38. Herbst RS, Sznol M (2016) Diminished but not dead: chemotherapy for the treatment of NSCLC. Lancet Oncol 17:1464–1465
39. Correale P, Del Vecchio MT, La Placa M et al (2008) Chemotherapeutic drugs may be used to enhance the killing efficacy of human tumor antigen peptide-specific CTLs. J Immunother 31:132–147
40. Galluzzi L, Buqué A, Kepp O, Zitvogel L, Kroemer G (2017) Immunogenic cell death in cancer and infectious disease. Nat Rev Immunol 17:97–111
41. Lynch TJ, Bondarenko I, Luft A et al (2012) Ipilimumab in combination with paclitaxel and carboplatin as first-line treatment in stage IIIB/IV non-small-cell lung cancer: results from a randomized, double-blind, multicenter phase II study. J Clin Oncol 30:2046–2054
42. Langer CJ, Gadgeel SM, Borghaei H et al (2016) Carboplatin and pemetrexed with or without pembrolizumab for advanced, non-squamous non-small-cell lung cancer: a randomised, phase 2 cohort of the open-label KEYNOTE-021 study. Lancet Oncol 17:1497–1508
43. Rizvi NA, Hellmann MD, Brahmer JR et al (2016) Nivolumab in combination with platinum-based doublet chemotherapy for first-line treatment of advanced non-small-cell lung cancer. J Clin Oncol 34:2969–2979
44. Kanda S, Goto K, Shiraishi H et al (2016) Safety and efficacy of nivolumab and standard chemotherapy drug combination in patients with advanced non-small-cell lung cancer: a four arms phase Ib study. Ann Oncol 27:2242–2250
45. Liu SV, Powderly JD, Camidge R et al (2015) Safety and efficacy of MPDL3280A (anti-PDL1) in combination with platinum-based doublet chemotherapy in patients with advanced

non-small cell lung cancer (NSCLC). In: 2015 ASCO annual meeting | abstracts | meeting library. http://meetinglibrary.asco.org/content/148182-156. Accessed 11 Apr 2017
46. Cappuzzo F, Reck M, Papadimitrakopoulou V et al (2017) P3.02c-038 first-line Atezolizumab plus chemotherapy in chemotherapy-Naïve patients with advanced NSCLC: a phase III clinical program. J Thorac Oncol 12:S1296–S1297
47. Larkin J, Hodi FS, Wolchok JD (2015) Combined Nivolumab and Ipilimumab or monotherapy in untreated melanoma. N Engl J Med 373:1270–1271
48. Hammers H, Plimack ER, Infante JR et al (2016) Updated results from a phase I study of nivolumab (Nivo) in combination with ipilimumab (Ipi) in metastatic renal cell carcinoma (mRCC): the CheckMate 016 study. Ann Oncol. doi:10.1093/annonc/mdw378.16
49. Gubens MA, Sequist LV, Stevenson J et al (2016) Phase I/II study of pembrolizumab (pembro) plus ipilimumab (ipi) as second-line therapy for NSCLC: KEYNOTE-021 cohorts D and H. In: 2016 ASCO annual meeting. http://meetinglibrary.asco.org/content/167103-176. Accessed 12 Mar 2017
50. Hellmann MD, Rizvi NA, Goldman JW et al (2017) Nivolumab plus ipilimumab as first-line treatment for advanced non-small-cell lung cancer (CheckMate 012): results of an open-label, phase 1, multicohort study. Lancet Oncol 18:31–41
51. Karakunnel JJ (2016) O2-8-1Safety and efficacy of durvalumab (MEDI4736) plus tremelimumab in advanced non-small-cell lung cancer (NSCLC). Ann Oncol. doi:10.1093/annonc/mdw521.045
52. Rizvi N, Balmanoukian A, Goldberg SB et al (2015) 418OPhase 1b study of the safety and antitumour activity of durvalumab (MEDI4736) tremelimumab in advanced NSCLC. Ann Oncol 26:ix126.1–ixix126
53. Rizvi N, Barlesi F, Brahmer J et al (2015) Phase III, randomized, open-label study of durvalumab (MEDI4736) in combination with tremelimumab or durvalumab alone versus platinum-based chemotherapy in first-line treatment of patients with advanced/metastatic NSCLC: MYSTIC. J Immunother Cancer 3:P171
54. Peters S, Antonia S, Goldberg SB, Heymach JV, Kim ES, Nakagawa K, Papadimitrakopoulou V, Mukhopadhyay P, McIntosh S, Rizvi NA (2016) 191TiP: MYSTIC: a global, phase 3 study of durvalumab (MEDI4736) plus tremelimumab combination therapy or durvalumab monotherapy versus platinum-based chemotherapy (CT) in the first-line treatment of patients (pts) with advanced stage IV NSCLC. J Thorac Oncol 11:S139–S140
55. Mok T, Schmid P, de Castro G et al (2016) 482TiP global, phase 3 study of first-line durvalumab (MEDI4736) tremelimumab vs standard of care platinum-based chemotherapy in advanced/metastatic NSCLC: NEPTUNE. Ann Oncol. doi:10.1093/annonc/mdw594.046
56. Juergens R, Hao D, Laurie S et al (2017) MA09.03 cisplatin/Pemetrexed Durvalumab /–Tremelimumab in pts with advanced non-squamous NSCLC: a CCTG phase IB study - IND.226. J Thorac Oncol 12:S392–S393
57. Frederick DT, Piris A, Cogdill AP et al (2013) BRAF inhibition is associated with enhanced melanoma antigen expression and a more favorable tumor microenvironment in patients with metastatic melanoma. Clin Cancer Res 19:1225–1231
58. Lee CK, Man J, Lord S, Links M, Gebski V, Mok T, Yang JC-H (2017) Checkpoint inhibitors in metastatic EGFR-mutated non–small cell lung cancer—a meta-analysis. J Thorac Oncol 12:403–407
59. Spigel DR, Schrock AB, Fabrizio D et al (2016) Total mutation burden (TMB) in lung cancer (LC) and relationship with response to PD-1/PD-L1 targeted therapies. In: 2016 ASCO annual meeting library. http://meetinglibrary.asco.org/content/165567-176. Accessed 11 Mar 2017
60. Rangachari D, VanderLaan PA, Shea M, Le X, Huberman MS, Kobayashi SS, Costa DB (2017) Correlation between classic driver oncogene mutations in EGFR, ALK, or ROS1 and 22C3-PD-L1 ≥50% expression in lung adenocarcinoma. J Thorac Oncol. doi:10.1016/j.jtho.2016.12.026

61. Gainor JF, Shaw AT, Sequist LV et al (2016) EGFR mutations and ALK rearrangements are associated with low response rates to PD-1 pathway blockade in non-small cell lung cancer: a retrospective analysis. Clin Cancer Res 22:4585–4593
62. Rudin C, Cervantes A, Dowlati A et al (2017) P3.02c-046 safety, clinical activity and biomarker results from a phase Ib study of Erlotinib plus Atezolizumab in advanced NSCLC. J Thorac Oncol 12:S1302–S1303
63. Gibbons DL, Chow LQ, Kim D-W, Kim S-W, Yeh T, Song X, Jiang H, Taylor R, Karakunnel J, Creelan B (2016) 57O efficacy, safety and tolerability of MEDI4736 (durvalumab [D]), a human IgG1 anti-programmed cell death-ligand-1 (PD-L1) antibody, combined with gefitinib (G): a phase I expansion in TKI-naïve patients (pts) with EGFR mutant NSCLC. J Thorac Oncol 11:S79
64. Mok TS, Wu Y-L, Ahn M-J et al (2017) Osimertinib or platinum-pemetrexed in EGFR T790M-positive lung cancer. N Engl J Med 376:629–640
65. Ahn M-J, Yang J, Yu H, Saka H, Ramalingam S, Goto K, Kim S-W, Yang L, Walding A, Oxnard GR (2016) 136O: osimertinib combined with durvalumab in EGFR-mutant non-small cell lung cancer: results from the TATTON phase Ib trial. J Thorac Oncol 11:S115
66. Motz GT, Santoro SP, Wang L-P, Garrabrant T, Lastra RR, Hagemann IS, Lal P, Feldman MD, Benencia F, Coukos G (2014) Tumor endothelium FasL establishes a selective immune barrier promoting tolerance in tumors. Nat Med 20:607–615
67. Ohm JE, Gabrilovich DI, Sempowski GD, Kisseleva E, Parman KS, Nadaf S, Carbone DP (2003) VEGF inhibits T-cell development and may contribute to tumor-induced immune suppression. Blood 101:4878–4886
68. Terme M, Pernot S, Marcheteau E, Sandoval F, Benhamouda N, Colussi O, Dubreuil O, Carpentier AF, Tartour E, Taieb J (2013) VEGFA-VEGFR pathway blockade inhibits tumor-induced regulatory T-cell proliferation in colorectal cancer. Cancer Res 73:539–549
69. Kandalaft LE, Motz GT, Busch J, Coukos G (2011) Angiogenesis and the tumor vasculature as antitumor immune modulators: the role of vascular endothelial growth factor and endothelin. Curr Top Microbiol Immunol 344:129–148
70. Ott PA, Hodi FS, Buchbinder EI (2015) Inhibition of immune checkpoints and vascular endothelial growth factor as combination therapy for metastatic melanoma: an overview of rationale, preclinical evidence, and initial clinical data. Front Oncol 5:202
71. Garon EB, Ciuleanu T-E, Arrieta O et al (2014) Ramucirumab plus docetaxel versus placebo plus docetaxel for second-line treatment of stage IV non-small-cell lung cancer after disease progression on platinum-based therapy (REVEL): a multicentre, double-blind, randomised phase 3 trial. Lancet 384:665–673
72. Herbst RS, Martin-Liberal J, Calvo E et al (2016) Interim safety and clinical activity in patients with advanced NSCLC from a multi-cohort phase 1 study of ramucirumab (R) plus pembrolizumab (P). Ann Oncol. doi:10.1093/annonc/mdw435.34
73. Rizvi NA, Antonia SJ, Shepherd FA, Chow LQ, Goldman J, Shen Y, Chen AC, Gettinger S (2014) Nivolumab (anti-PD-1; BMS-936558, ONO-4538) maintenance as monotherapy or in combination with Bevacizumab (BEV) for non-small cell lung cancer (NSCLC) previously treated with chemotherapy. Int J Radiat Oncol Biol Phys 90:S32
74. Formenti SC, Demaria S (2013) Combining radiotherapy and cancer immunotherapy: a paradigm shift. JNCI J Natl Cancer Inst 105:256–265
75. Dewan MZ, Galloway AE, Kawashima N, Dewyngaert JK, Babb JS, Formenti SC, Demaria S (2009) Fractionated but not single-dose radiotherapy induces an immune-mediated abscopal effect when combined with anti-CTLA-4 antibody. Clin Cancer Res 15:5379–5388
76. Golden EB, Demaria S, Schiff PB, Chachoua A, Formenti SC (2013) An abscopal response to radiation and ipilimumab in a patient with metastatic non-small cell lung cancer. Cancer Immunol Res 1:365–372
77. Golden EB, Chachoua A, Fenton-Kerimian MB, Demaria S, Formenti SC (2015) Abscopal responses in metastatic non-small cell lung cancer (NSCLC) patients treated on a phase 2 study of combined radiation therapy and Ipilimumab: evidence for the in situ vaccination hypothesis of radiation. Int J Radiat Oncol Biol Phys 93:S66–S67

78. Simon GR, Turrisi A, American College of Chest Physicians (2007) Management of small cell lung cancer: ACCP evidence-based clinical practice guidelines (2nd edition). Chest 132:324S–339S
79. von Pawel J, Jotte R, Spigel DR et al (2014) Randomized phase III trial of amrubicin versus topotecan as second-line treatment for patients with small-cell lung cancer. J Clin Oncol 32:4012–4019
80. Peifer M, Fernández-Cuesta L, Sos ML et al (2012) Integrative genome analyses identify key somatic driver mutations of small-cell lung cancer. Nat Genet 44:1104–1110
81. George J, Lim JS, Jang SJ et al (2015) Comprehensive genomic profiles of small cell lung cancer. Nature 524:47–53
82. Rizvi NA, Hellmann MD, Snyder A et al (2015) Cancer immunology. Mutational landscape determines sensitivity to PD-1 blockade in non-small cell lung cancer. Science 348:124–128
83. Reck M, Bondarenko I, Luft A, Serwatowski P, Barlesi F, Chacko R, Sebastian M, Lu H, Cuillerot J-M, Lynch TJ (2013) Ipilimumab in combination with paclitaxel and carboplatin as first-line therapy in extensive-disease-small-cell lung cancer: results from a randomized, double-blind, multicenter phase 2 trial. Ann Oncol 24:75–83
84. Reck M, Luft A, Szczesna A et al (2016) Phase III randomized trial of Ipilimumab plus etoposide and platinum versus placebo plus Etoposide and platinum in extensive-stage small-cell lung cancer. J Clin Oncol. doi:10.1200/JCO.2016.67.6601
85. Horn L, Reck M, Mok T et al (2016) PS01.57: IMpower133: a phase I/III study of 1L Atezolizumab with carboplatin and Etoposide in patients with extensive-stage SCLC: topic: medical oncology. J Thorac Oncol 11:S305–S306
86. Ready N, Owonikoko TK, Postmus PE, Reck M, Peters S, Pieters A, Selvaggi G, Fairchild JP, Govindan R (2016) CheckMate 451: a randomized, double-blind, phase III trial of nivolumab (nivo), nivo plus ipilimumab (ipi), or placebo as maintenance therapy in patients (pts) with extensive-stage disease small cell lung cancer (ED-SCLC) after first-line platinum-based doublet chemotherapy (PT-DC). In: 2016 ASCO annual meeting. http://meetinglibrary.asco.org/content/165269-176. Accessed 16 Mar 2017
87. Ott PA (2015) Pembrolizumab for ED SCLC: efficacy and relationship with PD-L1 expression. In: International association for the study of lung cancer. https://library.iaslc.org/search-speaker?search_speaker=28443. Accessed 20 Mar 2017
88. Ott P, Felip E, Hiret S, Kim D-W, Morosky A, Saraf S, Piperdi B, Mehnert J (2017) OA05.01 Pembrolizumab in patients with extensive-stage small cell lung cancer: updated survival results from KEYNOTE-028. J Thorac Oncol 12:S259
89. Ott PA, Fernandez MEE, Hiret S, Kim D-W, Moss RA, Winser T, Yuan Sammy Cheng Jonathan, Piperdi B, Mehnert JM (2015) Pembrolizumab (MK-3475) in patients (pts) with extensive-stage small cell lung cancer (SCLC): preliminary safety and efficacy results from KEYNOTE-028. In: 2015 ASCO annual meeting | abstracts | meeting library. http://meetinglibrary.asco.org/content/148558-15. Accessed 20 Mar 2017
90. Antonia SJ, López-Martin JA, Bendell J et al (2016) Nivolumab alone and nivolumab plus ipilimumab in recurrent small-cell lung cancer (CheckMate 032): a multicentre, open-label, phase 1/2 trial. Lancet Oncol 17:883–895
91. Goudar RK (2008) Review of pemetrexed in combination with cisplatin for the treatment of malignant pleural mesothelioma. Ther Clin Risk Manag 4:205–211
92. Ettinger DS, Wood DE, Akerley W et al (2016) NCCN guidelines insights: malignant pleural mesothelioma, version 3.2016. J Natl Compr Canc Netw 14:825–836
93. Bueno R, Stawiski EW, Goldstein LD et al (2016) Comprehensive genomic analysis of malignant pleural mesothelioma identifies recurrent mutations, gene fusions and splicing alterations. Nat Genet 48:407–416
94. Calabrò L, Morra A, Fonsatti E et al (2015) Efficacy and safety of an intensified schedule of tremelimumab for chemotherapy-resistant malignant mesothelioma: an open-label, single-arm, phase 2 study. Lancet Respir Med 3:301–309

95. Calabrò L, Morra A, Fonsatti E et al (2013) Tremelimumab for patients with chemotherapy-resistant advanced malignant mesothelioma: an open-label, single-arm, phase 2 trial. Lancet Oncol 14:1104–1111
96. Kindler HL, Scherpereel A, Calabrò L et al (2016) Tremelimumab as second- or third-line treatment of unresectable malignant mesothelioma (MM): results from the global, double-blind, placebo-controlled DETERMINE study. In: 2016 ASCO annual meeting I abstracts I meeting library. http://meetinglibrary.asco.org/content/162717-176. Accessed 21 Mar 2017
97. Hassan R, Thomas A, Patel MR et al (2016) Avelumab (MSB0010718C; anti-PD-L1) in patients with advanced unresectable mesothelioma from the JAVELIN solid tumor phase Ib trial: Safety, clinical activity, and PD-L1 expression. In: 2016 ASCO annual meeting I abstracts I meeting library. http://meetinglibrary.asco.org/content/164219-176. Accessed 17 Apr 2017
98. Alley EW, Lopez J, Santoro A, Morosky A, Saraf S, Piperdi B, van Brummelen E (2017) Clinical safety and activity of pembrolizumab in patients with malignant pleural mesothelioma (KEYNOTE-028): preliminary results from a non-randomised, open-label, phase 1b trial. Lancet Oncol. doi:10.1016/S1470-2045(17)30169-9
99. Nowak A, Kok P-S, Livingstone A, Lesterhuis WJ, Yip S, Donoghoe M, Lam W-S, Stockler M (2017) P2.06-025 DREAM - a phase 2 trial of DuRvalumab with first line chEmotherApy in mesothelioma with a safety run in. J Thorac Oncol 12:S1086–S1087
100. Calabrò L, Morra A, Giannarelli D, Annesi D, Bertocci E, Danielli R, Altomonte M, Di Giacomo AM, Maio M (2016) Tremelimumab and durvalumab (MEDI4736) combination for first and second-line treatment of mesothelioma patients: the NIBIT-MESO-1 study. In: 2016 ASCO annual meeting I abstracts I meeting library. http://meetinglibrary.asco.org/content/165621-176. Accessed 22 Mar 2017
101. Engels EA (2010) Epidemiology of thymoma and associated malignancies. J Thorac Oncol 5:S260–S265
102. Ströbel P, Hohenberger P, Marx A (2010) Thymoma and thymic carcinoma: molecular pathology and targeted therapy. J Thorac Oncol 5:S286–S290
103. Weksler B, Lu B (2014) Alterations of the immune system in thymic malignancies. J Thorac Oncol 9:S137–S142
104. Ettinger DS, Wood DE, Aisner DL et al (2017) NCCN clinical practice guidelines in oncology (NCCN guidelines®) thymomas and thymic Carcinomas. In: National comprehensive cancer network. https://www.nccn.org/professionals/physician_gls/pdf/thymic.pdf. Accessed 7 Apr 2017
105. Girard N, Ruffini E, Marx A, Faivre-Finn C, Peters S, Guidelines Committee ESMO (2015) Thymic epithelial tumours: ESMO clinical practice guidelines for diagnosis, treatment and follow-up. Ann Oncol 26(Suppl 5):v40–v55
106. Tiseo M, Damato A, Longo L et al (2017) Analysis of a panel of druggable gene mutations and of ALK and PD-L1 expression in a series of thymic epithelial tumors (TETs). Lung Cancer 104:24–30
107. Katsuya Y, Fujita Y, Horinouchi H, Ohe Y, Watanabe S-I, Tsuta K (2015) Immunohistochemical status of PD-L1 in thymoma and thymic carcinoma. Lung Cancer 88:154–159
108. Marchevsky AM, Walts AE (2017) PD-L1, PD-1, CD4, and CD8 expression in neoplastic and nonneoplastic thymus. Hum Pathol 60:16–23
109. Weissferdt A, Fujimoto J, Kalhor N, Rodriguez J, Bassett R, Wistuba II, Moran CA (2017) Expression of PD-1 and PD-L1 in thymic epithelial neoplasms. Mod Pathol. doi:10.1038/modpathol.2017.6
110. Padda SK, Riess JW, Schwartz EJ, Tian L, Kohrt HE, Neal JW, West RB, Wakelee HA (2015) Diffuse high intensity PD-L1 staining in thymic epithelial tumors. J Thorac Oncol 10:500–508
111. Yokoyama S, Miyoshi H, Nakashima K, Shimono J, Hashiguchi T, Mitsuoka M, Takamori S, Akagi Y, Ohshima K (2016) Prognostic value of programmed death ligand 1 and programmed death 1 expression in thymic carcinoma. Clin Cancer Res 22:4727–4734

112. Owen D, Chu B, Lehman A, Annamalai L, Yearley J, Shilo K, Otterson G (2017) P2.04-020 expression patterns and prognostic value of PD-L1 and PD-1 in thymoma and thymic carcinoma. J Thorac Oncol 12:S1008–S1009
113. Yokoyama S, Miyoshi H, Nishi T, Hashiguchi T, Mitsuoka M, Takamori S, Akagi Y, Kakuma T, Ohshima K (2016) Clinicopathologic and prognostic implications of programmed death ligand 1 expression in thymoma. Ann Thorac Surg 101:1361–1369
114. Naidoo J, Steele K, Sima CS, Yuan J, Robbins PB, Moreira AL, Pietanza MC, Wolchok JD, Riely GJ, Rizvi NA (2015) Defining the immunologic phenotype of thymic epithelial tumors. In: Journal of clinical oncology. http://ascopubs.org/doi/abs/10.1200/jco.2015.33.15_suppl.7516. Accessed 20 Apr 2017
115. Rajan A, Heery C, Mammen A, Pittaluga S, Lepone L, Donahue R, Grenga I, Schlom J, Gulley J, Hassan R (2017) OA18.03 safety and clinical activity of Avelumab (MSB0010718C; anti-PD-L1) in patients with advanced thymic epithelial tumors (TETs). J Thorac Oncol 12:S314–S315
116. Giaccone G, Thompson J, Crawford J, McGuire C, Manning M, Subramaniam D, Liu S (2016) A phase II study of pembrolizumab in patients with recurrent thymic carcinoma. In: 2016 ASCO annual meeting | abstracts | meeting library. http://meetinglibrary.asco.org/content/168922-176. Accessed 5 Apr 2017
117. Salama AKS, Moschos SJ (2017) Next steps in immuno-oncology: enhancing antitumor effects through appropriate patient selection and rationally designed combination strategies. Ann Oncol 28:57–74
118. Khan IS, Mouchess ML, Zhu M-L, Conley B, Fasano KJ, Hou Y, Fong L, Su MA, Anderson MS (2014) Enhancement of an anti-tumor immune response by transient blockade of central T cell tolerance. J Exp Med 211:761–768

Chapter 11
Melanoma Immunotherapy

Gregory A. Daniels

Abstract Two therapeutic pathways have driven the improvement in clinical outcomes for patients with melanoma, BRAF inhibition, and immune modulation. As clinical progress continues, there is a convergence of these therapeutic approaches as a dynamic interface between the tumor and the supporting environment. Immune therapy drives adaptive changes in tumor oncogenic pathways just as oncogenic pathways shape the tumor microenvironment. This chapter explores examples of current and developing therapies at the synapse between intrinsic oncogene signaling and the tumor microenvironment to improve patient outcomes.

Keywords Melanoma • Interleukin-2 • Aldesleukin • Proleukin • Ipilimumab • Pembrolizumab • Nivolumab • Dabrafenib • Vemurafenib • Talimogene laherparepvec • Coxsackievirus A21 • CAVATAK • CVA21 • NKTR214 • Indoleamine 2,3-dioxygenase

11.1 Introduction

This past decade has witnessed dramatic improvements in clinical outcomes for advanced cutaneous melanoma. The median overall survival for patients with metastatic disease has changed from 8 to 10 months in 2010 to greater than 24 months in current clinical trials [1, 2]. This improvement reflects advances in immune therapies and targeted agents (MAPK [mitogen-activated protein kinase] inhibitors). Appreciating opportunities for future immune therapeutics begins with understanding what we have learned and the current clinical challenges. This chapter provides a brief overview of current clinical care in immune therapy and highlights examples of novel immune therapeutic strategies in melanoma.

G.A. Daniels, MD, PhD (✉)
UC San Diego, Moores Cancer Center,
3855 Health Sciences Drive MC0987, La Jolla 92093-0987, 858-534-3804, CA, USA

VA San Diego Healthcare System,
3350 La Jolla Village Drive 111E, San Diego, CA 92161, USA
e-mail: gdaniels@ucsd.edu

S.P. Patel, R. Kurzrock (eds.), *Early Phase Cancer Immunotherapy*,
Current Cancer Research, DOI 10.1007/978-3-319-63757-0_11

Melanoma, like other tumors, develops in the context of a functioning immune system and utilizes mechanisms to both decrease an antitumor response and promote a protumor microenvironment [3]. While more than a century has passed since Paget proposed his seed and soil hypothesis regarding the relationship between intrinsic growth pathways and the extrinsic signals from the surrounding stroma, his insights have only recently been effectively translated to the clinic [4]. Ultraviolet light exposure not only drives melanomagenesis with a high mutation rate but likely also promotes chronic inflammatory changes selecting a tumor that often thrives within an immune response [5]. Understanding the dynamic synapse of intrinsic cancer cell pathways and extrinsic stromal support (including immune editing) has driven the development of more effective therapies [6].

The inflammatory state of primary melanoma lesions was recognized early as a prognostic marker (Clark) by the quantitative presence of a natural immune response to an antigenic tumor. Lymphocytic infiltration (inflamed or "brisk") is associated with better clinical outcomes and "nonbrisk" or "absent" infiltrated (noninflamed) lesions correlate with worse prognosis [7, 8]. Similarly, patients with recurrent or metastatic disease can be characterized as having inflamed and noninflamed tumors. This subdivision only begins to address the details necessary to direct therapy. One model groups melanomas into four categories—adaptive immune resistance (type I), immunological ignorance (type II), tolerance (type III) and intrinsic induction (type IV)—based on tumor infiltrating lymphocytes and PD-L1 expression (Fig. 11.1) [11]. Within these proposed functional categories will likely be multiple targetable mechanisms of clinical importance including additional immune regulatory steps and metabolic pathways.

Melanoma, like other malignancies, is subject to normal immune regulatory mechanisms of central (thymus) and peripheral tolerance that govern an antitumor response and shape a pro-tumor microenvironment. Current immune treatments (checkpoint and cytokine) utilize and expand an already present natural T cell response. A central challenge in following and understanding the T cell response is the identification of which antigen-specific T cells drive tumor regression. Melanoma antigen classes include differentiation-specific proteins involved in lineage specific functions (i.e., MART1, melanin), tumor testes antigens (i.e., NY-ESO), and neoantigens [12, 13]. Melanoma differentiation antigens and tumor testes antigens are subject to both peripheral and central tolerance. The driver mutations (MAPK activating mutations) and the genetic instability allowing melanocytes to gain functions necessary for the generation of tumors are often associated with novel mutations. These neoantigens would not be subject to central tolerance, and they rely on peripheral tolerance mechanisms and are likely the target of current checkpoint inhibitor therapy [14–16]. Naturally present tumor infiltrating T cells (TILs) fail to reject the melanoma tumors by the induction of several inhibitory pathways including programmed death ligands (PD-L1), indoleamine 2,3-dioxygenase (IDO), and regulatory T cells (Tregs). Understanding the T cell repertoire and these natural regulatory loops that interface between the adaptive and innate immune response will continue to improve the care of melanoma patients.

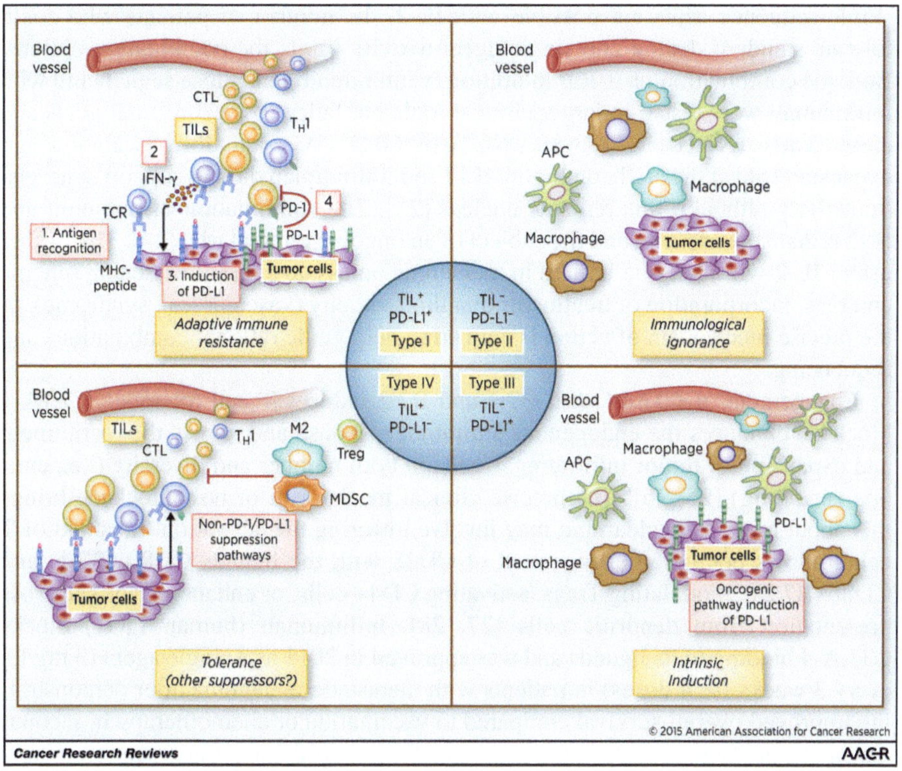

Fig. 11.1 Types of tumor microenvironment for tailoring cancer immunotherapeutic modules. Cancers have been categorized into four different tumor microenvironments based on the presence of TILs and PD-L1 expression [9, 10]. They are type I (adaptive immune resistance), type II (immunologic ignorance), type III (intrinsic induction), and type IV (tolerance). This proposed framework of stratifying tumors is simplistic but allows a platform to discuss the immunotherapeutic strategies best suited to targeting the four different tumor microenvironments. *APC*, antigen-presenting cell, *M2* M2 macrophage, *TH1* T helper 1

11.2 Current Immune Therapies in Melanoma

Interleukin-2 (aldesleukin, proleukin, IL-2) was the first cancer immunotherapy approved following the publication of a series of phase 2 trials from the National Cancer Institute (NCI) demonstrating durable drug free survival in a small percentage of patients [9]. Complete response occurs in approximately 5–10% of select metastatic melanoma patients with the majority of responses lasting decades without further treatment [10, 17]. High-dose IL-2 (600,000–720,000 U/kg every 8 h) is limited to select patients expected to tolerate the acute toxicity and multiorgan dysfunction [18–20]. Responders to interleukin-2 (IL-2) appear to be distinct from responders to cytotoxic T lymphocyte antigen 4 (CTLA-4) blocking antibody (ipilimumab) as response rates appear similar either following or preceding IL-2 [21, 22]. The position of IL-2 in the sequence of current therapeutic options is unclear.

While sequence trials are possible with IL-2, the number of patients who could tolerate standard dosing and single agent toxicity limits the combination options. Both the combination of B-Raf inhibition (vemurafenib) and close sequencing with ipilimumab were tested in larger clinical trials but failed to meet accrual goals and closed early (NCT01683188 and NCT01856023). A small dose escalation and expansion trial at the NCI combining IL-2 and ipilimumab did not support synergistic activity although this remains unclear [23]. The combination of radiation and IL-2 remains interesting and the subject of an ongoing clinical trial [24]. The further use of IL-2 will likely be limited in melanoma unless an alternative dosing scheme emerges, incorporation of treatments that limit toxicity (vascular leak syndrome), or the precise mechanism of action is defined to help guide rational combinations and sequencing.

Engagement of *CTLA4* with B7.1 and B7.2 induces T cell tolerance. CLTA-4 blockade enhances the endogenous antitumor response and allows the recruitment and expansion of tumor infiltrating T cells in both number and diversity (i.e., epitope spreading) [25, 26]. The precise clinical mechanism of how blockade brings this about remains unclear and may involve lowering the activation threshold of T cells (allows continued engagement of CD28 with the ligands CD80 (B7.1) and CD86 (B7.2)), modulating Tregs, activating CD4+ cells, or enhancing antigen cross presentation from dendritic cells [27, 28]. Ipilimumab (human IgG1) blocks CTLA-4 binding to its ligands and was approved in 2011 as a single agent (3 mg/kg every 3 weeks for 4 doses) in patients with metastatic melanoma after demonstrating improved overall survival compared to vaccination or chemotherapy in second- and first-line therapy [29, 30]. Long-term follow-up demonstrates approximately 20% of the treated patients maintain responses with a survival plateau evident around 3 years and extending beyond 10 years in the absence of continued therapy [31]. The clinical benefit of ipilimumab reflects the expansion of an antigen-specific immune response to tumor antigens. Interestingly, while the vaccines and chemotherapies utilized in the early clinical trials did not appear to improve response to ipilimumab, radiation as well as other tumor ablation strategies may add to the clinical benefit of ipilimumab therapy in melanoma (discussed later). Thus, strategies that promote productive antigen exposure may enhance ipilimumab activity.

Interfering with a central mechanism of peripheral tolerance has consequences—immune related adverse events (irAEs). These clinical events include inflammatory colitis, dermatitis, hepatitis, and endocrinopathies among others [32]. Autoimmune reactions reflect the breakdown of immune tolerance driven by the development of broader immune reactivity.

Despite some correlation between immune adverse events and clinical benefit, many more patients demonstrate enhanced tumor T cell infiltration without clinical response upon blocking CTLA-4 [33]. We are beginning to understand some of the innate and acquired limitations to an effective antitumor response in patients with ipilimumab [34, 35]. While a high tumor mutation burden favors response, genome analysis from responders and nonresponders to ipilimumab utilizing algorithms to predict specific neoantigen signatures associated with response have been conflicting

[15, 36]. One important step preventing clinical benefit appears to be mediated by a second checkpoint molecule—programed death 1 [37, 38].

Programed death 1 (PD-1) is present on T cells and engagement with ligand (PD-L1 or PD-L2) on tumor or stromal cells within the microenvironment decreases the antitumor response. Use of anti-PD-1 monotherapy (either pembrolizumab or nivolumab) demonstrates improved survival, overall response rates, and safety compared with either chemotherapy or ipilimumab monotherapy [39–41]. The phase 3 Keynote 006 showed response rates to pembrolizumab monotherapy to be approximately 37% with 1- and 2-year progression free survival of 38% and 28% [42]. Long-term safety and survival data with pembrolizumab from Keynote 001 demonstrated a grade 3–4 toxicity rate of about 17% with a 3-year progression free survival of 30% in previously untreated patients [43]. Of the patients who achieved a complete response, a percentage of them stopped therapy after an average of about 23 months and were observed. Most patients (59 of the 61) observed off pembrolizumab maintained a complete response at 10 months (Robert ASCO 2016). Continued follow up will better clarify the number of patients who ultimately transition to long-term disease-free and treatment-free survival with single agent PD-1 blocking therapy.

Predicting which melanoma patients will respond to PD-1 blockade monotherapy remains a clinical challenge. The presence of PD-L1 correlates with interferon-γ producing infiltrating tumor specific T cells (TILs) with only a small number of melanoma tumors that are PD-L1 positive and TIL negative [44]. Demonstrating PD-L1 by immune histochemistry would be expected to mark patients who would benefit from anti-PD-1 blocking therapy. However, while staining for PD-L1 does enrich for patients more likely to respond to PD-1 blocking antibodies, current assays show this to be neither sufficient nor necessary in melanoma [45]. Many factors likely contribute to poor assay predictability including the dynamic response of PD-L1, heterogeneous expression, detecting antibody variation, and the presence of additional immune checkpoints. As in other tumor types, high tumor mutation rates correlate with PD-1 blockade response in melanoma. Additionally, flow cytometry prior to and during therapy suggests patients with a high percentage of CD8+ TILs co-expressing high levels of surface PD-1 and CTLA-4 respond to anti-PD-1 monotherapy [46]. The absence or presence of additional surface markers including TIM-3 and LAG-3 divide lymphocytic populations into exhausted (but responsive to PD-1 blockade) and super exhausted (no longer responsive to PD-1 blocking therapy) [47]. Another approach uses the inflammatory signature focused upon IFN-γ signaling, T cell markers, and antigen presentation machinery to identify who would likely respond to PD-1 blockade alone [48]. Lack or loss of IFN-γ signaling is associated with a lack of PD-1 blockade response. Lastly, clinical parameters including LDH (lactate dehydrogenase), age, sex, extent of disease, and prior treatment history also reflect the likelihood of response [49]. Continued refinement with incorporation of other patient and tumor variables will improve the predictive power of these assays to identify those patients most likely to benefit from monotherapy PD-1 blockade.

Talimogene laherparepvec (Imlygic or TVEC) is an engineered oncolytic herpes simplex virus (HSV) type 1 expressing a transgene for human granulocyte macrophage colony-stimulating factor (GM-CSF) approved in 2015 for direct intralesional injection into accessible skin and lymph node metastasis in patients with advanced unresectable melanoma. Gene modifications promote selective tumor replication (lower expression of neurovirulence factor gene (*ICP34.5*)), antigen expression (deletion of *ICP47),* and dendritic cell activity (GM-CSF transgene) locally to promote an inflammatory T cell response [50]. Interestingly, tumor cells that loose IFN-γ signaling are more susceptible to oncolytic viral destruction and thus may partner well with immune check points (discussed later) [51].

Intralesional injections are associated with mild adverse events (AEs) with only 3% grade 3 or 4 events [52]. A randomized phase III trial of stage III and IV patients established a single agent durable response rate (CR [complete response] or PR [partial response] lasting >6 months) of 16% and an overall response rate of 26% [53]. Responses were observed in both injected and not injected lesions (15% of the evaluable not injected lesions decreased by 50% or more). No significant overall survival advantage was seen for patients with a median overall survival of 23.3 months for Talimogene laherparepvec and 18.9 months for GM-CSF. Unplanned subgroup analysis suggested that patients who were treatment naïve or had lower burden of disease had a higher clinical benefit. Talimogene laherparepvec is an option in patients with unresectable stage III or limited stage IV melanoma early in the treatment course but appears to have low clinical value in patients with a high burden of disease as a single agent.

11.3 Combination Checkpoint Therapy (CTLA-4 and PD-1)

The combination of ipilimumab plus nivolumab sets the current bar for treatment-free, cancer-free survival. Wolchok et al. reported a landmark phase 1 dose escalation study examining either sequenced or concurrent ipilimumab and nivolumab followed with dose expansion in metastatic melanoma patients between December 2009 and February 2013 [54]. The majority of treated patients responded and a large fraction achieved deep and durable responses. Toxicity was equally enhanced relative to sequential therapy or monotherapy with either ipilimumab or nivolumab. It should be noted in this phase 1 trial that some patients had nivolumab continued every 3 weeks for four doses after the combination was given and the combination could be repeated every 12 weeks.

The largest combination study, CheckMate 067, randomized 945 treatment naïve metastatic melanoma patients to either monotherapy with ipilimumab (3 mg/kg) or nivolumab (3 mg/kg) or concurrent ipilimumab (3 mg/kg) and nivolumab (1 mg/kg) followed by maintenance nivolumab (3 mg/kg every 2 weeks until progression or toxicity) [55]. Patients were stratified with respect to PD-L1 staining (Dako clone 28-8), BRAF mutation status, and extent of disease (M0, M1a, or M1b versus M1c). Eighteen-month follow up at ASCO 2016 demonstrated improvement in progression-free survival in the intent-to-treat population (primary endpoint) for ipilimumab plus nivolumab (46%) compared with nivolumab (39%) and ipilimumab (14%) monotherapy [56]. Similar progression-free survival was observed in patients expressing ≥5% tumor PD-L1 staining in patients treated with ipilimumab plus nivolumab or nivolumab monotherapy while the combination appeared superior in the PD-L1 negative tumor staining population for the endpoint of progression-free survival. As the toxicity of the combination treatment remains significantly higher than that with either monotherapy, it will be critical to further define the population of patients appropriate for combination therapy including which patients would likely respond (additional markers beyond PD-L1 immune histochemistry), the role of maintenance nivolumab, toxicity predictors, and the long-term outcomes.

A second large clinical trial, CheckMate 069, examined 142 treatment naïve patients randomized 2:1 to ipilimumab (3 mg/kg) plus either nivolumab (1 mg/kg) or placebo followed by continued maintenance nivolumab (3 mg/kg) or placebo [2, 57]. The combination again demonstrated improved response rate (64% versus 11%) and progression-free survival (Not Reached (NR) versus 4.4 months) over ipilimumab alone in BRAF wild type patients at a follow up period of 11 months. Patients who experienced a grade ≥3 drug-related adverse event and discontinued treatment had an overall survival in the ipilimumab plus nivolumab arm of 71% compared to 64% (total combination arm) or 54% with ipilimumab alone (Hodi ASCO 2016) [58]. Surprisingly, the 2-year progression-free survival was approximately 50% for combination therapy in patients regardless of continued nivolumab monotherapy versus 12% in the ipilimumab arm. These data suggest that up to half of patients who stop therapy due to significant dose-limiting irAEs require no additional therapy beyond the initial 1 to 4 doses of induction with the combination. This finding will need to be confirmed with the continued follow up of the larger data sets. The optimal dosing, schedule, and combinations of currently available immune checkpoint therapies in melanoma remain unknown.

11.4 Sequencing of Therapies

Melanoma patients have multiple treatment options and often have exposure to both targeted and immune therapies during the course of care. Targeted molecular agents have transformed oncology as much as immune modulators. BRAF gene activating mutations occur in roughly 50% of cutaneous melanoma patients and mitogen-activated protein kinase (MAPK) inhibition by either B-Raf inhibitors (vemurafenib or dabrafenib), Mek inhibitors (cobimetanib or trametanib), or a combination of B-Raf and Mek has relatively high response rates, rapid improvement in cancer-related symptoms and improvement in overall survival [59, 60]. Patients with high volume or symptomatic melanoma may not be appropriate candidates for upfront immune therapy and exposure to targeted agents is effective for providing clinical benefit and lowering the tumor burden for possible subsequent immune modulation.

Choosing between therapies not only depends upon the clinical goals of the patient but also that the order of therapies may influence outcomes to subsequent treatment. A brisk tumor lymphocytic infiltration occurs early in the treatment of melanomas containing an activating BRAF mutation exposed to MAPK pathway inhibitors [61]. The infiltration, predominantly T cells, decreases upon progression on MAPK inhibitor therapies. The dynamic changes in infiltration suggest that the clinical benefit of B-Raf-directed therapy may have an immune component and the development of resistance could alter response to subsequent immune treatments that rely on immune cell infiltration. Several lines of research outlined as follows support this concern.

Lo et al. evaluated the genomic, transcriptional, and phenotypic changes in melanoma patients undergoing MAPK directed therapy in two provocative studies [62, 63]. Patients who acquired MAPK inhibitor resistance experienced intratumoral T cell exhaustion and depletion correlating with CSF1R and CD163 expression on macrophages with loss of IFN-γ driven expression of CD8α+ T cells. In a second study, the group demonstrated a transcriptional signature correlating with innate anti-PD-1 resistance (IPRES) involving genes in mesenchymal transition, angiogenesis, hypoxia, and wound healing. These same signatures are induced in melanoma tumors treated with MAPK inhibitors. The authors suggest that targeted therapies could negatively impact sequential and concurrent immune therapy depending upon the timing and length of exposure.

If resistance to MAPK inhibitors is associated with resistance to subsequent immune modulation (at least PD-1 blockade), a possible solution would be to limit exposure to MAPK inhibition rather than treatment until the development of resistance. To this end, a phase 2 trial tested a 6-week induction with vemurafenib prior to ipilimumab (10 mg/kg induction and subsequent maintenance) in 46 patients [64]. The toxicities were as expected for the single agents but a suggestion of an improvement in response rate at the end of ipilimumab induction compared to historical controls. The size and follow up presented is not sufficient to assess the clinical value of this sequence. The sequential use of vemurafenib followed by ipilimumab was better tolerated than the combination of vemurafenib and ipilimumab [65]. A critically important study sponsored by the Eastern Cooperative Oncology Group (NCT02224781) randomizes metastatic melanoma patients with activating BRAF mutations to either dabrafenib plus trametanib followed by ipilimumab plus nivolumab at progression or to ipilimumab plus nivolumab followed by dabrafenib plus trametanib at progression. This trial will better define the clinical influence of sequencing targeted MAPK inhibitors with existing immune therapies.

Equally unclear is the influence the sequence of current immune checkpoints and cytokine therapy has upon patient outcomes. A randomized phase 2 trial suggested improved outcomes in patients with the sequential exposure of nivolumab followed by ipilimumab compared to the reverse with ipilimumab followed by nivolumab (CheckMate 064) [66]. The reason for this difference is unclear as all patients received subsequent nivolumab therapy and thus, the patients on the "nivolumab first arm" had two time points where they may have had significant exposure to both ipilimumab and nivolumab in combination compared to once on the "ipilimumab first arm." Further data is needed to clarify the optimal sequence of PD-1 and CTLA-4 blocking therapy.

11.5 Strategies to Manage Toxicity

A challenge for current immune checkpoints and cytokines is the overlap between the mechanism of antitumor response and immune related adverse events (irAEs). While novel combinations and agents will likely increase the number of responding patients with possibly improved toxicity profiles, a second strategy focuses upon current treatments including alternative dosing and routes of delivery to improve tolerability. Early recognition and management of irAEs limits toxicity and shortens the time of immune suppression required [32, 67]. Current strategies used to attenuate immune activation are broadly immune suppressive and rely on high doses of corticosteroids, mycophenolate mofetil, and TGFβ blocking antibodies (infliximab).

While immune suppression particularly with corticosteroids is effective in limiting most irAEs to 4 to 8 weeks, these agents may attenuate the anticancer response. Several strategies attempt to limit systemic immune suppression. The addition of the nonabsorbable steroid, budesonide, to ipilimumab treatment appears to have had little impact on the rates or severity of autoimmune colitis [68]. However, just as in inflammatory bowel management, earlier introduction of disease modifying steroid sparing agents may be a valid strategy. A trial to examine infliximab and lower dose steroid exposure compared to higher dose steroids is ongoing (NCT02763761). Hodi et al. reported a randomized phase II trial of ipilimumab (10 mg/kg dosing with maintenance) with or without systemic GM-CSF (sargramostim) in patients with metastatic melanoma enrolled between December 2010 and July 2011 with results reported in December 2012 [69]. This time frame is prior to the availability of PD-1 therapies. Interestingly, the investigators found that while overall progression-free survival was the same (3.1 months), the addition of GM-CSF resulted in improved overall survival and lower toxicity. This study raises several provocative questions regarding the mechanism of improved outcomes ranging from improved antigen presentation to improved toxicity driven survival. GM-CSF could limit toxicity due to the tolerizing impact on inducing myeloid-derived suppressor cells [70]. A similar trial is ongoing examining ipilimumab plus nivolumab combination therapy with GM-CSF (NCT02339571).

Other strategies to manage irAEs include examining agents used in allograft rejection or autoimmune disease management that may have a more selective immune suppression. For example, toclilizumab (anti-IL6R antibody) is used to treat moderate to severe rheumatoid arthritis and was used successfully to treat a patient with Crohn's disease exacerbation due to anti-PD-1 therapy [71]. While the changes in treatments and outcomes in the last 10 years for melanoma patients is nothing short of revolutionary, more needs to be done to understand and manage the toxicities associated with treatments.

11.6 Acquired and Innate Resistance to Immune Therapy

Identifying the mechanisms of both innate and acquired resistance will be critical to improve patient outcomes. Long-term disease-free survival is achieved only in a fraction of patients by adoptive cell therapy, high-dose interleukin-2, or checkpoint blockade. At least half of melanoma patients who initially achieve a response to PD-1 monotherapy acquire resistance [43]. Resistance mechanisms include target antigen loss, immune exclusion, and induction of other resistance pathways (Fig. 11.1). Loss of interferon responsiveness occurs in some patients progressing with either CTLA-4 or PD-1 blockade with changes observed in expression or mutations in beta 2 microglobulin and JAK1 or JAK2 [47, 72, 73]. Analysis of ipilimumab (CTLA-4) responders and nonresponders samples identified genomic changes in the IFN-γ pathway genes including IFNGR1, IRF1, JAK2 and IFNGR2. Defects in the IFN-γ pathway genes have been similarly observed in patients progressing after adoptive cellular therapy, high-dose interleukin-2 and PD-1 blockade [74–76]. Interestingly, changes in JAK1 or JAK2 are associated with primary resistance to PD-1 treatment suggesting that selection occurred in the development of the expanding tumor. Tumors that lack interferon receptor signaling may have a selective advantage in avoiding activated T cells. Loss of JAK1 or JAK2 may also decrease T cell migration to the tumor. T cell mediated tumor killing involves the IFN-γ pathway and defects in this pathway allows tumor progression. Strategies to reverse interferon resistance (i.e., epigenetic, intralesional treatments) may overcome primary and acquired resistance to immune therapy in some patients. An additional challenge will be the heterogeneous nature of solid tumors and ongoing dynamic adaptive changes (immunoediting). While monitoring IFN-γ pathway signatures may function as a biomarker directing therapy choices; this will be challenging. Improved techniques to monitor the tumor adaptive responses to treatment will ultimately guide rational combinations to improve the percentage of long-term responders.

11.7 Novel Therapeutics

Novel agents provide an opportunity to expand the number of patients not addressed by current therapies and improve outcomes with lower toxicity. A fraction of melanoma tumors are resistant to current checkpoints due to poor immunologic response (innate resistance) or acquired resistance as outlined earlier (Fig. 11.1). Strategies to enhance immune recognition of tumors lacking a natural immune response could improve outcomes and provide additional partners with current checkpoints. Critical to this will be the understanding of why some melanomas lack immune cell infiltration. This could be due to lack of tumor recognition or by active immune exclusion. Tumors lack T cell recognition due to central and peripheral tolerance mechanisms. Most current and developing immune treatments focus on interrupting peripheral tolerance mechanisms employed by tumors [77]. Cell-based therapy including chimeric antigen receptors, TCRs, bispecific antibodies, and neoantigen enriched products may allow us to address central tolerance.

Adoptive T cell therapy (ACT) mediates tumor regression in melanoma that can be durable and complete with up to 40% percent of patients achieving cancer control at 5 years. Current protocols pioneered at the NCI surgery branch by Rosenberg et al. employ autologous TILs from surgical resections that are expanded ex vivo to generate a patient specific product. To date, the best activity has been with unselected bulk TILs infused following lymphodepletion and subsequent high-dose bolus interleukin 2 [78]. However, several areas limit the number of patients appropriate for treatment including efficient generation of cells and the intensity of therapy. Strategies to improve adoptive cell therapy include enrichment of tumor reactive cells and subsequent treatments.

Identification of antigens associated with tumor regression and particularly the identification of the critical tumor reactive T cells has been elusive. Functional identification may allow for improvement in cell product generation by enriching for naturally occurring tumor reactive T cells. Characterization of CD8+ TILs expressing exhaustion markers (PD-1, LAG-3, and TIM-3) identifies clones targeting mutated tumor antigens [79]. A second approach relies upon reactivity selection by tumor sequencing and identification of neoantigens to enrich for tumor reactive TILs [80]. Treatment of patients prior to TIL harvest with therapies that promote an increase in TIL-engraftment could improve the number of patients who have successful product or lower the amount of material needed for TIL treatment. These could include intralesional treatments, radiation, targeted agents, or checkpoint exposure.

Conditioning or subsequent therapy may improve adoptive cell therapy (ACT) activity. Lymphodepletion with chemotherapy prior to cell infusion enhances adoptive cell activity but the mechanism remains poorly understood [81, 82]. While many mechanisms have been suggested, including elimination of a cytokine sink or providing space to allow for proliferation and activation of T cells, lymphodepletion likely decreases the natural regulatory loops including regulatory cell populations and checkpoint stimulation. As TILs represent a selected product dependent on the infiltrating natural T cell immunity, the same adaptive checkpoints may ultimately limit T cell product activity. To this end, blocking PD-1 (or IDO or Tregs) may allow for further enhancement of autologous cell therapy. The surgery branch is examining the safety and activity of PD-1 blockade following standard TIL (NCT01174121). To date, autologous ACT requires treatment with bolus HD IL2 following infusion. Alternative IL2 dosing, formulations, or cell modification could improve tolerability.

11.8 Cytokines

Proinflammatory cytokines provide a "third" signal in the immune response and may be an important tool to expand and activate the natural immune infiltrate (T and NK cells) particularly in tumors with low infiltration. Optimal cytokine dosing, alternative formulations, and combinations with checkpoints are being explored.

11.8.1 Interleukin-2

Recombinant high-dose interleukin-2 leads to durable immune mediated responses likely by driving the development of effector T cells but at the cost of low response rates and high acute toxicity. Several strategies have attempted to improve this narrow therapeutic window.

The prodrug NKTR214 consists of interleukin-2 (aldesleukin) conjugated to polyethylene glycol (PEG), which decreases the binding of IL-2 to the high-affinity receptor IL2αR (CD25) [83]. Response to bolus IL-2 is associated with a relative decrease in circulating Tregs [84]. NKTR214 undergoes hydrolysis of the PEG moieties to generate an active single PEG-conjugated molecule that favors T effector memory cell stimulation over Treg generation. As Tregs depend upon growth signals from IL-2 via the high-affinity IL-2 receptor, limiting the generation or survival of Tregs by differential binding may be a strategy to increase the response to IL-2.

A phase 1 dose escalation study in a variety of solid tumors including melanoma and renal cell carcinoma was presented at SITC 2016 by Bernatchez et al. [85] While hypotension was observed, toxicities were modest relative to high-dose bolus IL2. Biomarker evaluation demonstrated a transient increase in circulating but not tumor Treg cells and an increase in infiltrating PD-1+, CD8+ T cells, and NK cells at 3 weeks. The demonstration of increases in TILs and PD-1+ cells has prompted clinical evaluation of NKTR214 in combination with the PD-1 blocking antibody nivolumab (NCT02983045).

Ipilimumab may deplete Tregs and thus may be a rational partner for interleukin-2. The NCI performed a dose escalation of ipilimumab with bolus IL-2 at 720,000 IU/kg/dose [23]. Responses were observed in all cohorts and in 5 of 24 patients (21%) in the ipilimumab 3 mg/kg group. The investigators concluded that the response rate was similar to what one would expect for each of the single agents and toxicity was moderate with an overlap of immune related adverse events. This small study however leaves open the question of alternative dosing in this combination. A larger study examining the sequencing of ipilimumab and bolus interleukin-2 in melanoma was terminated due to lack of accrual (NCT01856023).

11.8.2 Interleukin-12

Interleukin-12 mediates antitumor response and stimulates T helper 1, NK, NKT, and CD8 T cells [86]. However, the toxicity of this proinflammatory cytokine has limited its clinical development to intralesional approaches (see local therapy discussion with plasmid IL-12) and to activate cell products with gene transfection into autologous TILs [87, 88]. While gene transfer effectively enhanced T cell activity, transfected cells were difficult to produce, showed poor persistence, and patients experienced systemic toxicities.

11.8.3 Interleukin-15

Interleukin-15 shares the β−chain (CD122) and γ−chain (CD132) receptors with IL-2 but has a unique α−receptor (CD215) [89]. Interleukin-15 has a similar proinflammatory profile as IL-2 without the induction of Treg cells. A phase 1 trial of human recombinant IL-15 demonstrated redistribution and expansion of NK, γδ T cells and CD8+ effector memory cells with dosing of 3 mcg/kg/day bolus for 12 days [90]. Stable disease was the best response in this safety trial of metastatic melanoma and renal cell cancer patients. However, toxicity was limiting and alternative dosing schemes are being pursued. In addition, the complex of IL-15 and IL-15αR (hetIL-15) is in phase 1 trials (NCT02452268); so is IL-15 complex (ALT-803) for melanoma and other solid tumors (NCT01946789) [91].

11.8.4 Interleukin-21

Similar to interleukin-2 and interleukin-15, interleukin-21 stimulates both innate and adaptive immune cells mediating antitumor responses dependent on NK and CD8+ T cells [92]. Like interleukin-15, interleukin-21 lacks Treg stimulation and may enhance the generation of T effector memory cells. Both phase I and II trials have been completed utilizing an outpatient regimen of between 30 mcg and 50 mcg/day bolus infusions three times per week [93, 94]. Toxicity was generally grade 2 or less at these doses and included flu-like reactions, pruritus, and rash. Single agent activity was modest with overall response rate in the 40 patients reported in phase II of 23% and a duration of response around 5 months [94]. Unfortunately, interleukin-21 failed to show a benefit over dacarbazine in a randomized trial [95].

11.9 Local Ablative Techniques

Metastatic melanoma often affords the opportunity to access tumors in the skin or lymph nodes for local therapy [96]. Intralesional therapy provides an opportunity to improve antigen release by cell killing, increase innate stimulation, and promote a broader adaptive response. T cells recognize antigen in the context of MHC and co-stimulation. Density, avidity, and context of antigen presentation influence T cell quantitative and qualitative responses. Several strategies focus on shifting antigen release to generate or enhance antitumor T cell response. Critical to this process is presenting antigen in the correct context to promote priming and activation of T cells. Successful intralesional strategies in melanoma promote antigen release in the context of "danger signals" and promote acute inflammation.

Therapeutics for local unresectable melanoma have two goals: (1) control local tumor spread and (2) generate or enhance systemic immunity as local and distant recurrence is common. Clinical trials of local ablation in melanoma include infectious agents, DNA-encoded immune stimulants, chemotherapy, cytokines, and other danger signals including endogenous and pathogen-associated molecular patterns. The examples highlighted include a few of the agents that utilize inflammatory killing to activate innate pathways to promote an in situ adaptive immune response. In situ vaccination can promote T cell expansion or trafficking of tumors that lack sufficient natural immunity needed for checkpoint or cytokine agents due to low antigenicity or immune exclusion.

11.9.1 Rose Bengal

Intralesional injections of rose bengal (PV-10 = 10% solution in 0.9% saline) has clinical activity in patients with injectable lesions leading to lysis of tumor cells and induction of tumor-specific T cell response [97]. Used medically since the 1920s, this xanthine dye appears to mediate tumor cell killing by generating reactive oxygen species and inducing autolysis. Adverse events include local injection site reactions as well as skin discoloration, vesicles, pruritus, pain, and edema. Like many local injection strategies, injected and nearby lesions had a high rate of response but distant disease control was modest [98]. PV-10 is being evaluated as a single agent and in combination with checkpoint inhibitors (NCT02288897 and NCT02557321). As a noninfectious, nonbiologic agent, rose bengal and other small molecule stimulants (i.e., TLR agonist) have an ease of use and potential cost advantage relative to biologic injectable agents.

11.9.2 Cytokines

Several cytokines (IL-2, IL-12, IL-15, and IL-21) enhance the activation and expansion of naïve T cells undergoing TCR binding and co-stimulation, and have been examined as intralesional therapy. Intralesional cytokines have been used as either direct protein injections or as intralesional gene therapy products. Intralesional interleukin-2 promotes frequent regression of melanoma with injected lesion but requires frequent injection and clinically significant impact on distant disease is rare [99]. Plasmid encoded IL-2 injected in lipid nanoparticles was designed to provide sustained IL-2 exposure with improved local control and possible systemic disease benefit [100]. The lipid component likely also provided local innate immune stimulation.

Intralesional IL-12 similarly utilized a plasmid construct but relied on electroporation for gene delivery [101]. Again, local tumor regression was observed correlating with enhanced intratumoral immune response marked by IFN-γ and CD8+ T cell infiltration. A phase 1 study found therapy well tolerated (transient pain at the treated site) with increased lymphocytic infiltration associated with target lesion necrosis. Both near and distant sites of melanoma were noted to respond. A subsequent trial combining IL-12 electroporation and pembrolizumab was associated with increased IFN-γ expression as well as T cell and NK cell trafficking to tumors in responders [102]. Responders demonstrated an increase in T cell clonality relative to nonresponders with investigator assessed response in the 22 patients examined of 43% at 12 weeks. It is interesting to note that the study utilized pretreatment biopsies to identify patients with a low percentage of CD8+ TILs coexpressing high levels of surface PD-1 and CTLA-4, who were therefore unlikely to respond to PD-1 blockade monotherapy.

11.9.3 Intralesional Biologic Agents

Talimogene laherparepvec in combination with either ipilimumab or pembrolizumab appears well tolerated in early clinical reports with toxicity similar to single agent therapies [103]. A phase 1b/2 trial of TVEC combined with standard ipilimumab (3 mg/kg for 4 infusions) reported preliminary data in 18 patients at ASCO 2015 with responses in injected and uninjected lesions along with a progression-free survival of greater than 50% at 18 months. The randomized phase 2 of combination therapy compared to ipilimumab alone is ongoing (NCT01740297) with interim analysis reported for 82 patients having an overall response rate of approximately 36% for combination and 18% with ipilimumab alone. Similarly, the phase 1b portion of TVEC in combination with pembrolizumab in unresectable stage IIIB to IVM1c (MASTERKEY-265) reported an overall response rate of 57% with 24% complete responders in the first 21 patients discussed at ASCO 2016. The phase III portion is ongoing with a planned 660 patients randomized to either TVEC and pembrolizumab or pembrolizumab alone (NCT02263508). A second oncolytic herpes type 1 virus in clinical testing, HF-10, is also undergoing phase 2 evaluation in combination with ipilimumab (NCT02272855) with similar safety reports as the individual agents and response rates (43 patients assessed at 24 weeks) of approximately 42%.

Coxsackievirus A21 (CAVATAK or CVA21) is a naturally occurring nongenetically modified bioselected virus with oncolytic activity [104, 105]. CVA21 has been administered either intratumoral or intravenously in melanoma patients in several phase 1 studies and a completed open label phase II trial involving 70 patients with advanced unresectable or metastatic melanoma [106, 107]. Intratumoral injection has been well tolerated with no grade 3 or higher toxicities. The primary endpoint of progression-free survival at 6 months was 38.6% with complete and partial responses of approximately 21%. Pre- and post-injection biopsies documented increased intratumoral immune cell infiltration characteristic of an interferon driven response with expression of PD-L1 and other checkpoint markers (LAG-3, TIM-3 and IDO). The induction of CD8+ infiltration along with chemokines and checkpoints correlated with response [108]. Ongoing combination trials include a phase I study examining intravenous CVA21 and pembrolizumab in solid tumors (including melanoma) and a phase I/II study of intratumoral CVA21 and ipilimumab. Curti et al., reported data on 22 patients at AACR 2017 with the combination of virus and ipilimumab. Two patients experienced grade 3 adverse events of fatigue and liver enzyme elevation consistent with ipilimumab induced irAEs while demonstrating a best overall response rate of 50% including 4 responses in the 11 patients previously treated with checkpoint blockade. The phase 2 study is ongoing (NCT02307149).

Generation of a robust T cell response depends upon the activity of the innate immune cells. While many other intralesional agents are in clinical development not discussed here, a fraction of patients with unresponsive non-T-cell-inflamed tumors appear to lack innate cell activation due to low stimulation in the recently identified stimulator of IFN genes (STING) pathway. Agonists of STING (cyclic dinucleotides) have been identified and are entering clinical trials [109]. Intralesional STING agonists would be expected to enhance an adaptive immune response but may also induce adaptive resistance. Thus, STING could offer a rational partner with checkpoint inhibitors in patients lacking an adequate antitumor response due to low innate immune engagement. Lack of innate stimulation may however be only one of many barriers preventing tumor inflammation. Other mechanisms preventing the generation of a natural immune response may be more challenging to overcome and include lack of unique tumor antigens and immune exclusion by the activation of metabolic pathways including the WNT/β−catenin pathway [110]

11.9.4 Other Tumor Ablation Strategies

Not all lesions are amenable to intralesional injection and other ablative techniques including external beam radiation, ultrasound and thermal ablation can be utilized. External beam techniques are attractive, noninvasive strategies to induce antigen release. As the context of antigen release is likely critical, the timing, dose, and location of ablation need to be biologically optimized [111]. Radiation dosage will influence the balance of apoptotic cell death (relatively immune tolerizing) and necrosis (immune stimulatory). Stereotactic body radiotherapy (SBRT) or hypofractioned radiation would be expected to promote more tumor necrosis than apoptosis. SBRT was applied to patients with metastatic melanoma and RCC immediately prior to standard high-dose interleukin-2 therapy demonstrating safety and possible improved clinical response rates [24]. A larger confirmatory study is ongoing (NCT02306954). Similarly, retrospective analysis suggests that combining radiation with checkpoint therapy (particularly anti-CTLA-4) improves patient outcome with many ongoing studies looking to confirm.

11.10 Combination Metabolic and Immune Modulation

The approval of vemurafenib and ipilimumab revolutionized melanoma care and combination studies quickly evaluated the possible benefits of concurrent therapy [112]. As mentioned earlier, treatment of BRAF mutated tumors with oral tyrosine kinase inhibitors (vemurafenib or dabrafenib) alone or in combination with Mek inhibitors (cobimetanib or trametanib) results in early clinical response, improvement in symptoms, and extension of survival in patients whose melanoma tumors poses an activating BRAF mutation. Activating mutations occur in B-Raf to drive tumor growth via MAPK signaling in approximately half of all cutaneous melanomas. While some patients continue to benefit beyond 3 years of therapy, resistance generally develops with a medium progression free survival of 7 to 11 months [59, 60]. Thus, the hope was to combine the early and robust response of targeted agents with the durable benefits seen with immune therapies. Several combination studies have been completed or are ongoing to explore the optimal use of these agents with some early limiting toxicity combining vemurafenib with ipilimumab observed [65, 113]. Combining pembrolizumab (PD-1) with dabrafenib plus trametanib appears tolerable and safe in phase 1. There are two ongoing phase 2 trials examining different dose exposures to MAPK inhibition (NCT02130466 and NCT02625337).

11.11 Developing Checkpoints

Indoleamine 2,3-dioxygenase (IDO) is a metabolic enzyme originally identified as immune modulatory in fetal protection from maternal T cells and more recently as a barrier to cancer immune therapy in a variety of tumors including melanoma [114]. IDO expression in primary tumors, draining lymph nodes, and metastatic deposits correlates with tumor progression and worse outcome in patients with melanoma [115]. Depletion of tryptophan promotes the conversion of naïve T cells to Treg cells. However, treatment of metastatic melanoma patients with inhibitors of IDO alone has shown little clinical activity [116]. IDO expression is induced in tumor cells and antigen presenting cells (macrophages and dendritic cells) by inflammatory signaling including IFN-γ and appears to be induced with either anti-CTLA-4 or anti-PD-1 therapy [117].

Indoximod (NewLink genetics) appears to be safe and have clinical activity when combined with immune checkpoint inhibitors in a phase Ib/II trial (NCT02073123) with indoximod 1200 mg twice daily concurrent with either CTLA-4 or PD-1 blockade. Interim data at the annual meeting of the American Association of Cancer Research (AACR) 2017 showed an overall response rate of 52% (31/60) and 10% complete responses. Most patients were treated with standard pembrolizumab 3 mg/kg every 3 weeks and approximately doubled the monotherapy response rate previously reported in Keynote 006 of 33% [42].

As discussed in detail in other chapters, numerous other checkpoints mark the presence of an antitumor immune response and are possible targets for modulation [27, 118]. Both T cell immunoglobulin and mucin-3 (TIM-3) and lymphocyte activation gene 3 (LAG-3) appear co-expressed in tumor T cell samples with preclinical support as targets to enhance an antitumor immune response particularly in combination with PD-1 blockade. TIM-3 is expressed on monocytes, activated T cells, and NK cells and appears coincident with PD-1 to mark a more exhausted TIL population [119]. Antibodies to TIM-3 promote autoimmunity and enhanced tumor rejection in preclinical models. Trials are ongoing (NCT02817633). Preclinical studies suggest improved antitumor responses in combination with anti-PD-1 and anti-LAG-3 compared to anti-PD-1 monotherapy [120]. Many other blocking antibodies of checkpoints and stimulatory antibodies of proinflammatory signaling are just entering trials but clinical data is not available.

11.12 Adjuvant Therapy

Adjuvant therapy treats microscopic disease to lower the risk of recurrence with the goal of improving not just disease-specific but also overall survival of patients. Systemic administration of IFN-α2b was approved after demonstrating both improved disease-free and overall survival in high-risk patients although subsequent trials have suggested that this clinical benefit modest [121]. Vaccines from a variety of sources and targets (peptide, glycoproteins, autologous cells, and allogeneic cells) are well tolerated but to date lack significant clinical benefit in metastatic and adjuvant therapy [122]. The inhibitory checkpoints in metastatic disease are now moving into adjuvant care.

Ipilimumab was approved in 2015 for the adjuvant treatment of resected node positive patients following lymphadenectomy at 10 mg/kg based on the European Organisation for Research and Treatment of Cancer (EORTC) 18071 trial randomizing between placebo and ipilimumab [123]. Ipilimumab improved both disease-free and overall survival. However, the dose of 10 mg/kg is associated with higher irAEs compared to the 3 mg/kg dosing and current trials are focused on optimal dosing and the role of the other checkpoints in the adjuvant setting. The Eastern Cooperative Oncology Group completed enrollment in a randomized three arm trial examining IFN-α2b (1 year) or ipilimumab at 3 mg/kg or ipilimumab at 10 mg/kg in resected stage IIIB to IV melanoma patients (NCT01274338). The study is ongoing. A second intergroup adjuvant trial examined IFN-α2b or ipilimumab 10 mg/kg compared to pembrolizumab 3 mg/mg in resected stage IIIA (N2) to IV melanoma patients and continues enrollment as of May 2017. A similar trial, CheckMate 238, completed enrollment comparing resected stage IIIB to IV melanoma patients randomized between nivolumab 3 mg/kg every 2 weeks or ipilimumab 10 mg/kg every 3 weeks for 4 doses and then every 12 weeks starting at week 24 until disease recurrence, toxicity, or up to 1 year (NCT02388906). A 40 patient study reported at ASCO 2016 evaluated two dosing cohorts of ipilimumab plus nivolumab followed by nivolumab in resected stage IIIC to IV melanoma patients [124]. Toxicities were lower in the lower dose ipilimumab arm, and overall similar to those reported in the metastatic setting. A larger combination trial of ipilimumab plus nivolumab in the adjuvant setting is ongoing (NCT03068455).

11.13 Conclusion

Targeted and immune based treatments have meaningfully changed the clinical outcomes for many patients with melanoma. Melanoma remains a challenge as a heterogeneous group of tumors that have both interpatient variability and intrapatient diversity. Tumor growth pathways both shape and respond to the extrinsic pressure of the natural immune response. Some tumors depend upon the proinflammatory reaction to drive tumor growth while others have little inflammation present. Appreciating and monitoring the interface between intrinsic and extrinsic growth pathways will be critical to personalizing therapy, lowering toxicity, and ultimately benefiting more patients. Ongoing clinical trials will better define the dosing, sequencing, and combination of existing agents as well as guide new agent discovery to achieve cancer-free, treatment-free survival.

References

1. Long GV, Weber JS, Infante JR et al (2016) Overall survival and durable responses in patients with BRAF V600-mutant metastatic melanoma receiving Dabrafenib combined with Trametinib. J Clin Oncol 34(8):871–878
2. Hodi FS, Chesney J, Pavlick AC et al (2016) Combined nivolumab and ipilimumab versus ipilimumab alone in patients with advanced melanoma: 2-year overall survival outcomes in a multicentre, randomised, controlled, phase 2 trial. Lancet Oncol 17(11):1558–1568
3. Dunn GP, Bruce AT, Ikeda H, Old LJ, Schreiber RD (2002) Cancer immunoediting: from immunosurveillance to tumor escape. Nat Immunol 3(11):991–998
4. Paget S (1889) The distribution of secondary growths in cancer of the breast. Lancet 133(3421):571–573
5. Zaidi MR, Davis S, Noonan FP et al (2011) Interferon-gamma links ultraviolet radiation to melanomagenesis in mice. Nature 469(7331):548–553
6. Balkwill F, Mantovani A (2001) Inflammation and cancer: back to Virchow? Lancet 357(9255):539–545
7. Clark WH Jr, Elder DE, Guerry D et al (1989) Model predicting survival in stage I melanoma based on tumor progression. J Natl Cancer Inst 81(24):1893–1904
8. Eriksson H, Frohm-Nilsson M, Jaras J et al (2015) Prognostic factors in localized invasive primary cutaneous malignant melanoma: results of a large population-based study. Br J Dermatol 172(1):175–186
9. Rosenberg SA (2014) IL-2: the first effective immunotherapy for human cancer. J Immunol 192(12):5451–5458
10. Rosenberg SA, Yang JC, White DE, Steinberg SM (1998) Durability of complete responses in patients with metastatic cancer treated with high-dose interleukin-2: identification of the antigens mediating response. Ann Surg 228(3):307–319
11. Teng MW, Ngiow SF, Ribas A, Smyth MJ (2015) Classifying cancers based on T-cell infiltration and PD-L1. Cancer Res 75(11):2139–2145
12. Hunder NN, Wallen H, Cao J et al (2008) Treatment of metastatic melanoma with autologous CD4+ T cells against NY-ESO-1. N Engl J Med 358(25):2698–2703
13. Weide B, Zelba H, Derhovanessian E et al (2012) Functional T cells targeting NY-ESO-1 or Melan-A are predictive for survival of patients with distant melanoma metastasis. J Clin Oncol 30(15):1835–1841
14. Gubin MM, Zhang X, Schuster H et al (2014) Checkpoint blockade cancer immunotherapy targets tumour-specific mutant antigens. Nature 515(7528):577–581
15. Snyder A, Makarov V, Merghoub T et al (2014) Genetic basis for clinical response to CTLA-4 blockade in melanoma. N Engl J Med 371(23):2189–2199
16. van Rooij N, van Buuren MM, Philips D et al (2013) Tumor exome analysis reveals neoantigen-specific T-cell reactivity in an ipilimumab-responsive melanoma. J Clin Oncol 31(32):e439–e442
17. Rosenberg SA, Lotze MT, Yang JC et al (1993) Prospective randomized trial of high-dose interleukin-2 alone or in conjunction with lymphokine-activated killer cells for the treatment of patients with advanced cancer. J Natl Cancer Inst 85(8):622–632
18. Alva A, Daniels GA, Wong MK et al (2016) Contemporary experience with high-dose interleukin-2 therapy and impact on survival in patients with metastatic melanoma and metastatic renal cell carcinoma. Cancer Immunol Immunother 65(12):1533–1544
19. Payne R, Glenn L, Hoen H et al (2014) Durable responses and reversible toxicity of high-dose interleukin-2 treatment of melanoma and renal cancer in a community hospital biotherapy program. J Immunother Cancer 2:13
20. Schwartzentruber DJ (2001) Guidelines for the safe administration of high-dose interleukin-2. J Immunother 24(4):287–293

21. Downey SG, Klapper JA, Smith FO et al (2007) Prognostic factors related to clinical response in patients with metastatic melanoma treated by CTL-associated antigen-4 blockade. Clin Cancer Res 13(22 Pt 1):6681–6688
22. Buchbinder EI, Gunturi A, Perritt J et al (2016) A retrospective analysis of high-dose interleukin-2 (HD IL-2) following Ipilimumab in metastatic melanoma. J Immunother Cancer 4:52
23. Maker AV, Phan GQ, Attia P et al (2005) Tumor regression and autoimmunity in patients treated with cytotoxic T lymphocyte-associated antigen 4 blockade and interleukin 2: a phase I/II study. Ann Surg Oncol 12(12):1005–1016
24. Seung SK, Curti BD, Crittenden M et al (2012) Phase 1 study of stereotactic body radiotherapy and interleukin-2--tumor and immunological responses. Sci Transl Med 4(137):137ra174
25. Neville KL, Dal Canto MC, Bluestone JA, Miller SD (2000) CD28 costimulatory blockade exacerbates disease severity and accelerates epitope spreading in a virus-induced autoimmune disease. J Virol 74(18):8349–8357
26. van Elsas A, Hurwitz AA, Allison JP (1999) Combination immunotherapy of B16 melanoma using anti-cytotoxic T lymphocyte-associated antigen 4 (CTLA-4) and granulocyte/macrophage colony-stimulating factor (GM-CSF)-producing vaccines induces rejection of subcutaneous and metastatic tumors accompanied by autoimmune depigmentation. J Exp Med 190(3):355–366
27. Topalian SL, Drake CG, Pardoll DM (2015) Immune checkpoint blockade: a common denominator approach to cancer therapy. Cancer Cell 27(4):450–461
28. Wistuba-Hamprecht K, Martens A, Heubach F et al (2017) Peripheral CD8 effector-memory type 1 T-cells correlate with outcome in ipilimumab-treated stage IV melanoma patients. Eur J Cancer 73:61–70
29. Robert C, Thomas L, Bondarenko I et al (2011) Ipilimumab plus dacarbazine for previously untreated metastatic melanoma. N Engl J Med 364(26):2517–2526
30. Hodi FS, O'Day SJ, McDermott DF et al (2010) Improved survival with ipilimumab in patients with metastatic melanoma. N Engl J Med 363(8):711–723
31. Schadendorf D, Hodi FS, Robert C et al (2015) Pooled analysis of long-term survival data from phase II and phase III trials of Ipilimumab in unresectable or metastatic melanoma. J Clin Oncol 33(17):1889–1894
32. Weber JS, Dummer R, de Pril V, Lebbe C, Hodi FS, Investigators MDX (2013) Patterns of onset and resolution of immune-related adverse events of special interest with ipilimumab: detailed safety analysis from a phase 3 trial in patients with advanced melanoma. Cancer 119(9):1675–1682
33. Huang RR, Jalil J, Economou JS et al (2011) CTLA4 blockade induces frequent tumor infiltration by activated lymphocytes regardless of clinical responses in humans. Clin Cancer Res 17(12):4101–4109
34. Hamid O, Schmidt H, Nissan A et al (2011) A prospective phase II trial exploring the association between tumor microenvironment biomarkers and clinical activity of ipilimumab in advanced melanoma. J Transl Med 9:204
35. Brueggemann C, Weide B, Goldinger SM, Konrad A, Erdmann M, Schadendorf D, Croner RS, Kraehenbuehl L, Kaehler KC, Hafner C, Leisgang W, Kiesewetter F, Dummer R, Schuler G, Stürzl M, Heinzerling L (2015) Association of PD-L1 expression in melanoma with response and prognosis to ipilimumab. Paper presented at: J Clin Oncol
36. Van Allen EM, Miao D, Schilling B et al (2015) Genomic correlates of response to CTLA-4 blockade in metastatic melanoma. Science 350(6257):207–211
37. Tumeh PC, Harview CL, Yearley JH et al (2014) PD-1 blockade induces responses by inhibiting adaptive immune resistance. Nature 515(7528):568–571
38. Brahmer JR, Drake CG, Wollner I et al (2010) Phase I study of single-agent anti-programmed death-1 (MDX-1106) in refractory solid tumors: safety, clinical activity, pharmacodynamics, and immunologic correlates. J Clin Oncol 28(19):3167–3175
39. Weber JS, D'Angelo SP, Minor D et al (2015) Nivolumab versus chemotherapy in patients with advanced melanoma who progressed after anti-CTLA-4 treatment (CheckMate 037): a randomised, controlled, open-label, phase 3 trial. Lancet Oncol 16(4):375–384

40. Ribas A, Puzanov I, Dummer R et al (2015) Pembrolizumab versus investigator-choice chemotherapy for ipilimumab-refractory melanoma (KEYNOTE-002): a randomised, controlled, phase 2 trial. Lancet Oncol 16(8):908–918
41. Freeman-Keller M, Kim Y, Cronin H, Richards A, Gibney G, Weber JS (2016) Nivolumab in resected and Unresectable metastatic melanoma: characteristics of immune-related adverse events and association with outcomes. Clin Cancer Res 22(4):886–894
42. Robert C, Schachter J, Long GV et al (2015) Pembrolizumab versus Ipilimumab in advanced melanoma. N Engl J Med 372(26):2521–2532
43. Ribas A, Hamid O, Daud A et al (2016) Association of pembrolizumab with tumor response and survival among patients with advanced melanoma. JAMA 315(15):1600–1609
44. Garcia-Diaz A, Shin DS, Moreno BH et al (2017) Interferon receptor signaling pathways regulating PD-L1 and PD-L2 expression. Cell Rep 19(6):1189–1201
45. Daud AI, Wolchok JD, Robert C et al (2016) Programmed death-ligand 1 expression and response to the anti-programmed death 1 antibody Pembrolizumab in melanoma. J Clin Oncol 34(34):4102–4109
46. Daud AI, Loo K, Pauli ML et al (2016) Tumor immune profiling predicts response to anti-PD-1 therapy in human melanoma. J Clin Invest 126(9):3447–3452
47. O'Donnell JS, Long GV, Scolyer RA, Teng MW, Smyth MJ (2017) Resistance to PD1/PDL1 checkpoint inhibition. Cancer Treat Rev 52:71–81
48. Ayers M, Lunceford J, Nebozhyn M et al (2015) Relationship between immune gene signatures and clinical response to PD-1 blockade with pembrolizumab (MK-3475) in patients with advanced solid tumors. J Immunother Cancer 3(Suppl 2):P80–P80
49. Nosrati A, Tsai KK, Goldinger SM et al (2017) Evaluation of clinicopathological factors in PD-1 response: derivation and validation of a prediction scale for response to PD-1 monotherapy. Br J Cancer 116(9):1141–1147
50. Kaufman HL, Kim DW, DeRaffele G, Mitcham J, Coffin RS, Kim-Schulze S (2010) Local and distant immunity induced by intralesional vaccination with an oncolytic herpes virus encoding GM-CSF in patients with stage IIIc and IV melanoma. Ann Surg Oncol 17(3):718–730
51. Xia T, Konno H, Barber GN (2016) Recurrent loss of STING signaling in melanoma correlates with susceptibility to viral oncolysis. Cancer Res 76(22):6747–6759
52. Senzer NN, Kaufman HL, Amatruda T et al (2009) Phase II clinical trial of a granulocyte-macrophage colony-stimulating factor-encoding, second-generation oncolytic herpesvirus in patients with unresectable metastatic melanoma. J Clin Oncol 27(34):5763–5771
53. Andtbacka RH, Kaufman HL, Collichio F et al (2015) Talimogene Laherparepvec improves durable response rate in patients with advanced melanoma. J Clin Oncol 33(25):2780–2788
54. Wolchok JD, Kluger H, Callahan MK et al (2013) Nivolumab plus ipilimumab in advanced melanoma. N Engl J Med 369(2):122–133
55. Larkin J, Chiarion-Sileni V, Gonzalez R et al (2015) Combined nivolumab and Ipilimumab or monotherapy in untreated melanoma. N Engl J Med 373(1):23–34
56. Wolchok JD, Chiarion-Silen V, Gonzalez R, Rutkowski P, Grob JJ, Lance Cowey C, Lao C, Schadendorf D, Ferrucci PF, Smylie M, Dummer R, Hill A, Haanen JBAG, Maio M, McArthur GA, Walker D, Jiang J, Horak CE, Larkin JMG, Stephen Hodi F (2016) Updated results from a phase III trial of nivolumab (NIVO) combined with ipilimumab (IPI) in treatment-naive patients (pts) with advanced melanoma (MEL) (CheckMate 067). Paper presented at: J Clin Oncol
57. Postow MA, Chesney J, Pavlick AC et al (2015) Nivolumab and ipilimumab versus ipilimumab in untreated melanoma. N Engl J Med 372(21):2006–2017
58. Stephen Hodi F, Postow MA, Chesney JA, Pavlick AC, Robert C, Grossmann KF, McDermott DF, Linette GP, Meyer N, Giguere JK, Agarwala S, Shaheen MF, Ernstoff MS, Minor DR, Salama AK, Taylor MH, Ott PA, Jiang J, Gagnier P, Wolchok JD (2016) Overall survival in patients with advanced melanoma (MEL) who discontinued treatment with nivolumab (NIVO) plus ipilimumab (IPI) due to toxicity in a phase II trial (CheckMate 069). Paper presented at: J Clin Oncol

59. Ascierto PA, McArthur GA, Dreno B et al (2016) Cobimetinib combined with vemurafenib in advanced BRAF(V600)-mutant melanoma (coBRIM): updated efficacy results from a randomised, double-blind, phase 3 trial. Lancet Oncol 17(9):1248–1260
60. Long GV, Flaherty KT, Stroyakovskiy D et al (2017) Dabrafenib plus trametinib versus dabrafenib monotherapy in patients with metastatic BRAF V600E/K-mutant melanoma: long-term survival and safety analysis of a phase 3 study. Ann Oncol
61. Wilmott JS, Long GV, Howle JR et al (2012) Selective BRAF inhibitors induce marked T-cell infiltration into human metastatic melanoma. Clin Cancer Res 18(5):1386–1394
62. Hugo W, Shi H, Sun L et al (2015) Non-genomic and immune evolution of melanoma acquiring MAPKi resistance. Cell 162(6):1271–1285
63. Hugo W (2016) Genomic and transcrioptomic features of response to anti-PD-1 therapy in metastatic melanoma. Cell 165(1):35–44. PMID 26997480
64. Amin A, Lawson DH, Salama AK et al (2016) Phase II study of vemurafenib followed by ipilimumab in patients with previously untreated BRAF-mutated metastatic melanoma. J Immunother Cancer. 4:44
65. Ribas A, Hodi FS, Callahan M, Konto C, Wolchok J (2013) Hepatotoxicity with combination of vemurafenib and ipilimumab. N Engl J Med 368(14):1365–1366
66. Jeffrey S, Weber GTG, Sullivan RJ, Sosman JA, Slingluff CL, Lawrence DP, Logan TF, Schuchter LM, Nair S, Buchbinder EI, Berghorn E, Jiang J, Horak CE, Stephen Hodi F (2016) Survival outcomes of nivolumab (NIVO) given sequentially with ipilimumab (IPI) in patients with advanced melanoma (CheckMate 064). J Clin Oncol 34:9517
67. Weber JS, Postow M, Lao CD, Schadendorf D (2016) Management of adverse events following treatment with anti-programmed death-1 agents. Oncologist 21(10):1230–1240
68. Weber J, Thompson JA, Hamid O et al (2009) A randomized, double-blind, placebo-controlled, phase II study comparing the tolerability and efficacy of ipilimumab administered with or without prophylactic budesonide in patients with unresectable stage III or IV melanoma. Clin Cancer Res 15(17):5591–5598
69. Hodi FS, Lee S, McDermott DF et al (2014) Ipilimumab plus sargramostim vs ipilimumab alone for treatment of metastatic melanoma: a randomized clinical trial. JAMA 312(17):1744–1753
70. Ma N, Liu Q, Hou L, Wang Y, Liu Z (2017) MDSCs are involved in the protumorigenic potentials of GM-CSF in colitis-associated cancer. Int J Immunopathol Pharmacol 30(2):152–162
71. Uemura M, Trinh VA, Haymaker C et al (2016) Selective inhibition of autoimmune exacerbation while preserving the anti-tumor clinical benefit using IL-6 blockade in a patient with advanced melanoma and Crohn's disease: a case report. J Hematol Oncol 9(1):81
72. Zaretsky JM, Garcia-Diaz A, Shin DS et al (2016) Mutations associated with acquired resistance to PD-1 blockade in melanoma. N Engl J Med 375(9):819–829
73. Shin DS, Zaretsky JM, Escuin-Ordinas H et al (2017) Primary resistance to PD-1 blockade mediated by JAK1/2 mutations. Cancer Discov 7(2):188–201
74. Restifo NP, Marincola FM, Kawakami Y, Taubenberger J, Yannelli JR, Rosenberg SA (1996) Loss of functional beta 2-microglobulin in metastatic melanomas from five patients receiving immunotherapy. J Natl Cancer Inst 88(2):100–108
75. Hicklin DJ, Wang Z, Arienti F, Rivoltini L, Parmiani G, Ferrone S (1998) beta2-microglobulin mutations, HLA class I antigen loss, and tumor progression in melanoma. J Clin Invest 101(12):2720–2729
76. Gao J, Shi LZ, Zhao H et al (2016) Loss of IFN-gamma pathway genes in tumor cells as a mechanism of resistance to anti-CTLA-4 therapy. Cell 167(2):397–404. e399
77. Gajewski TF, Woo SR, Zha Y et al (2013) Cancer immunotherapy strategies based on overcoming barriers within the tumor microenvironment. Curr Opin Immunol 25(2):268–276
78. Dudley ME, Gross CA, Somerville RP et al (2013) Randomized selection design trial evaluating CD8+–enriched versus unselected tumor-infiltrating lymphocytes for adoptive cell therapy for patients with melanoma. J Clin Oncol 31(17):2152–2159
79. Gros A, Robbins PF, Yao X et al (2014) PD-1 identifies the patient-specific CD8(+) tumor-reactive repertoire infiltrating human tumors. J Clin Invest 124(5):2246–2259

80. Robbins PF, Lu YC, El-Gamil M et al (2013) Mining exomic sequencing data to identify mutated antigens recognized by adoptively transferred tumor-reactive T cells. Nat Med 19(6):747–752
81. Dudley ME, Yang JC, Sherry R et al (2008) Adoptive cell therapy for patients with metastatic melanoma: evaluation of intensive myeloablative chemoradiation preparative regimens. J Clin Oncol 26(32):5233–5239
82. Klebanoff CA, Khong HT, Antony PA, Palmer DC, Restifo NP (2005) Sinks, suppressors and antigen presenters: how lymphodepletion enhances T cell-mediated tumor immunotherapy. Trends Immunol 26(2):111–117
83. Charych DH, Hoch U, Langowski JL et al (2016) NKTR-214, an engineered cytokine with biased IL2 receptor binding, increased tumor exposure, and marked efficacy in mouse tumor models. Clin Cancer Res 22(3):680–690
84. Cesana GC, DeRaffele G, Cohen S et al (2006) Characterization of CD4+CD25+ regulatory T cells in patients treated with high-dose interleukin-2 for metastatic melanoma or renal cell carcinoma. J Clin Oncol 24(7):1169–1177
85. Bernatchez C, Haymaker C, Tannir NM, Kluger H, Tetzlaff M, Bentebibel SE, Jackson N, Gergel I, Tagliaferri M, Zalevsky J, Hoch U, Imperiale U, Aung S, Hwu P, Sznol M, Hurwitz M, Diab A (2016) A CD122-biased agonist increases CD8+T Cells and natural killer cells in the tumor microenvironment; making cold tumors hot with NKTR-214. Paper presented at: SITC
86. Lasek W, Zagozdzon R, Jakobisiak M (2014) Interleukin 12: still a promising candidate for tumor immunotherapy? Cancer Immunol Immunother 63(5):419–435
87. Leonard JP, Sherman ML, Fisher GL et al (1997) Effects of single-dose interleukin-12 exposure on interleukin-12-associated toxicity and interferon-gamma production. Blood 90(7):2541–2548
88. Zhang L, Morgan RA, Beane JD et al (2015) Tumor-infiltrating lymphocytes genetically engineered with an inducible gene encoding interleukin-12 for the immunotherapy of metastatic melanoma. Clin Cancer Res 21(10):2278–2288
89. Jakobisiak M, Golab J, Lasek W (2011) Interleukin 15 as a promising candidate for tumor immunotherapy. Cytokine Growth Factor Rev 22(2):99–108
90. Conlon KC, Lugli E, Welles HC et al (2015) Redistribution, hyperproliferation, activation of natural killer cells and CD8 T cells, and cytokine production during first-in-human clinical trial of recombinant human interleukin-15 in patients with cancer. J Clin Oncol 33(1):74–82
91. Xiaoyue Chen BL, Han K, Kong L, Noel T, Jeng EK, Alter S, Rubinstein M, Rhode PR, Wong HC (2016) Combination therapy of an IL-15 superagonist complex, ALT-803, and a tumor targeting monoclonal antibody promotes direct antitumor activity and protective vaccinal effect in a syngenic mouse melanoma model. Paper presented at: SITC
92. Davis MR, Zhu Z, Hansen DM, Bai Q, Fang Y (2015) The role of IL-21 in immunity and cancer. Cancer Lett 358(2):107–114
93. Thompson JA, Curti BD, Redman BG et al (2008) Phase I study of recombinant interleukin-21 in patients with metastatic melanoma and renal cell carcinoma. J Clin Oncol 26(12):2034–2039
94. Petrella TM, Tozer R, Belanger K et al (2012) Interleukin-21 has activity in patients with metastatic melanoma: a phase II study. J Clin Oncol 30(27):3396–3401
95. Petrella TM, Mihalcioiu CLD, McWhirter E, Belanger K, Savage KJ, Song X, Hamid O, Cheng T, Davis ML, Lee CW, Spatz A, Monzon JG, Hagerman L, Chen BE, Dancey J (2013) Final efficacy results of NCIC CTG IND.202: A randomized phase II study of recombinant interleukin-21 (rIL21) in patients with recurrent or metastatic melanoma (MM). J Clin Oncol 31:9032
96. Sloot S, Rashid OM, Sarnaik AA, Zager JS (2016) Developments in Intralesional therapy for metastatic melanoma. Cancer Control 23(1):12–20
97. Thompson JF, Hersey P, Wachter E (2008) Chemoablation of metastatic melanoma using intralesional Rose Bengal. Melanoma Res 18(6):405–411
98. Thompson JF, Agarwala SS, Smithers BM et al (2015) Phase 2 study of Intralesional PV-10 in refractory metastatic melanoma. Ann Surg Oncol 22(7):2135–2142

99. Weide B, Derhovanessian E, Pflugfelder A et al (2010) High response rate after intratumoral treatment with interleukin-2: results from a phase 2 study in 51 patients with metastasized melanoma. Cancer 116(17):4139–4146
100. Galanis E, Hersh EM, Stopeck AT et al (1999) Immunotherapy of advanced malignancy by direct gene transfer of an interleukin-2 DNA/DMRIE/DOPE lipid complex: phase I/II experience. J Clin Oncol 17(10):3313–3323
101. Daud AI, DeConti RC, Andrews S et al (2008) Phase I trial of interleukin-12 plasmid electroporation in patients with metastatic melanoma. J Clin Oncol 26(36):5896–5903
102. Alain Algazi KT, Rosenblum M, Nandoskar P, Andtbacka RHI, Li A, Takamura T, Dwyer M, Browning E, Talia R, Twitty C, Gargosky S, Campbell J, Ballesteros-Merino C, Bifulco CB, Fox BA, Le MH, Pierce RH, Daud A (2017) An intratumoral treatment modality to address an unmet medical need: results from a phase ii combination study with pil-12 plus pembrolizumab in melanoma patients predicted to not respond to anti-pd-1 therapy. ASCO-SITC Poster No 78
103. Dummer R, Hoeller C, Gruter IP, Michielin O (2017) Combining talimogene laherparepvec with immunotherapies in melanoma and other solid tumors. Cancer Immunol Immunother 66(6):683–695
104. Shafren DR, Au GG, Nguyen T et al (2004) Systemic therapy of malignant human melanoma tumors by a common cold-producing enterovirus, coxsackievirus a21. Clin Cancer Res 10(1 Pt 1):53–60
105. Au GG, Lindberg AM, Barry RD, Shafren DR (2005) Oncolysis of vascular malignant human melanoma tumors by Coxsackievirus A21. Int J Oncol 26(6):1471–1476
106. Andtbacka RHI, Curti BD, Kaufman H, Daniels GA, Nemunaitis JJ, Spitler LE, Hallmeyer S, Lutzky J, Schultz SM, Whitman ED, Zhou K, Karpathy R, Weisberg JI, Grose M, Shafren D (2015) Final data from CALM: a phase II study of Coxsackievirus A21 (CVA21) oncolytic virus immunotherapy in patients with advanced melanoma. Paper presented at: J Clin Oncol
107. Hardev S. Pandha KJH, Ralph C, Melcher A, Mansfield D, Grose M, Davies B, Karpathy, Shafren D (2016) Phase I STORM study (KEYNOTE 200): intravenous delivery of a novel oncolytic immunotherapy agent, Coxsackievirus A21 in combination with pembrolizumab in advanced cancer patients. Paper presented at: J Clin Oncol
108. Andtbacka RHI, Curti BD, Kaufman H, Nemunaitis JJ, Daniels GA, Hallmeyer S, Whitman ED, Lutzky J, Schultz SM, Spitler LE, Feng Z, Paustian C, Fox BA, Bifulco CB, Zhou K, Grose M, Shafren D (2016) Dynamics of tumor response in advanced melanoma patients treated with Coxsackievirus A21. Paper presented at: J Clin Oncol
109. Corrales L, McWhirter SM, Dubensky TW Jr, Gajewski TF (2016) The host STING pathway at the interface of cancer and immunity. J Clin Invest 126(7):2404–2411
110. Malladi S, Macalinao DG, Jin X et al (2016) Metastatic latency and immune evasion through autocrine inhibition of WNT. Cell 165(1):45–60
111. Weichselbaum RR, Liang H, Deng L, Fu YX (2017) Radiotherapy and immunotherapy: a beneficial liaison? Nat Rev Clin Oncol 14(6):365–379
112. Luke JJ, Hodi FS (2013) Ipilimumab, vemurafenib, dabrafenib, and trametinib: synergistic competitors in the clinical management of BRAF mutant malignant melanoma. Oncologist 18(6):717–725
113. Deniger DC, Kwong ML, Pasetto A et al (2017) A pilot trial of the combination of Vemurafenib with adoptive cell therapy in patients with metastatic melanoma. Clin Cancer Res 23(2):351–362
114. Godin-Ethier J, Hanafi LA, Piccirillo CA, Lapointe R (2011) Indoleamine 2,3-dioxygenase expression in human cancers: clinical and immunologic perspectives. Clin Cancer Res 17(22):6985–6991
115. Speeckaert R, Vermaelen K, van Geel N et al (2012) Indoleamine 2,3-dioxygenase, a new prognostic marker in sentinel lymph nodes of melanoma patients. Eur J Cancer 48(13):2004–2011
116. Beatty GL, O'Dwyer PJ, Clark J et al (2017) First-in-human phase I study of the oral inhibitor of Indoleamine 2, 3-Dioxygenase-1 Epacadostat (INCB024360) in patients with advanced solid malignancies. Clin Cancer Res 23:3269–3276

117. Holmgaard RB, Zamarin D, Munn DH, Wolchok JD, Allison JP (2013) Indoleamine 2,3-dioxygenase is a critical resistance mechanism in antitumor T cell immunotherapy targeting CTLA-4. J Exp Med 210(7):1389–1402
118. Sharma P, Allison JP (2015) Immune checkpoint targeting in cancer therapy: toward combination strategies with curative potential. Cell 161(2):205–214
119. Fourcade J, Sun Z, Benallaoua M et al (2010) Upregulation of Tim-3 and PD-1 expression is associated with tumor antigen-specific CD8+ T cell dysfunction in melanoma patients. J Exp Med 207(10):2175–2186
120. Woo SR, Turnis ME, Goldberg MV et al (2012) Immune inhibitory molecules LAG-3 and PD-1 synergistically regulate T-cell function to promote tumoral immune escape. Cancer Res 72(4):917–927
121. Davar D, Kirkwood JM (2016) Adjuvant therapy of melanoma. Cancer Treat Res 167:181–208
122. Rosenberg SA, Yang JC, Restifo NP (2004) Cancer immunotherapy: moving beyond current vaccines. Nat Med 10(9):909–915
123. Eggermont AM, Chiarion-Sileni V, Grob JJ et al (2016) Prolonged survival in stage III melanoma with Ipilimumab adjuvant therapy. N Engl J Med 375(19):1845–1855
124. Weber J, Grob J-J, Margolin KA, Ascierto PA, Sznol M, Ott PA, Lejeune C, de Pril V, Ruisi MM, Stephen Hodi F (2015) A phase III study (CheckMate 238) of adjuvant immunotherapy with nivolumab (NIVO) versus ipilimumab (IPI) after complete resection of stage IIIb/c or stage IV melanoma (MEL) in patients (pts) at high risk for recurrence. Paper presented at: J Immunother Cancer

MIX
Papier aus verantwortungsvollen Quellen
Paper from responsible sources
FSC® C105338

If you have any concerns about our products,
you can contact us on
ProductSafety@springernature.com

In case Publisher is established outside the EU,
the EU authorized representative is:
Springer Nature Customer Service Center GmbH
Europaplatz 3, 69115 Heidelberg, Germany

Printed by Libri Plureos GmbH
in Hamburg, Germany